Echocardiology

with Doppler applications and Real time imaging

edited by N. Bom

Thoraxcentrum

Erasmus University Rotterdam

SPRINGER-SCIENCE+BUSINESS MEDIA, B.V. 1977

Design: Audiovisual Center,
        Erasmus University Rotterdam

Springer Science+Business Media Dordrecht
Originally published by Martinus Nijhoff, P.O.B. 269, The Hague, The Netherlands
ISBN 978-94-010-1105-1   ISBN 978-94-010-1103-7 (eBook)
DOI 10.1007/978-94-010-1103-7

Softcover reprint of the hardcover 1st edition 1977

Foreword

Echocardiology comprises all aspects of diagnostic application of ultrasound to cardiac patients. It is probably the fastest growing non-invasive technique today. Almost all progress in this young and exciting field has been the positive result of close co-operation between medical and technical scientists.

This book contains a series of lectures held at Erasmus University Rotterdam in June 1977 and is divided in three sections:

- clinical echocardiology, consisting of both an introduction to the basic principles as well as a wide variety of applications aimed at the clinically oriented reader.
- Doppler methods, where in addition to its clinical applications also the engineering of new developments will be presented.
- the two dimensional real-time imaging where many new techniques including computer methods, holography and acousto-optical systems will be discussed.

We hope that this book will stimulate communication between scientists of various disciplines and nationalities.

N. Bom
J. Roelandt
P.G. Hugenholtz

Rotterdam, June 1977

Preface

The last three decades have seen a remarkable advance in diagnostic instrumentation in diseases of the circulation. In the 1940's the only diagnostic aids were the electrocardiogram and simple X-ray. These were quickly followed by the cardiac catheter, phonocardiography, radio isotope methods and angiocardiography. The development of cardiac surgery provided the impetus to developing more accurate methods of diagnosis, preferably those that did not need invasion of the patient. The introduction of ultrasound has contributed towards this aim in the last few years.

To some extent this latter technique remains a mixture of science and art. The science is well established but it needs considerable experience and skill on the part of the operator to position the ultrasound generator and interpret the results. However, at the present time echocardiography has proved itself to be of undoubted clinical value in interpreting disease of the mitral and aortic valves, in detecting pericardial effusions and improving the diagnosis of congenital heart disease. More recent work has been directed to wall thickness, ventricular volume and ventricular function, and it would appear more research and rigorous testing is necessary to firmly establish the accuracy of these methods. Multihead generators combined with cine recording give a moving picture of the heart; time will tell whether this method has an advantage over the more simple methods of recording in M-mode, certain is that much research is carried out in this area.

The non-invasive measurement of blood flow has been the dream of physiologists and clinicians for many years. The recent development of methods using the Doppler effect has opened up the possibility of looking at flow waveforms in a qualitative, if not a quantitative way.

Echocardiography in clinical heart disease has come to stay and should be an integral part of any cardiac diagnostic laboratory, Future development will include improvement of instrumentation but above all improved skill in using the technique and interpreting the results. It is our sincere hope that this lecture series will contribute to further understanding of Echocardiography, particularly here in Europe, where so many original ideas in echo were started.

J.P. Shillingford

Chairman of the working group on
Monitoring the Seriously ill. (CRM).
Commission of the European Communities.

L. Donato

Chairman of the Committee on Medical and
Public Health Research. (CRM).
Commission of the European Communities.

The lecture series contained in this book

Was initiated by

the working groups on Biomedical-Engineering and Monitoring the Seriously ill. Committee on Medical and public health research (CRM).

In association with

- Inter-university Cardiology Institute of the Netherlands
- Dutch Society of Ultrasound in Medicine and Biology
- Netherlands Heart Foundation
- European Society of Cardiology.

With contributions from

P. Alais, R.H. Anderson, D.W. Baker, A.E. Becker, A. Bloch, N. Bom, J.S. Borrer, M. Brandestini, E. Bridoux, C. Bruneel, F.J. ten Cate, H.J.M. Dohmen, W.G. van Dorp, D. Durrer, F.C. van Egmond, D. Gibson, J.M. Griffith, W.J. Gussenhoven, F. Hagemeijer, W.L. Henry, H. Hertz, A. Hoeks, P.G. Hugenholtz, F.E. Kloster, C.T. Lancée, G.J. Leech, L.H. Light, C.M. Ligtvoet, G. Lorch, P. Péronneau, L. Pourcelot, R.S. Reneman, J. Ridder, H. Rinke, J. Roelandt, J.M. Rouvaen, S.A. Rubenstein, D.J. Sahn, P.W. Serruys, A. Shaw, J. Somer, R. Torguet, M.J. Tynan, R. Vermeulen, W.B. Vletter, J.A. Vogel, W. Walsh, H.J.J. Wellens, J.W. Wladimiroff, G. van Zwieten.

Acknowledgement

Without the excellent co-operation of all lecturers, the members, and in particular the chairmen of committees of the commission of the European Communities which initiated this concerted activity, this book would not exist. In addition we would like to express our sincere gratitude to Joop van Dijk and Bea Grashoff of the Audiovisual Center, Erasmus University, who, together with our secretaries Ineke de Deckere and Ria Willemstein cheerfully invested many hours in the preparation of this book.

V

CONTENTS

Clinical Echocardiology

Chapter 1

CLINICAL ECHOCARDIOLOGY

The future of echocardiography as scanned by an outsider

by Dirk Durrer,
Department of Cardiology and Clinical Physiology,
University of Amsterdam, Wilhelmina Gasthuis and the
Interuniversity Cardiology Institute,
Amsterdam, The Netherlands.

Echocardiography, a priceless gift of physics and technology to medicine and patients alike, has made it possible to explore the heart and its interior by delineating the structures of this organ, using methods found in nature and applied for comparable purposes. What happened yesterday and happens today may give us a clue as to what we can expect from this technique in the future. Nine years after the method was introduced in 1945 in its rudimentary state 1), two scientists, recognizing its clinical potential and thereby becoming prime movers in this field, have adapted it sufficiently to make it suitable for clinical use 2). I saw these humble beginnings but, like many other cardiologists at that time, I remained uncommitted, being preoccupied with the fascinating developments following the introduction of cardiac catheterization. The hazy pictures, which were difficult to interpret, gave rise to expressions of doubt, which were to be confounded three years later when a left atrial myxoma - hardly an easy thing for cardiologists to diagnose in those days - was recognized with the echo technique 3), 4).

The usual resistance to innovative procedures, particularly those of a fundamental nature, meant that progress was slow, although the time-lag in this case between introduction and acceptance was relatively short, as within a decade there was a small but growing band of clinicians who had joined the prophets who appreciated the method's unique diagnostic potential 5), 6).

Along with a rapid growth in technology and the advent of better display techniques and sophisticated electronics diagnostic successes began to accumulate, gradually convincing an increasing number of cardiologists that the method was one of great importance. What might be termed the 'extrovert' character of heart action, which is depicted so clearly by this technique, may of itself have been partly responsible for this increasing momentum, which led to a full-blown clinical gold rush, resulting in the rapid accumulation of diagnostic knowledge.

The rate of expansion of echocardiography in the clinic is well illustrated by the increase in size of Feigenbaum's work on the subject: the first edition in 1972 had 129 pages and 157 references; less than five years later the second edition came out with 512 pages and 590 references 7). Echocardiography, which has greatly simplified the diagnosis of many cardiac diseases and in some cases is now looked upon as the only answer to the problem, has made obsolete many expensive, time-consuming

3

Echocardiology, N. Bom editor, published by Martinus Nijhoff, the Hague 1977.

and painful procedures. It can be applied with equal success in critically ill patients, for example, in the CCU, and in the newborn with congenital heart disease. That it has proved such a resounding success is due in no small measure to the excellent work performed in centres such as Rotterdam.

Physiological and pathophysiological results
The application of echocardiography has meant that many physiological aspects of cardiac activity can now be seen in a new light. Results obtained with this inertia-free method have indicated that generally accepted views concerning the intricate movement of the valves, based on the work of Wiggers and Dean with threads and levers, are now no longer entirely tenable. Pressure changes across the valves are only partly responsible for their closure, a finding given credence by the valvular movements in the isolated, Langendorff-perfused heart, which does not propel blood. Movements which were neither foreseen nor expected from cineangiographic studies have been demonstrated in the ventricular septum.

Wall thickness in systole and diastole can now be measured with acceptable accuracy and a quantitative approach to pump function may even become possible. However, without a significant improvement in resolution and the opening up of as yet inaccessible regions of the heart - apical half, left lateral wall - it will not be easy to solve the problems associated with the fact that endocardial and epicardial points do not only move radially during contraction but also exhibit complex torque. I sometimes have the impression that it is not yet universally recognized that ventricular filling and contraction is not comparable to inflation and deflation of a balloon.

One of the most interesting developments is the possibility of correlating the electrical and mechanical activity of the heart. As the time sequence in which the heart cells begin to contract is identical to that of depolarization, one might assume that a similar relationship exists between repolarization and relaxation in the normal heart.

In the W-P-W syndrome echocardiography has shown that the pre-excited region, activated by the anomalous pathway, contracts before the rest of the ventricle and causes slight enlargement of the latter, due to displacement of blood in the ventricular cavity. During relaxation of the region activated by the bypass the reverse holds true, and the contraction which is still present in the remainder of the ventricle now causes an outward movement. One might therefore say that pre-excitation causes precontraction and early repolarization, early relaxation.

It is hoped that high-resolution echo techniques will make it possible to study these slight or more pronounced dissimilarities in contraction patterns caused by differences in the time course of electrical activity, and may, for example, throw light on disturbances in electrical activity such as papillary muscle disfunction.

Major breakthroughs may confidently be expected in such investigative techniques as phonocardiography and the recording of external pulsations if echocardiography is combined with these procedures and with single-stimulation techniques.

4

Consequences of growth, education and research

Being bowled over backwards by echocardiography without a proper and thorough grounding in this misleadingly simple technique is clearly something which needs to be avoided at all costs. The words of Wilson 8), one of the founders of modern electrocardiography, are as applicable in this field as they ever were to the interpretation of ECGs, and should accordingly be taken to heart.

Discussing the explosive growth in the use of the electrocardiograph, he wrote: "In 1914 there was only one instrument of this kind in the State of Michigan, and this was not in operation; there were probably not more than a dozen electrocardiographs in the whole of the US. Now there is one or more in every village of any size, and there are comparatively few people who are not in greater danger of having their peace and happiness destroyed by an erroneous diagnosis of cardiac abnormality based on a faulty interpretation of the electrocardiogram, than of being injured or killed by an atomic bomb." Wilson then went on to say that the number of physicians with electrocardiographs and comparatively little knowledge of their proper use would doubtless increase by leaps and bounds, along with a proliferation of works offering nothing more than the elements of clinical electrocardiography or an introduction to this subject.

The avoidance of heart disease of echocardiographic origin is only possible with assiduity and expert tuition, and I am pleased to say that teaching is currently of a very high order. The challenge facing echocardiographists remains formidable, however, as the intelligent interpretation of signs is dependent upon a proper appreciation of the causative mechanism, which is one reason why atlases alone are insufficient. Let us hope that the near future will see the birth of 'deductive echocardiography'.

Improvement of techniques

Better resolution is clearly one of the most important desiderata for the future. Two-dimensional systems, which are very helpful for the partly initiated and which are comparable to ultrasound tomography, are currently represented on the market by several types, including the multi-element linear scanner, e.g., the Rotterdam 20 transducer version 9), yielding real-time cross-sectional images, which has impressed many people. Other models are based on the phased-array pinciple which generates an electronically controlled sector scan. In most systems resolution is being improved.

Many other types testify to the ingenuity of workers in this field. In many groups physicists, technologists and doctors are working closely together in their attempts to develop clinically optimal apparatus, and it seems to me important that non-medical people in this field should understand, as a result of direct observation, the problems facing the clinician and the consequences for the patient of diagnoses made with their instruments. Only in this way will innovative processes lose their esoteric character and become human-oriented.

5

Epilogue

There are many reasons why an outsider should congratulate echocardiographists on their work and achievements. The time has now come to put echocardiography on a sound physiological basis, a major task which the clinician cannot delegate to the physiologist. And while clinicians may sometimes be reluctant to accept this view it is only in this way that echocardiography will remain a scientific method and continue to grow healthily. One of the consequences of a discipline devoted to hypothesizing and the collection of information and lacking an experimental foundation would be great harm to the patient.

I accept echocardiography as part of science in its own right, but I sincerely hope that its ultimate goal will remain the care of the patient. By remaining linked to cardiology it will be assured of a bright future.

References

1) Firestone FA: *The supersonic reflectoscope, an instrument for inspecing the interior of solid parts by means of sound waves.*
J. Acoust. Soc. Am., 17: 287, 1945.

 The supersonic felectoscope for interior inspection.
 Metal Prog., 48: 505, 1945.

2) Edler I, and Hertz CH: *Use of ultrasonic reflectoscope for continuous recording of movements of heart walls.*
Kung. Fysiograf. Sallsk. Lund. Fordhandl., 24: 40, 1954.

3) Edler I: *Diagnostic use of ultrasound in heart disease.*
Acta Med. Scand., 308: 32, 1955.

4) Effert S, Domanig E, and Erkens H: *Moglichkeiten des Ultraschall-echo-verfahrens in der Herzdiagnostik.*
Cardiologia, 34: 73, 1959.

5) Morison EM: *Men, Machines and Modern Times.*
Cambridge, MIT Press, 1968.

6) Durrer D: *About Wampanoag, Tigerstedt, Science and Scientists, and Karl Marx's son-in-law.*
European Journal of Cardiology, 5, 1, 7-15, 1977.

7) Feigenbaum H: *Echocardiography.*
Philadelphia, Lea and Febiger, 1st edition 1973, 2nd edition 1976.

8) Wilson FN in Lepeschkin E: *Modern Electrocardiography.*
Williams and Wilkins, Baltimore 1952.

9) Bom N: *New concepts in Echocardiography.*
Stenfert Kroese, Leiden 1972.

Principles of ultrasound in medical diagnosis.

Hellmuth Hertz,
Dept of Electrical Measurements
Lund Institute of Technology - LUND/Sweden

During the last decade ultrasound has been increasingly used in different fields of medical diagnosis. In most cases the so called echo principle has been used (cf. fig. 1). As is well known from echo sounding this method allows the determination of the distance to the bottom of the sea by measuring the transit time of a short sound pulse from the boat to the bottom of the sea and back to the boat again.

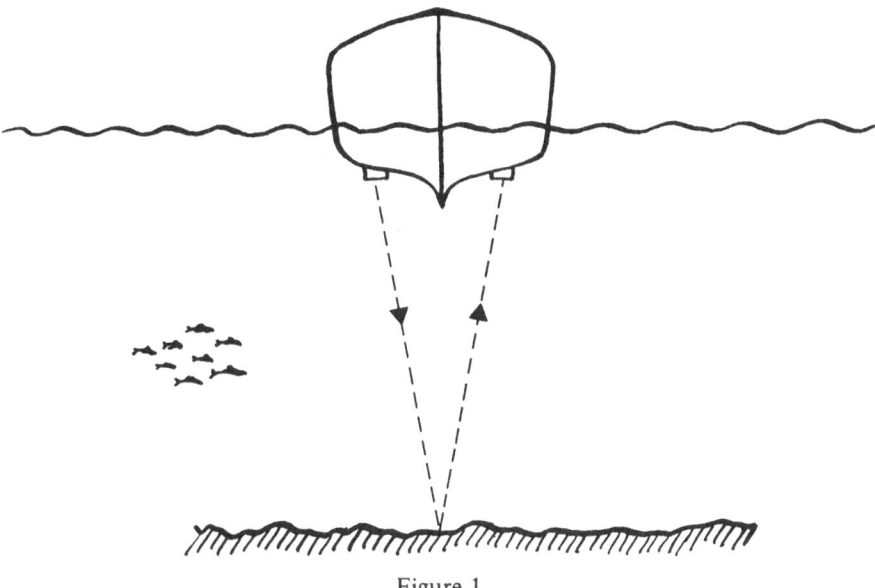

Figure 1

This echo method is extensively used also in medical diagnosis since many interfaces between biological tissues reflect sound. However, since the distances between the surface of the patient and some organ inside the body is much smaller than in the case shown in fig. 1, it is necessary to use very short sound pulses to ensure good resolution. This is due to the fact that the physical length of the sound pulse must be shorter than the minimum distance between two adjacent reflecting surfaces which one wants to discern separately. Because of this in medical diagnosis so called ultrasound is used.

7

Echocardiology, N. Bom editor, published by Martinus Nijhoff, the Hague 1977.

The ultrasound employed here differs from normal sound (longitudinal waves) only in frequency. According to definition all sound having frequencies higher than 20.000 Hz is called ultrasound. However, in the medical field frequencies between 1 and 10 MHz are used for reasons shown below. Since the speed of sound in biological tissue and water is about 1500 m/sec the wavelength at 2 MHz is 0.75 mm. Since sound pulses used in medical equipment usually consist of about 3 wavelengths the physical length of such a sound pulse is about 2.5 mm. For this reason the minimum resolution obtainable with medical ultrasonic equipment is of the same order.

These short pulses are generated by a so called transducer. The transducer consists of a disc of ferroelectric material, e.g. barium titanate, the diameter of which is about 10 mm and the thickness 1 mm. Both faces of this disc are covered by electric conducting layers. If a sudden electric voltage pulse - about 30-300 V large and 1 μs long - is applied to these two layers the ferromagnetic material vibrates for a few microseconds. These vibrations consist mainly of periodic changes of the thickness of the disc the frequency of which is dependent on that thickness. The disc described above will vibrate with a frequency of about 2 MHz.

If this vibrating disc is brought into mechanical contact with some other medium, e.g. biological tissue, a sound pulse is sent into that tissue. Since it is important to keep these sound pulses short the other side of the ferroelectric disc is usually damped by a special backing material which stops the vibrations of the crystal after a few oscillations.

Inversely, if a sound pulse hits such a transducer an electric signal will be generated between the conducting layers on the ferroelectric disc. Thus, the transducer acts as a generator for sound pulses as well as a microphone for the detection of sound pulses.

Echoscope principle

Instruments using the ultrasonic echo method for medical diagnosis are generally called *echoscopes*. The block diagram shown in fig. 2a represents a simplified version of such an instrument while the time sequences of the electrical voltages appearing at different points of the diagram are given in fig. 2b.

Every measurement made with the instrument is initiated by a timer, which normally generates about 1000 pulses per second (curve A in fig. 2b). Thus 1000 measurements are made per second. Each of these pulses starts a measuring cycle by causing the transmitter to generate a short pulse which is applied to the transducer. This output from the transmitter is normally 50 to 500 V high and about 1 μs long and causes the transducer to generate a short acoustic wave pulse which propagates into the medium between the transducer and the reflecting boundaries the position of which is to be measured. In many medical applications this acoustic pulse consists of about 3 wavelengths of a 2 MHz acoustic wave and thus has an actual length of about 2.5 millimeters in biological tissue.

8

The acoustic pulse generated by the transducer is partly reflected back to the transducer at the reflecting boundaries 1 and 2 shown in fig. 2a. Thus, if the velocity of sound in the medium is v, echo pulses will return to the transducer after the time $t_1 = \frac{2l_1}{v}$ and $t_2 = \frac{2l_2}{v}$.

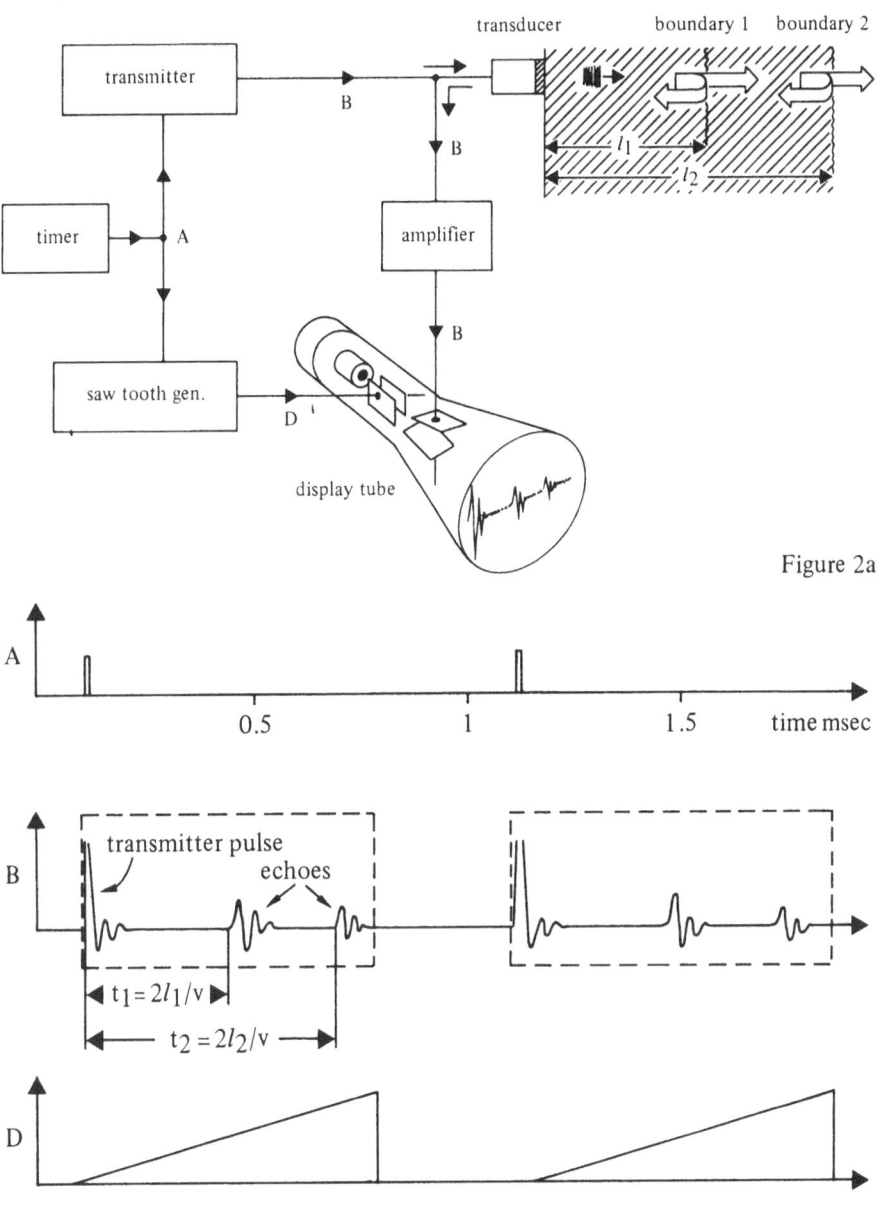

Figure 2a

Figure 2b

Since the transducer also acts as a microphone, the acoustic energy of the returning echoes is transformed back into electrical signals when the echoes arrive at the transducer. Curve B in fig, 2b shows the voltage signals generated on the connecting line to and from the transducer.

Hence, by measuring the transit times t_1 and t_2 the distance between the face of the transducer and the boundaries can be determined, if v is known and constant throughout the medium. Luckily this is practically true for all biological tissues and fluids except for bone (cf. tabel 1). This fact is essential for the use of ultrasound in medicine.

These transit times and thus the distance to the boundaries are most easily measured with a cathode ray tube (CRT) which will be called *display tube* in the following. To this end a sawtooth generator is started by the timer simultaneously with the transmitter pulse. The output voltage from the sawtooth generator (curve D in fig. 2b) is used to deflect the electron beam of the display tube in the horizontal x-direction with constant speed. In this way a horizontal line is generated on the screen of the display tube each time an acoustic pulse is transmitted into the medium. This horizontal line actually can be used as a time base so measure the transit time of the sound pulse as shown in the following.

If the echo signals returning to the transducer are amplified and then applied to the y-deflection plates of the display tube, every echo signal will displace the electron beam in the vertical direction and thus create a vertical mark on the screen (cf. fig. 2a and b). The trace inside the dotted lines of fig. 2b shows the actual picture appearing on the display screen. Since $l_1 \sim t_1$, $l_2 \sim t_2$ etc., the distance of these marks from the start of the trace will be proportional to l_1 and l_2, i.e. the true distance of the reflecting boundaries from the transducer. In the present instrument, the start of the trace is also marked by a strong vertical mark due to the transmitter pulse applied to the transducer at the beginning of each measuring cycle. Hence, the trace shown on the screen of the display tube is equal to those parts of curve D in fig. 2b. which lie within the dotted rectangles.

By calibrating the instrument the true distances l_1 and l_2 can be measured. This can be achieved by measuring an echo from a reflector immersed in water at a known distance from the transducer. Normally echoscopes are supplied with an internal pulse generator which creates small markers along the display trace. These markers represent a centimeter or millimeter scale which facilitates orientation and depth measurements in biological tissue.

Properties of ultrasound important in medical diagnosis

For the successful use of an echoscope certain principles of ultrasound physics are of importance. In the following these properties will be considered shortly.

a) Reflection.
Obviously the echo method can only detect reflecting boundaries in media.

10

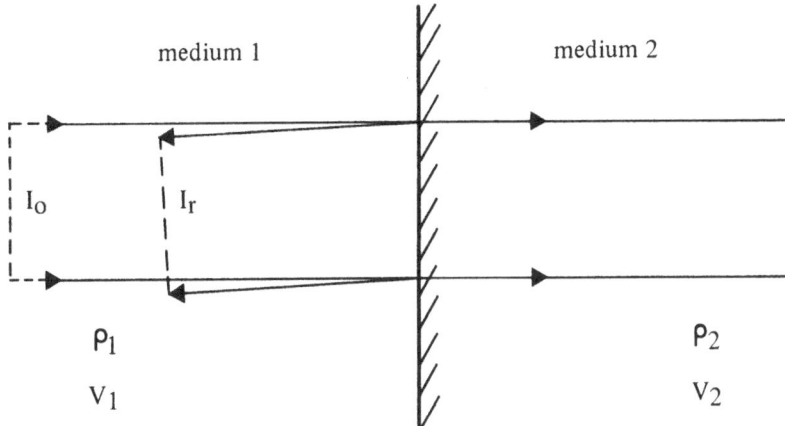

medium 1   medium 2

ρ_1 ρ_2

v_1 v_2

The reflection of sound from such a boundary between medium 1 and medium 2 (cf. fig. 3) is governed by the equation

$$I_r = I_0 \left(\frac{v_1\rho_1 - v_2\rho_2}{v_1\rho_1 + v_2\rho_2} \right)^2$$

under the condition that the sound beam impinges on the boundary at right angles. In this equation I_0 is the sound intensity impinging on the boundary while I_r is the reflected sound intensity. ρ_1 and ρ_2 are the densities and v_1 and v_2 are the sound velocities in the two media respectively. It can be seen from the equation that the product $\rho \cdot v$ is important for the intensity of the reflected echo pulse. If this product is very similar in both media nearly no sound is reflected, on the other hand large differences give rise to strong echoes. The product $\rho \cdot v$ is called the characteristic impedance of the material and is not dependent on frequency.

Table 1. Sound velocity and characteristic impedances of some common materials.

	Material	Sound velocity $(m \cdot s^{-1})$	Characteristic impedance $(g \cdot cm^{-2}sec^{-1}) \cdot 10^{-5}$
Non-biological	Air 0°C	331	0.004
	Water 25°C	1497	1.48
	Perspex	2670	3.20
	Aluminium	6260	18.0
	Brass	4430	38.0
Biological	Fat	1450	1.38
	Brain	1541	1.58
	Blood	1570	1.61
	Kidney	1561	1.62
	Liver	1549	1.65
	Muscle	1585	1.70
	Skull-bone	4080	7.80

From tabel 1 we see that the characteristic impedance does not differ too much between different biological tissues because of which only small echoes from tissue boundaries can be expected. On the other hand ultrasound is heavily reflected at boundaries between biological tissue and air. Because of the latter fact ultrasound does not readily penetrate lung tissue which makes the investigation of the heart by ultrasound difficult.

If the reflecting boundary is not placed at right angles to the impinging ultrasonic beam the beam will be reflected like light on a mirror as shown in fig. 4.

Figure 4

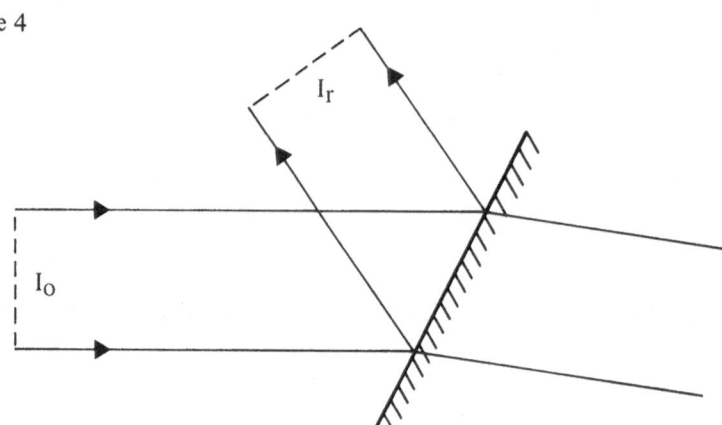

If the inclination of the boundary is large enough this means that the sound pulse will not return to the transducer (cf. fig. 2a) and therefore no echo is recorded. Thus such a boundary will not be observed at all by the simple echo method as described above. Since most of the boundaries of biological organs do not lie perpendicular to the sound beam direction this seems to diminish the usefulness of the echoscope very much. However, it will be explained in the next lecture how this difficulty can be circumvented by the use of the so called compound scan technique.

Even if this compound scan technique would not exist some useful information could be obtained from biological tissue in spite of the difficulty described here, since small inhomogenities inside biological tissue tend to scatter ultrasound in all directions. Some of this scattered sound is always reflected back to the transducer and can thus be detected even if its intensity is much lower than the echoes from boundaries between different kinds of tissues.

b) Absorption.
When transversing biological tissue the energy of the ultrasonic pulse is absorbed in the tissue. Thus the intensity of the sound pulse decreases with the distance transversed in the tissue. This decrease is given by the formula

$$I_x = I_o \; e^{-2 \, \alpha \, f \, x}$$

where I_0 and I_x are the intensities of the sound at the surface and the depth x in the tissue respectively. Further the absorption is approximately dependent on the frequency f and a constant α which is typical for different kinds of tissues as shown in table 2.

Table 2.

Tissue	$\alpha \cdot 10^2$ cm^{-1} MHz^{-1}	Frequency range MHz
Blood	2	1
Fat	7.5	0.8 - 7
Brain	10	0.9 - 3.4
Liver	11	0.3 - 3.4
Kidney	12	0.3 - 4.5
Muscle along fibers	15	0.8 - 4.5
Muscle across fibers	38	0.8 - 4.5
Skull bone	230	1.6

As can be seen from this expression the absorption of ultrasound increases strongly with frequency. Since it is important that the returning echoes should be strong, this seems to indicate that a sound frequency as low as possible should be used. However, it was already pointed out in the introduction that sound pulses should be kept short to ensure good resolution and we will see in the following paragraph that this is even more true for the lateral resolution. Thus a suitable compromise has to be reached between good resolution and the intensity of the returning echoes because of which different frequencies are often used in different types of patients e.g. adults or children.

c) Diffraction.
According to the laws of physics waves do not travel as a well-defined beam through large distances if the beam diameter is comparable to the wavelength. Instead such a beam diverges with an angle β due to the so called diffraction phenomenon as shown in fig. 5.

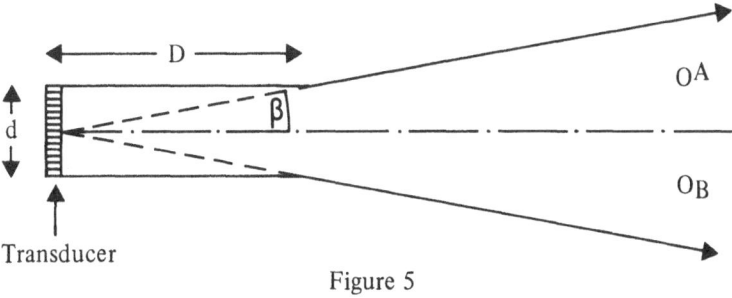

Figure 5

13

The angle β is approximately given above according to the formula $\sin \beta = 1.22 \frac{\lambda}{d}$ where d is the diameter of the transducer and λ is the wavelength of the sound. As can be seen from the picture the beam diameter increases over distance $D = \frac{d^2}{4\lambda}$ which is called the near zone. Because of this increase in beam diameter ouside of the near zone it is obvious that the resolution vertical to the beam direction, i.e. the lateral resolution, will decrease with distance. Thus it will not be possible to distinguish the two objects A and B in fig. 5 since they will both reflect sound echoes back to the transducer.

To obtain good lateral resolution it is obvious that the beam diameter should be as small as possible. Therefore one would tend to keep the diameter d of the transducer small. However, we can see from the diffraction equation given above that this would increase the angle β and thereby actually decrease the resolution. Alternatively the frequency could be increased. However, this is possible only within certain limits because of the strong dependence of absorption on frequency pointed out above. Because of this it is in fact much harder to obtain good lateral resolution with the echoscope compared to the resolution along the axis of the sound beam. Many different devices have been designed to circumvent this difficulty, the most common of these is again the compound scan method.

d) Doppler effect.

Finally it should be mentioned that the frequency of an ultrasonic beam reflected from a boundary moving along the axis of the sound beam is changed by an amount Δf according to the formula $\frac{\Delta f}{f} = \frac{2w}{v}$

Here Δf is the frequency change of the frequency f of the ultrasound being used, v the speed of the sound in the tissue and w the velocity of the moving boundary. Since this frequency change Δf can be detected by suitable electronic circuits it is obvious that the velocity w of the boundary can be measured. This so called Doppler method is well known from radar control of automobile speeds by the police, where microwaves are used instead of ultrasound. In ultrasonic applications both continuous ultrasound and pulsed ultrasound are used for doppler measurements. However, the continuous wave methods are still predominant in hospital routine.

Summary

In this article a short description of the principle of an echoscope was given as well as the main physical parameters which influence its use in medical diagnosis. However, it should be observed that actual echoscopes are much more sophisticated in order to accomodate the special requirements for medical diagnosis. Also the Doppler method for measuring the speed of moving structures has been touched upon.

Echocardiographic examination techniques

by Frank E. Kloster
University of Oregon Health Science Center
Portland, Oregon 97201, U.S.A.

The most critical and difficult part of echocardiography is obtaining an echocardiographic record of the best possible technical quality which accurately represents the patient's cardiac anatomy and physiology. When a satisfactory record is obtained, interpretation is not difficult in the majority of cases. Accurate interpretation is often impossible with technically poor or incomplete records, even when the underlying cardiac disease is straightforward and uncomplicated. Three major and interrelated factors contribute to consistent success in obtaining satisfactory records: a firm understanding of cardiac anatomy, development of the technical ability to direct the probe at important cardiac structures and knowledge of proper adjustment of the instrumentation to obtain optimal records.

The importance of a thorough understanding of cardiac anatomy and three-dimensional anatomic relationships in performing and interpreting echocardiograms cannot be over-emphasized. During performance of the examination the operator must have a clear three-dimensional mental image of the structures being examined and of geometric relationships between them. This is for the purposes of both locating structures and correctly recording normal or abnormal relationships. The technical ability to identify and properly record important cardiac structures is closely related to this, and technical success is more often limited by lack of anatomic and physiologic insight than by lack of manual dexterity. Proper instrument settings vary between individuals and with different instrument design characteristics, but are relatively straightforward for most examiners after initial instruction.

Most of the important diagnostic information in a cardiac examination is obtained by directing the transducer along a sagittal plane following the long axis of the heart (fig. 1).
The mitral valve is the landmark and central structure for orientation in this plane. Once the position of this landmark is identified other valves, chambers and structures are visualized by tilting the transducer cephalad or caudad along the plane of the long axis of the heart, as shown diagrammatically in fig. 1. The anterior heart wall and right ventricular (RV) cavity are anterior in the chest closest to the transducer. When the echo beam is directed through the landmark mitral valve it passes anteriorly to posteriorly through these structures, the ventricular septum (IVS), the left ventricular (LV) cavity, mitral valve (MV) leaflets and posterior left ventricular wall (pLVW). The aorta (Ao) is superior, with the anterior wall a direct upward ex-

15

Echocardiology, N. Bom editor, published by Martinus Nijhoff, the Hague 1977.

tension of the IVS and the posterior wall an indirect upward continuity with the anterior MV leaflet. The left atrium (LA) lies posterior and the pulmonary outflow tract anterior to the Ao.

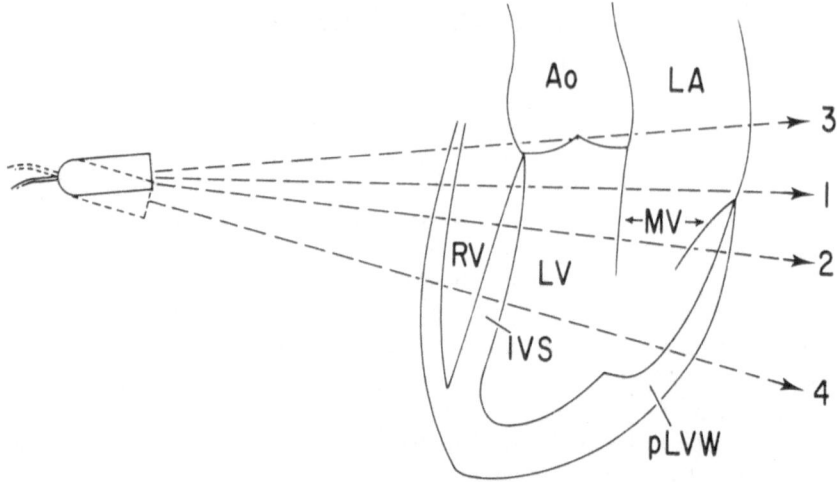

fig. 1. Transducer positions for examining different areas of the heart: see text for description.

Patients are examined in the supine or shallow left lateral position: comparative studies in our laboratory and others have shown no difference in findings in the two positions, but slightly greater success in the left lateral position. The transducer is initially placed in the left third intercostal space immediately adjacent to the sternum and the landmark structure, the MV, is located. Once the location of the MV is established the *standard position* of the transducer on the chest wall for recording the echographic study is determined. This is in the intercostal space and position on the chest where an optimal MV echo image is recorded with the transducer perpendicular to the chest wall. This position may vary in different individuals between the second and fifth intercostal space, but recording from the standard position is critical in obtaining reproducible, accurate echo data. A number of studies have clearly demonstrated that recording from nonstandard positions can give misleading pattern information, such as false discontinuity between Ao and IVS or false MV prolapse, and inconsistent quantitative information, such as chamber dimensions.

Mitral Valve Study

With the transducer in the standard position on the chest, indicated as Position 1 in fig. 1, the typical motion pattern of the anterior leaflet of the MV will be recognized directly under the transducer (fig. 2).

The characteristic "M-shaped" pattern begins with opening of the MV at the onset of ventricular diastole, which is seen as an initial anterior movement of the anterior

16

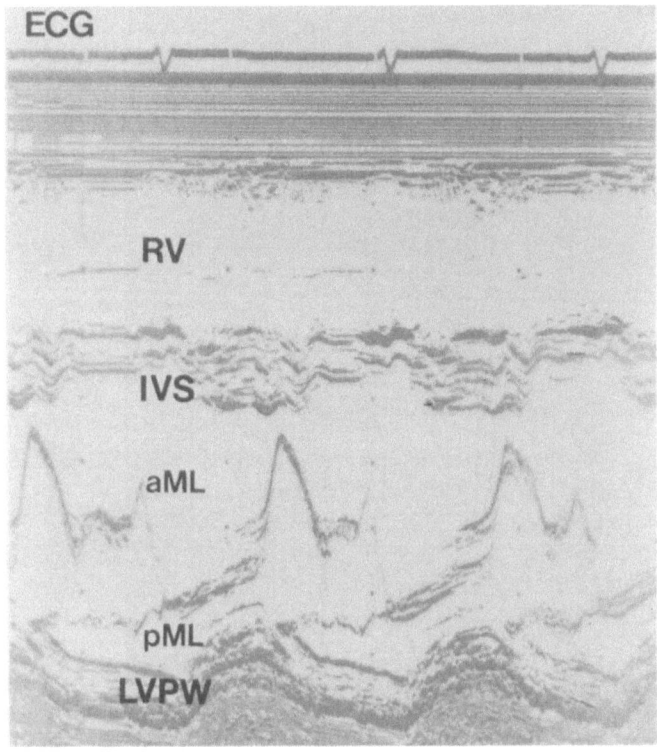

fig. 2. Mitral valve echogram showing the characteristic "M-shaped" pattern of the anterior mitral leaflet (aML) and mirror-image "W-shaped" pattern of the posterior mitral leaflet (pML). Right ventricle (RV), ventricular septum (IVS) and left ventricular posterior wall (LVPW) are labeled.

leaflet toward the chest wall. In early- to middiastole the MV partially closes and moves away from the chest wall, then reopens anteriorly with atrial contraction and closes posteriorly at the end of diastole. During ventricular systole the MV echo image normally moves slowly toward the chest wall. This represents anterior movement of the entire MV apparatus, including the leaflets and annulus, related to LV emptying and LA filling.

A complete study of the mitral valve must also include a recording of posterior mitral leaflet (PMV) motion. If the PMV is not visualized in Position 1, it can be seen by directing the transducer slightly caudad and toward the left (fig. 1, Position 2). The normal PMV is a "W-shaped" image with a smaller amplitude of motion than the anterior leaflet. It is helpful to sweep the transducer between Positions 1 and 2 while recording the echogram to include both maximal excursions of the AMV and simultaneous AMV and PMV images.

17

Aortic and Left Atrial Study

To record Ao and LA images the transducer is directed caphalad and medially (fig. 3). In this position (Position 3, fig. 1) the echo beam traverses in sequence the chest wall, anterior heart wall, RV outflow tract, Ao and LA. The position is most easily recognized by the parallel motion of the anterior and posterior Ao walls (fig. 4).

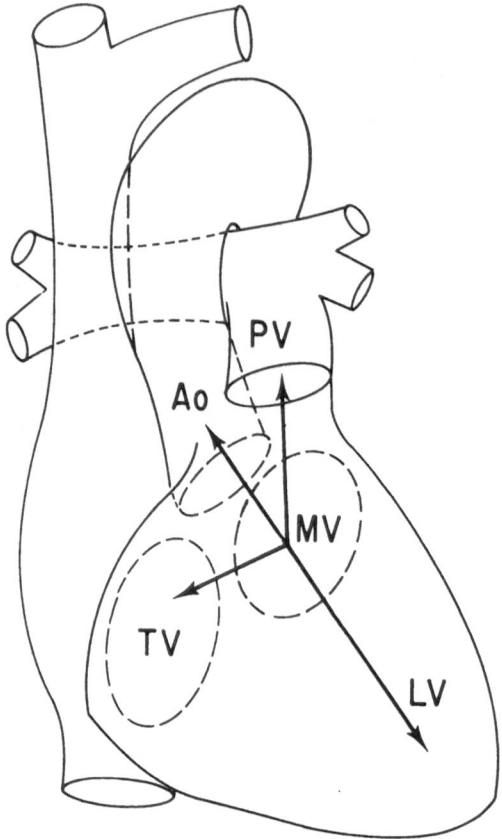

fig. 3. Relationship of the aorta (Ao), left ventricle (LV), pulmonary and tricuspid valves (PV and TV) to the landmark mitral valve (MV).

The Ao moves toward the transducer during ventricular systole and away from the transducer during diastole. The normal Ao valve cusps are seen as fine echo images which are joined in the center of the Ao during diastole and separate, opening in opposite directions toward the Ao walls, during systole. The anterior echo represents the right coronary cusp and the posterior echo the noncoronary cusp.

The LA cavity is bounded by the posterior Ao wall and the posterior LA wall, which usually does not move significantly at this level. If the transducer is gradually direct-

18

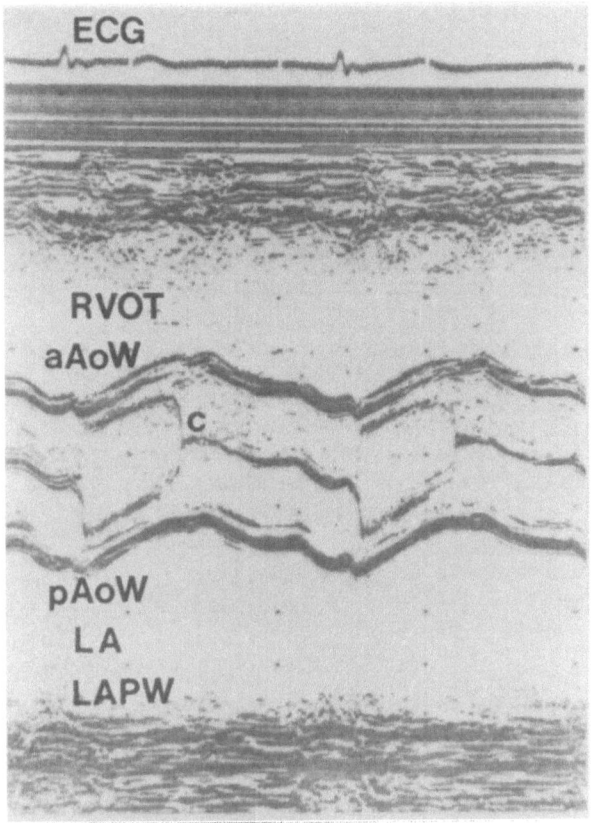

fig. 4. Aortic and left atrial echogram. The right ventricular outflow tract (RVOT), anterior and posterior aortic walls (aAoW and pAoW), aortic valve cusps (c), left atrial cavity (LA) and left atrial posterior wall (LAPW) are identified.

ed slightly caudad, increasing movement of the LA posterior wall will be apparent as the mitral annulus is approached. An optimal Ao/LA study is obtained when the echogram displays nearly equal parallel movement of the Ao walls and good visualization of the valve cusps.

Left Ventricular Study

Images of the ventricular chambers are obtained by directing the transducer caudad and toward the left (fig. 3). The standard position for ventricular studies is indicated as Position 4 in fig. 1, where the echo beam traverses the anterior heart wall, RV cavity, IVS, LV cavity at the level of the chordae tendineae and posterior LV wall (fig. 5).

Correct identification of the proper position is best accomplished by sweeping the echo beam downward from the MV to the level of the posteriomedial papillary

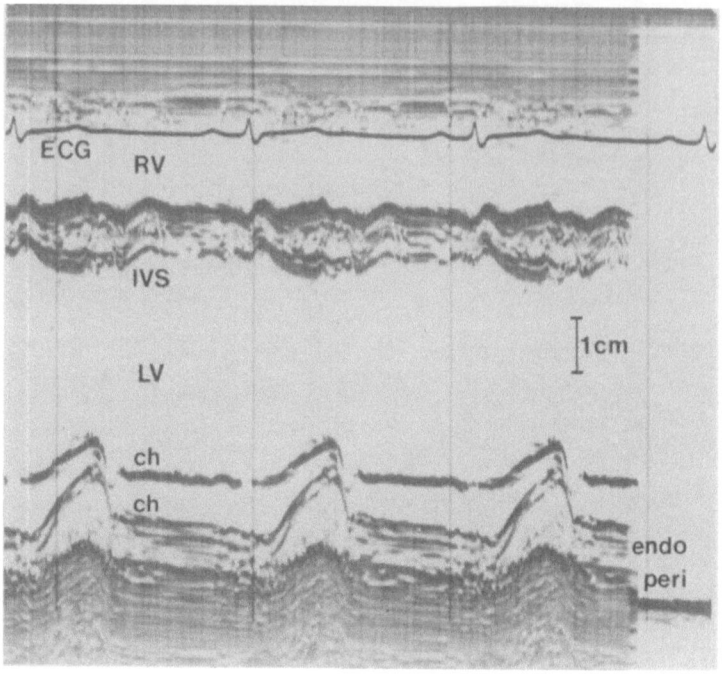

fig. 5. Ventricular echogram at the level of the chordae tendineae (ch) identifying the right ventricle (RV), ventricular septum (IVS), left ventricular cavity (LV), endocardium (endo) and pericardium (peri) of the posterior LV wall.

muscle near the apex of the LV. As the transducer is directed downward the high amplitude "M-shaped" motion pattern of the anterior mitral leaflet disappears as the sound beam passes below the free edges of the valve and is replaced by the more flat images of the chordae which float over the top of the normally moving posterior wall. Caudad the chordal images merge with a thick posterior band of echoes which represent the posterior papillary muscle.

A satisfactory image for LV evaluation and dimension measurements must include the right and left surfaces of the IVS, the endocardial and pericardial surfaces of the posterior wall and chordae tendineae in the LV cavity. The LV transverse dimension recorded should be the largest dimension discernible as defined by a transverse scan of the chamber. When all of these criteria are met, the study is restricted to a very discrete portion of the LV which can be reproduced with a high degree of consistency by different examiners and on multiple occasions. Such reproducibility is obviously crucial in obtaining meaningful quantitative measurements of ventricular dimensions and function.

Simultaneous recording of the septum and posterior wall is frequently the most difficult part of the entire echo procedure. This is accomplished more easily with

20

the patient in a left lateral position and sometimes requires slight movement of the transducer from the standard position on the chest wall toward the sternum. In addition to careful identification of the correct echo direction through the heart, special care is necessary in adjusting the instrument to avoid introducing spurious echoes or eliminating meaningful echoes, particularly the right side of the septum. At some point during each ventricular recording it is important to positively identify the pericardium by damping the echo signal or reducing the gain until only the posterior pericardium, the strongest reflecting interface, is seen.

M-mode Scan

To clearly demonstrate anatomic relationships between cardiac structures and to provide an overall assessment of cardiac geometry and anatomy it is important to record an M-mode scan of the heart in addition to isolated studies of the above three interest areas. To accomplish this the transducer is directed through the Ao and LA (fig. 1, Position 3) and swept downward through the MV and body of the LV to the apex, while the resulting images are continuously recorded (fig. 6). Such scans are particularly helpful in patients with abnormal anatomic relationships due to congenital heart disease, such as aortic-septal discontinuity.

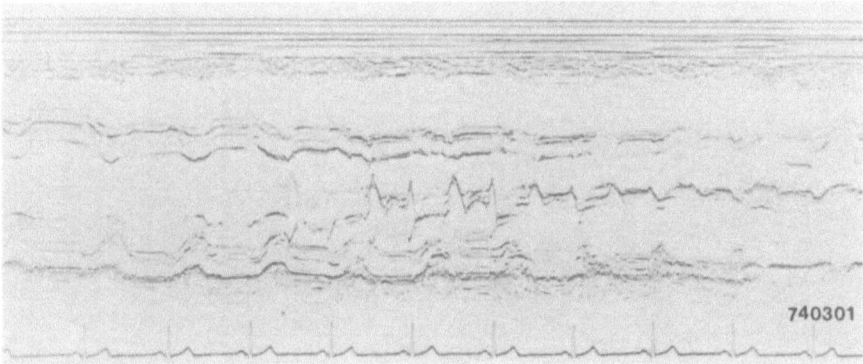

fig. 6. M-mode scan of the heart, beginning near the cardiac apex on the left and sweeping across the mitral valve in the center to the aorta and left atrium on the right.

Studies of Other Structures

Echographic recordings of other cardiac structures, particularly the pulmonary and tricuspid valves (PV and TV) can be obtained in many patients and are sometimes critical in evaluating children or patients with suspected congenital heart disease. The PV lies directly superior to the MV (fig. 3) and is examined by directing the transducer cephalad from the standard position. The echo beam passes obliquely through the chest wall and anterior heart wall, along the RV outflow tract and through the posteriorly located PV cusp, which is usually the only cusp visualized.

21

The TV is located directly to the right of the MV and is located by directing the transducer medially from the standard position. If this is unsuccessful the TV can be located by finding the Ao root, then directing the transducer medially and inferiorally. The anterior TV leaflet is the one routinely recorded and is recognized by a motion pattern similar to that of the anterior MV leaflet. Anatomic relationships between the MV and TV, which are important in some congenital malformations, are established by scanning back and forth between the two valves.

Echocardiographic examination of the aortic root and aortic valve

by H. Rinke
II Medizinische Klinik der Universität München

Echocardiography allows display of the moving anatomy of the heart 1). Qualitative as well as quantitative information concerning functional, congenital and acquired changes can be obtained by examining the aortic root and the aortic valves. The normal anatomic relations are represented in the echocardiogramme as follows. A sectional view of the heart along the longitudinal axis using the multi-element technique according to Bom 2), 3) shows continuity between the anterior aortic wall and the interventricular septum as well as between the posterior aortic wall and the anterior mitral cusp (fig. 1).

The aortic valves produce a reflection in the middle of the aortic lumen. The symmetrical valves make contact with one another in the center of the aortic lumen near the noduli arantii during diastole so that, even if the angle of incidence of the ultrasound varies, the impingement of the ultrasound is perpendicular and thus reflection can occur. During systole the valves lie against the aortic wall. The opening movement toward the anterior aortic wall corresponds to the opening of the right coronary cusp, movement toward the posterior wall corresponds to the opening of the acoronary cusp. The left coronary cusp moves transversely relative to the propagation of the ultrasound and is displayed in the form of an intermediate echo during systole only if it is thickened 4), 10).

If the information of one crystal is recorded continuously either by interposing an element of the multi-element transducer or by a single element transducer an improved evaluation of the movements is possible (M-mode registration). In systole the cusps show a box-like configuration with a fine fluttering at the aortic walls. In diastole the cusps are represented by an echo trace in the middle of the aortic root performing the motion of the aortic walls. The opening and closing speed as well as the opening amplitude can be measured in this way (fig. 2).

23

Echocardiology, N. Bom editor, published by Martinus Nijhoff, the Hague 1977.

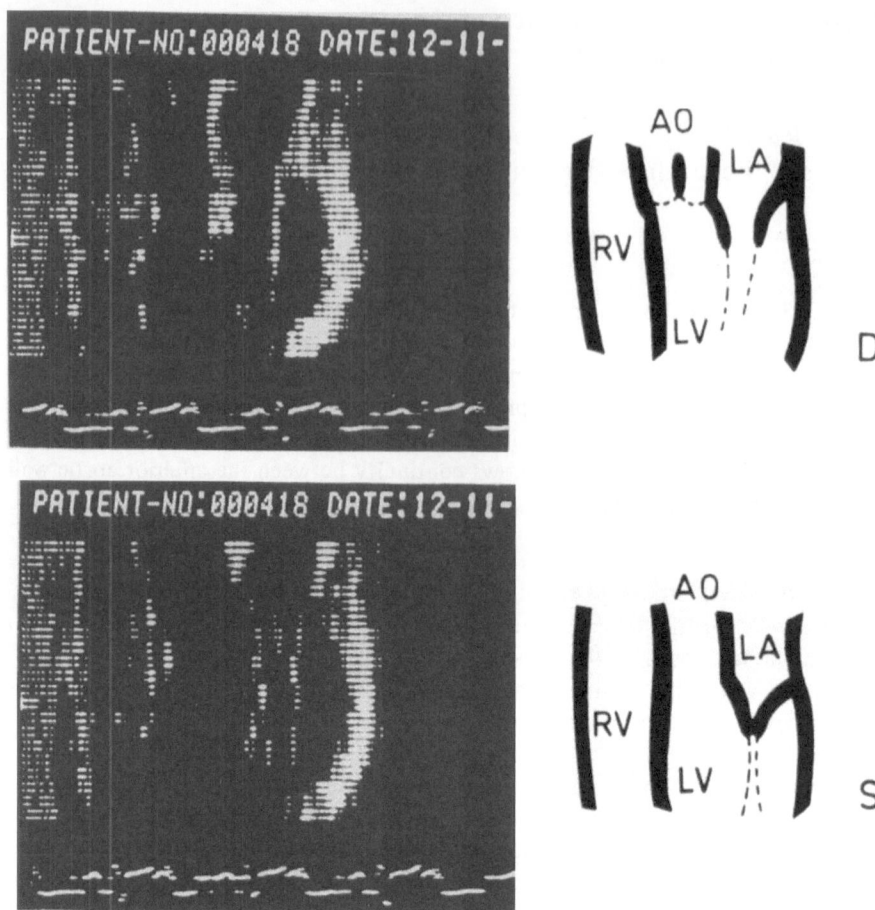

fig. 1. Cross-section of a normal heart with the multi-element system. AO: aorta, LA: left atrium, LV: left ventricle, RV: right ventricle, D: diastole, S: systole.

The movement of the aortic root is similar to the movement of the mitral ring. An anterior movement occurs during systole which exceeds the duration of the ejection time of the blood and which recedes in two phases in the form of a fast and slow rear movement corresponding to the fast and slow cardiac filling phases. Renewed dorsal movement coinciding with the atrial contraction phase occurs during presystole 6).

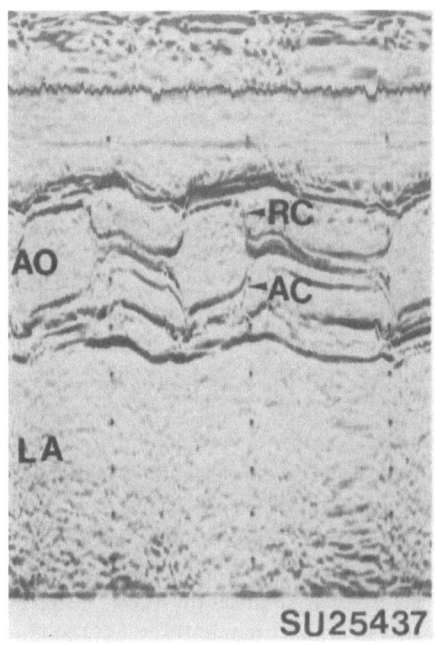

fig. 2. Normal movement of a thickened aortic valve (M-mode registration). RC: right coronary cusp, AC: acoronary cusp.

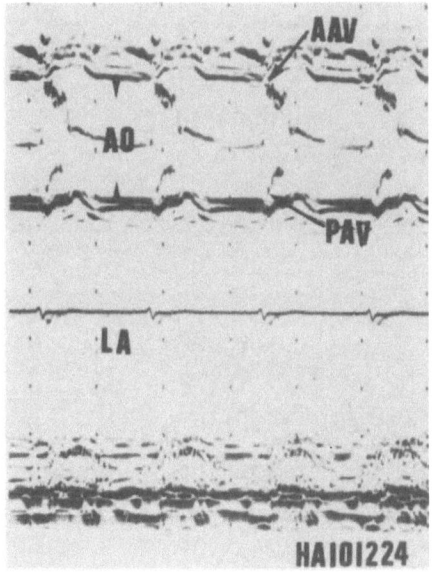

fig. 3. Aortic valve in low cardiac output (congestive cardiomyopathy). AAV: right coronary cusp, PAV: acoronary cusp.

Functional changes

The apparent mobility of the aortic valves is determined to a decisive extent by the way in which blood is discharged from the left ventricle. Changes in the stroke volume and changes in the output due to subvalvular stenoses cause a change in aortic valve mobility. When analysing the aortic valve mobility in patients with markedly reduced cardiac index, it is found that the valves do not remain in the wide open position after regular systolic opening as is normally the case, but rather display a closing movement during systole with the valves executing a more coarse fluttering (fig. 3).

Restricted initial opening amplitudes are registered predominantly during premature incidence of ventricular contraction. Further the ejection time is shortened when measured on the basis of the time which elapses from the opening to the closing of the valve 7), 8). As for the amplitude of the forward movement of the aortic root during systole, this is depressed, which has been explained to be a direct function of low cardiac output 9), 6). However, comparing the systolic amplitude of aortic root motion and cardiac output with different size of left atrium we feel that besides the cardiac output and hence the left atrial volume changes 10) the size of the left atrium is of considerable influence.

In the case of discrete subvalvular stenosis the valves, after opening wide initially, lean against the blood stream which frequently is only as thick as a pencil due to the subvalvular stenosis. In the echocardiogramme an initial rapid opening and closing movement can be seen. Afterwards the valves execute a coarse fluttering in an almost closed position during systole (fig. 4) 10)-13).

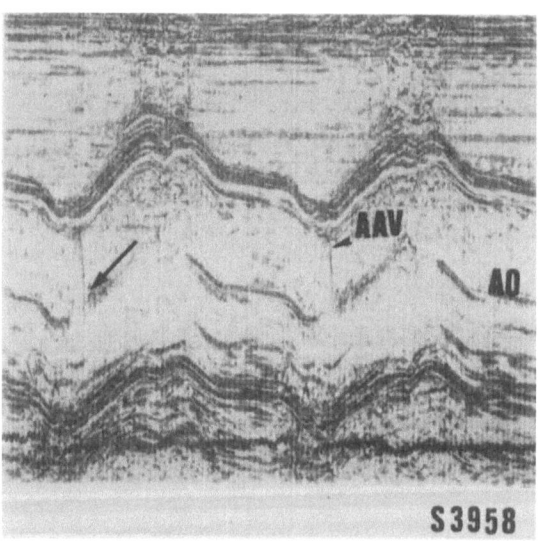

fig. 4. Discrete subaortic stenosis. Arrow: rapid closing movement of the right coronary cusp after the initial opening.

26

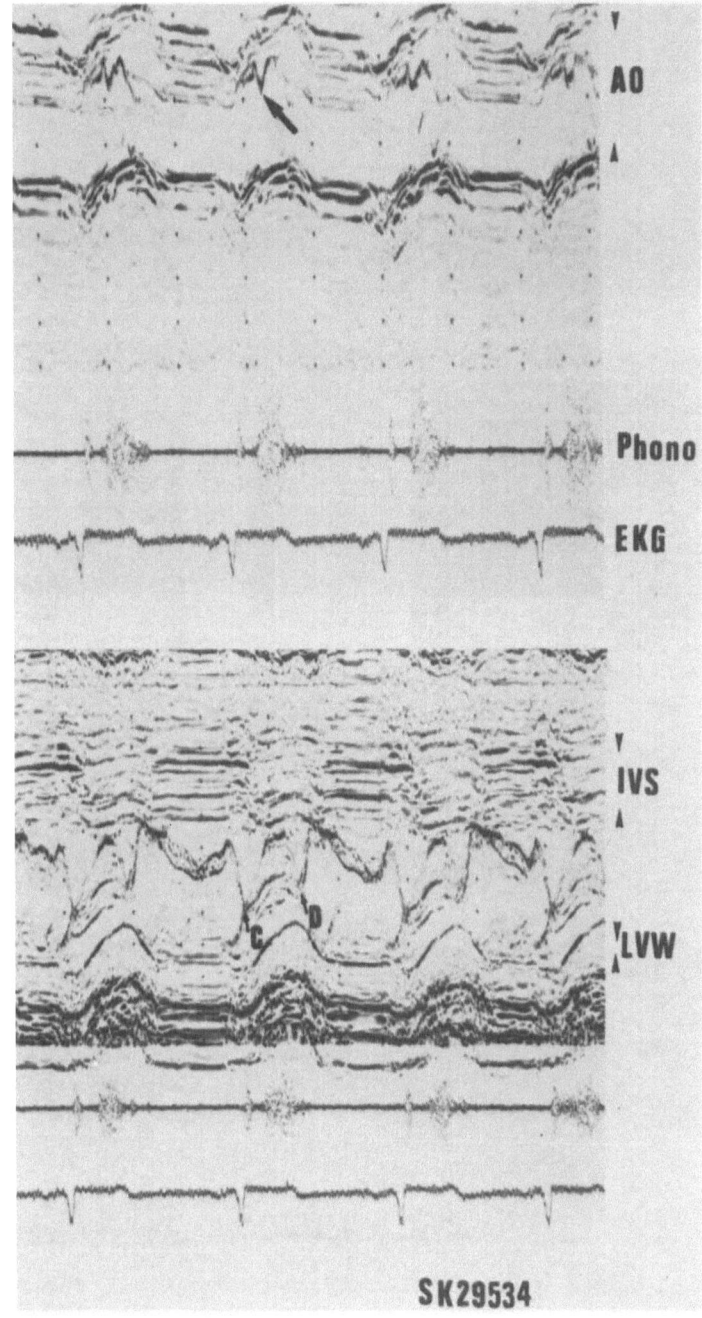

fig. 5. Hypertrophic obstructive cardiomyopathy. Arrow: midsystolic closure of the right coronary cusp.

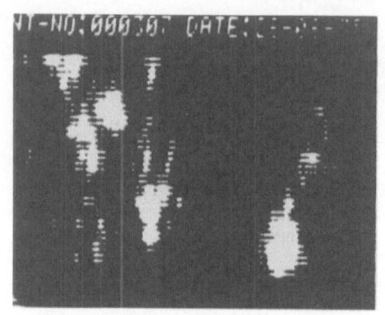
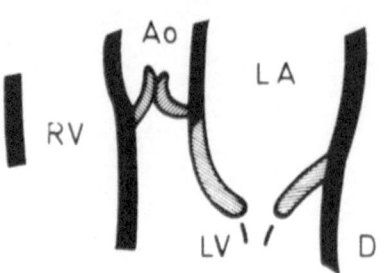

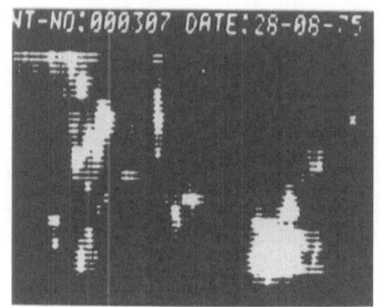
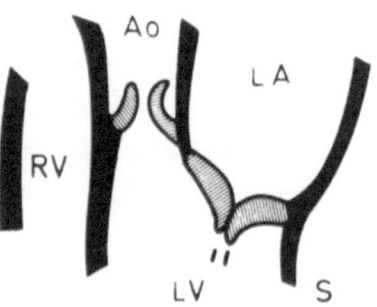

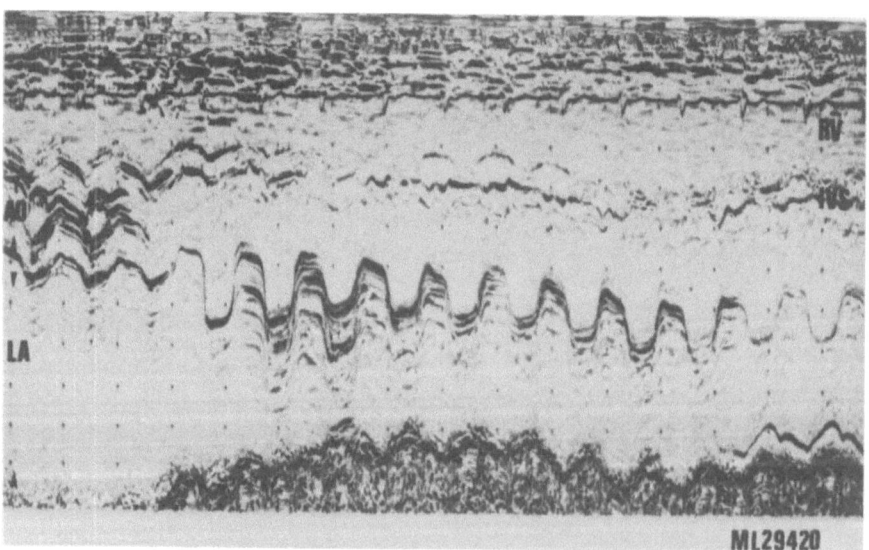

fig. 6. Combined aortic and mitral valve lesion. Cross-section and M-mode.

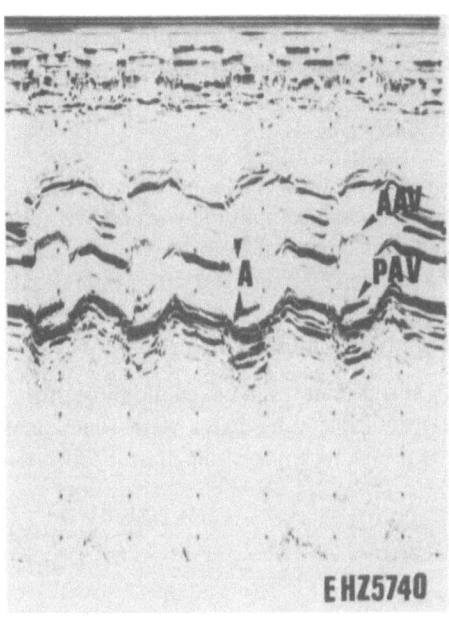

fig. 7. Aortic stenosis with reduced mobility of the right coronary cusp. A: restricted opening amplitude.

In the case of hypertrophic obstructive cardiomyopathy, the obstruction develops during the course of systole due to the abnormal mitral valve mobility 14)-16). The obstruction reaches a maximum approximately in the middle of systole and recedes again during late systole. According to the changes in the flow conditions the aortic valve, after opening initially, displays a closing movement which attains its maximum in the middle of systole (fig. 5). A renewed opening movement can be observed during late systole. This closing movement in the middle of systole is frequently only vaguely displayed due to the marked turbulence formation and the associated coarse enttering of the cusps.

Aortic stenosis
Rheumatic endocarditis results in an intensified reflection of the valve due to fibrosis and calcification. Mobility is restricted due to fusion of the commissures 4), 5), 17)-21). In the case of the multi-element display (fig. 6), strong reflection are shown in the lumen of the aortic root which demonstrate only slight mobility during systole. M-mode registration is capable to detect the restricted opening amplitude which has to be measured at the beginning of systole to minimize the influence of low cardiac output.

If only one commissure is fused, a restriction of movement of the adjacent cusp occurs, the cusp opposite the commissure not being impaired in its mobility (fig. 7).

A comparison of valve mobility of 60 patients with aortic stenoses with the finding at operation (20 pat.) and with hemodynamically obtained parameters such as pressure gradient and aperture area showed that three groups can be differentiated with respect to valve mobility (fig. 8) 20):

1) Aortic stenoses with restricted opening amplitude (dots) demonstrated a clinically useful correlation of opening amplitude with respect to the hemodynamically obtained parameters such as pressure gradient and aperture area. An opening amplitude below 0.6 cm corresponds to a serious aortic stenosis, from 0.6 - 1.2 cm to a moderate stenosis and from 1.2 - 1.8 cm to a minor stenosis. These data are in accordance with those published by Yeh 19).

2) A second group with aortic stenoses in which mobility of the cusps was no longer detectable (triangles). Multiple echo paths were found in the aortic lumen in these cases which did not show any systolic-diastolic difference in the pattern of

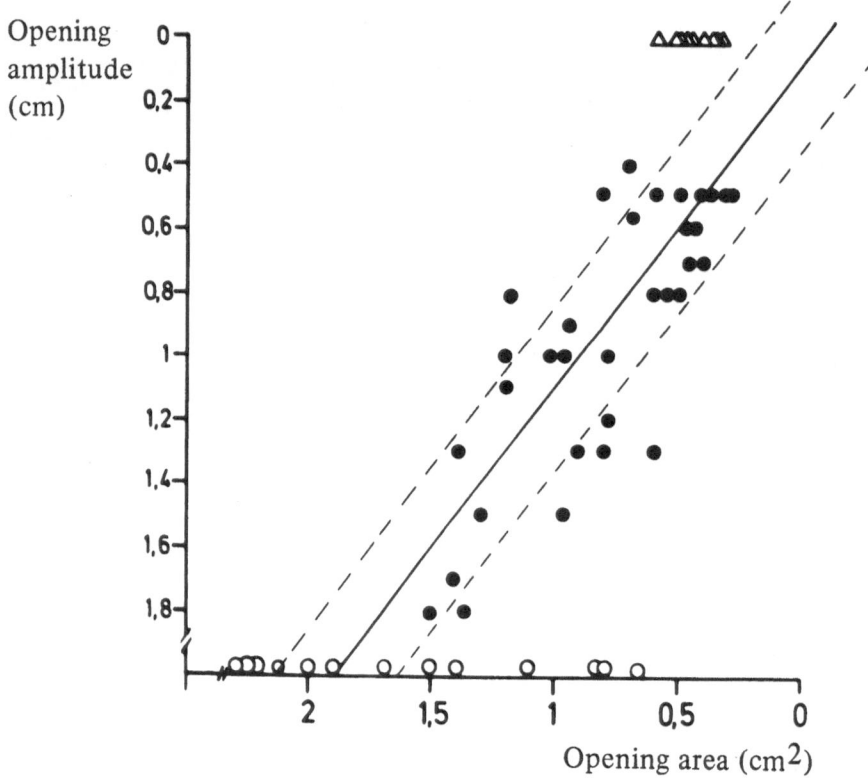

fig. 8. Correlation of the opening amplitude (cm) in the echocardiogramme with the opening area (cm^2). Dots: aortic stenosis with minimal regurgitation, triangles: aortic stenosis with immobile cusps and regurgitation grad 1-2, circles: congenital bicuspid aortic valves. (From H. Rinke et al., Verh. Dtsch. Ges. Inn. Med. 81: 247, 1975).

movement. This picture is associated predominantly with high-grade aortic stenoses. During surgery markedly calcified and immobile valves were found.

3) In the case of the third group (circles), there is no restriction of the opening amplitude in spite of a considerable pressure gradient, so that no graduation of the stenosis can be made on the basis of the analysis of mobility. During surgery congenital bicusped aortic valves were found.

By echocardiography congenital bicuspid aortic stenoses can be detected by a loss of the central echo trace during diastole, because the symmetry of the valve is destroyed (fig. 9) 21)-24). The echo trace evident during diastole is displaced more toward the anterior or posterior aortic wall. A differentiation with respect to the normal population is possible using the eccentricity index cited by Nanda 22). However, in few cases with diseased tricuspid aortic valve eccentric diastole echo traces can be observed. The unrestricted opening amplitude of these valves is due to the fact that they show a domeshaped pattern during systole. Since perpendicular impingement of the ultrasound is thus only possible in the area of the base, a regular opening amplitude occurs since the valve parts near the base lie against the aortic wall during systole. Due to the increased diastolic folding of the valve multiple echoes in the aortic lumen may frequently occur. Depending on the position of the transducer an alternating trace during diastole is often registered.

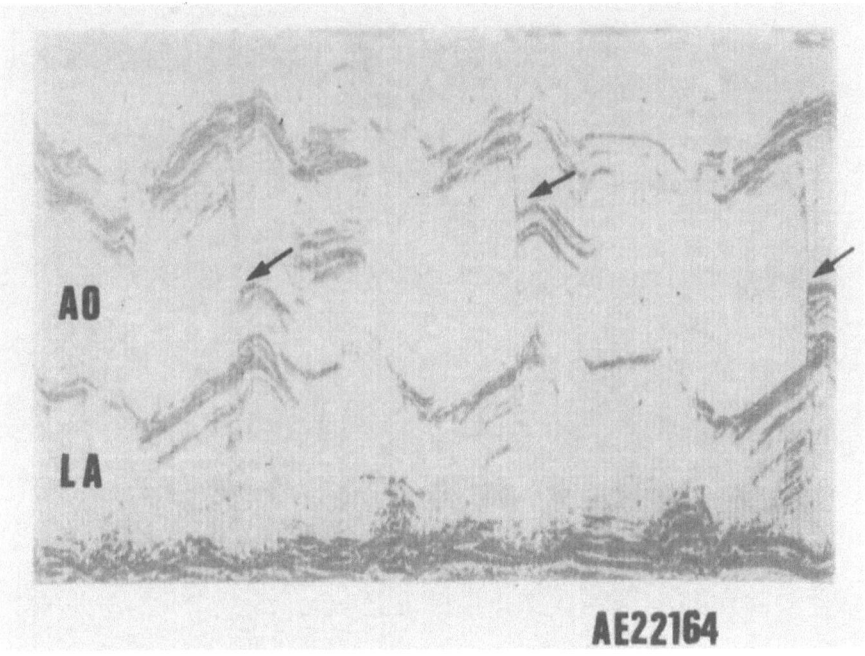

fig. 9. Congenital bicuspid aortic valve. Arrow: variable diastolic echo trace.

Aortic insufficiency

The mechanism which produces the leakage of the aortic valves can be recognized by echo-cardiographic means. Aortic insufficiencies due to rheumatic 4), 5), 17)-22) or bacterial endocarditis 25)-32), as well as aortic dilatation 33), are accompanied by a typical echo-cardiographic picture.

In the case of rheumatic endocarditis the insufficiency can be explained by the shrinking of the valves and the resultant loss of diastolic overlap. The valves then appear thickened in the echo-cardiogram and usually demonstrate a separated trace during diastole (fig. 10). The extent of this separation during diastole, however, does not give any indication of the degree of regurgitation 20). An additional stenotic component due to a restriction of cusp mobility is registered frequently.

Acute endocarditis results in the formation of vegetation on the valves. The valve tissue is destroyed during the course of the disease. Perforations can be observed and the valves often loose their stability and droop into the outflow tract during diastole (flail aortic valve).
Due to the deposits the reflectivity of the valves is higher and demonstrates a thickened echo trace. Fine to coarse oscillating echo traces are frequently detectable and are caused by the fact that the deposits and the affected parts of the cusps which have lost their stability due to the inflammatory process execute fluttering movements 25)-32).

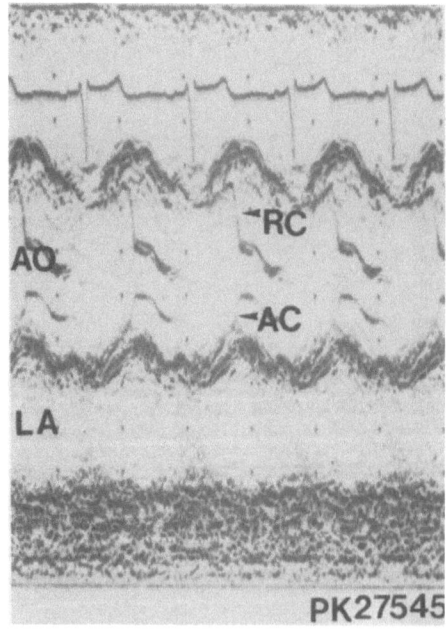

fig. 10. Aortic regurgitation caused by a shrinkage of the acoronary cusp.

32

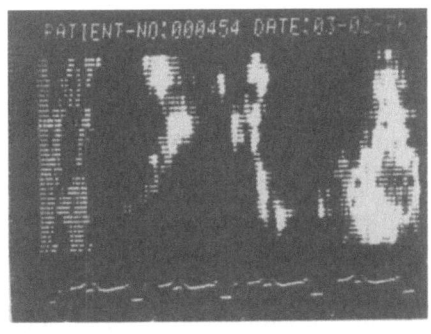

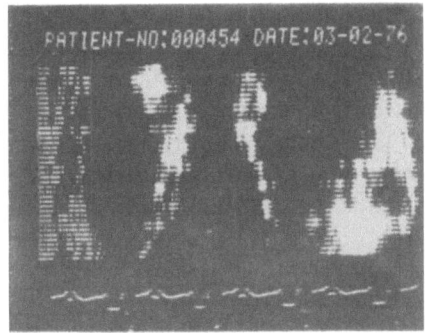

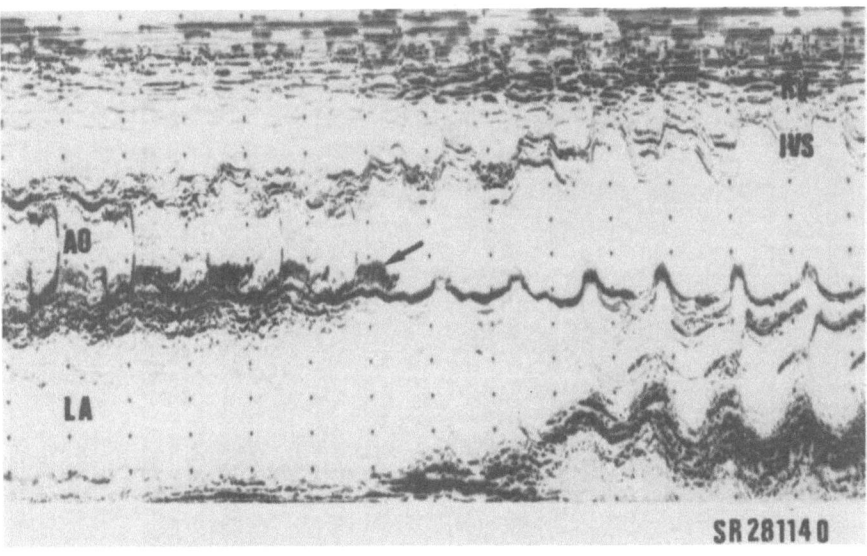

fig. 11. Bacterial endocarditis of the acoronary cusp and dissecting aneurisma of the posterior aortic wall. (M-mode and cross-section).

If the acoronary cusp is affected (fig. 11), these changes are evident during systole in the valve area near the posterior aortic wall and in the subvalvular area during diastole. This means that cusp parts with deposits are displaced into the valve area by the discharged blood during systole and into the subvalvular area by the returning blood during diastole. This movement along the longitudinal axis of the aortic root can be shown by the multi-element method (fig. 11).

If the left coronary cusp is diseases, the changes are located in the center of the aortic lumen (fig. 12) and if the right coronary cusp is affected, on the anterior aortic wall (fig. 13). If perforations of the cusp occur, regular mobility is shown in only slightly thickened cusps. Oscillating echo traces are not detectable.

Comparing the echocardiographic picture with the findings gained during surgery, in 13 patients with bacterial endocarditis we were able to confirm, that the extent of valve damage can be detected sufficiently. Hence, the course of the disease can also be evaluated well. However, we could not distinguish the acute endocarditis from the healed because vegetations could not be distinguished from those healed lesions, especially if there was a flail aortic valve in addition.

Aneurysms
The diameter of the aortic root can be calculated and the aortic wall evaluated exactly with the aid of echo-cardiography. Abnormal root dilatations can lead to aortic insufficiencies. This is especially frequent in the case of Marfan's syndrom (fig. 14) 33) with the associated mitral valve prolapse syndrom.

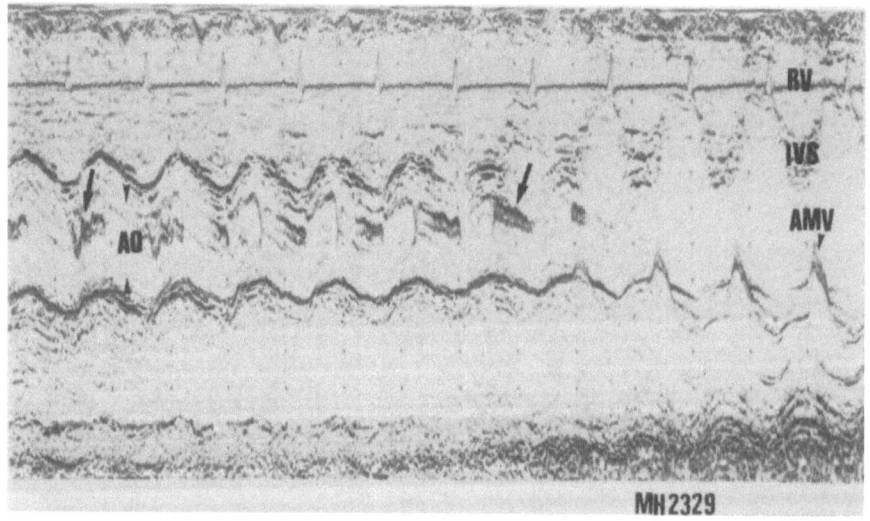

fig. 12. Bacterial endocarditis of the left coronary cusp. Left arrow: systolic oscillations of the left coronary cusp in the valve area, right arrow: diastolic oscillations in the subvalvular area.

34

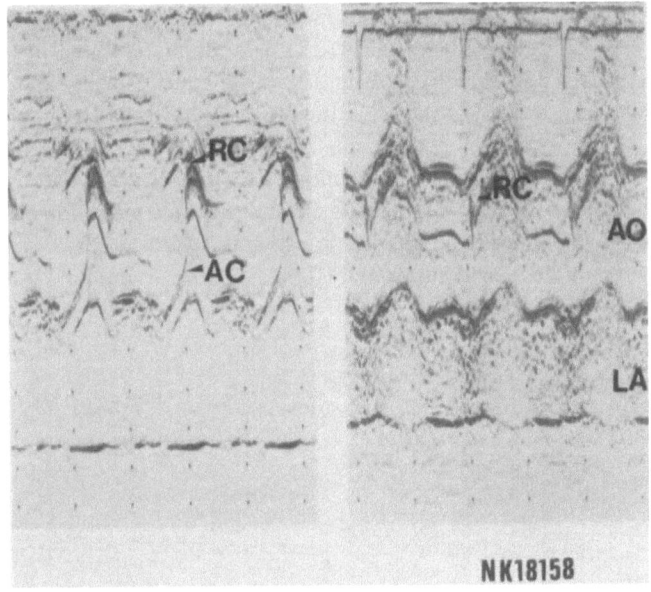

fig. 13. Bacterial endocarditis of the right coronary cusp.

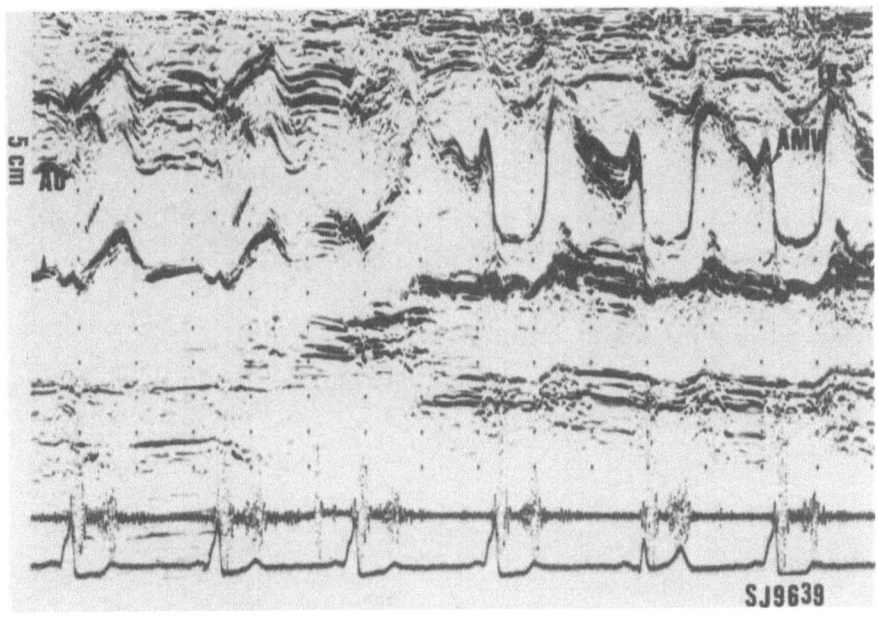

fig. 14. Aortic root dilatation with aortic regurgitation and mitral valve prolaps in a patient with Marfan's syndrom. AMV: anterior mitral valve, IVS: interventricular septum.

35

An increase in the root diameter with simultaneous double wall contours supports the finding of a dissecting aneurysm 34)-37). If doubling is found in the posterior aortic wall area (fig. 15), thereby making the atrium appear smaller and revealing no continuity between the mitral valve and the posterior aortic wall, this is a dissection in the area of the posterior aortic wall. A dissection affecting the entire circumference of the aorta correspondingly demonstrates double wall contours in the anterior and posterior wall area. Diagnosis is difficult in those cases in which dissection is limited to the lateral wall and in those in which it is formed only discretely, thereby revealing only a thickened aortic wall (fig. 11).

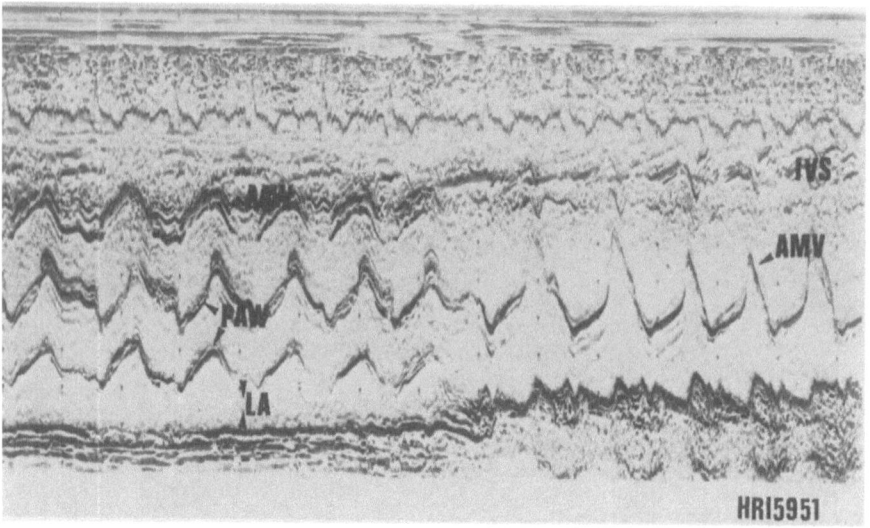

fig. 15. Dissecting aneurisma of the posterior aortic wall.

References

1) Rinke H, and Rudolph W: *Echokardiographie*.
   Fortschr. Med. 12: 94, 1976.

36

2) Bom N, Lancée CT, van Zwieten G, Kloster SE, and Roelandt J: *Multiscan-Echocardiography, I. Technical description.*
Circulation 48: 1066, 1973.

3) Roelandt J, Kloster SE, ten Cate FJ, van Dorp WG, Honkoop J, Bom N, and Hugenholtz PG: *Multidimensional Echocardiography an Appraisal of its Clinical Usefulness.*
Brit. Heart J. 36: 29, 1974.

4) Feizi O, Symons C, and Yacoub M: *Echocardiography of the aortic valve. I. Studies of normal aortic valve, aortic stenosis, aortic regurgitation, and mixed aortic valve disease.*
Brit. Heart J. 36: 341, 1974.

5) Gramiak R, and Shah PM: *Echocardiography of the aortic root.*
Invest. Radiology 3: 356, 1968.

6) Pratt RC, Parisi AF, Harrington JJ, and Sasahara AA: *The influence of left ventricular stroke volume on aortic root motion.*
Circulation 53: 947, 1976.

7) Hirschfeld S, Meyer R, Schwartz DC, Korfhagen J, and Kaplan S: *Measurement of right and left ventricular systolic time intervals by echocardiography.*
Circulation 51: 304, 1975.

8) Stefadouros MA, and Witham AC: *Systolic time intervals by echocardiography.*
Circulation 51: 114, 1975.

9) Gehrke J, Maldonado J, Goht V, and Leeman S: *Neue echographische Beurteilungsmöglichkeiten der Aortenwurzel: Hämodynamische Zusammenhänge und klinische Bedeutung.*
Z. Kardiol. Suppl. 2: 47, 1975.

10) Biamino G. (in press).

11) Popp RL, Silvermann JS, French JW, Stinson EB, and Harrison DC: *Echocardiographic findings in discrete subvalvular aortics stenoses.*
Circulation 49: 226, 1974.

12) Davis HR, Feigenbaum H, Chang S, Koneke L, and Dillon JC: *Echocardiographic manifestations of discrete subaortic stenoses.*
Amer. J. Cardiology 33: 277, 1974.

13) Weyman AE, Feigenbaum H, Hurwitz RA, Girod DA, Dillon JC, and Chang S: *Cross-sectional echocardiography in evaluating patients with discrete subaortic stenosis.*
Am. J. Cardiol. 37: 358, 1976.

14) Henry WK, Chester EC, and Ebstein S: *Asymmetric septal hypertrophy, echocardiographic identification of the pathogmonic anatomic abnormality of IHSS.*
Circulation 157: 225, 1973.

15) Rinke H, Späth, and Rudolph W: *Die Mitralklappenbeweglichkeit im UKB bei der hypertrophen Kardiomyopathie mit Obstruktion (IHSS) und ihre Veränderung nach Betarezeptorenbehandlung.*
Z. Kardiol. Suppl. II, 15, 1975.

16) Hanrath B, Schweither I, Bleifeld W, and Effert S: *Echokardiographisch diagnostische Kriterien der idiopathischen hypertrophen subaortalen stenose.*
Dtsch. Med. Wschr. 36: 1759, 1975.

17) Hernberg J, Weiss B, and Keegan A: *The ultrasonic recording of aortic valve motion.*
Radiologie 94: 361, 1970.

18) Winsberg F, and Mercer EN: *Echocardiography in Combined Valve Disease.*
Radiology 105: 405, 1972.

19) Yeh HCh, Winsberg F, and Mercer EN: *Echographic aortic valve oriface dimension: its use in evaluating aortic stenosis and cardiac output.*
J. Clin. Ultrasound, 1: 182, 1973.

20) Rinke H, Stahlbauer W, Dacian S, and Rudolph W: *Echokardiographische Beurteilung von Aortenklappenfehlern.*
Verh. Dtsch. Ges. Inn. Med. 81: 247, 1975.

21) Rinke H, Dacian S, and Stahlbauer W, et al: *Echocardiographic evaluation of aortic stenosis and regurgitation.*
2nd Europ. Congr. Ultrasonics in Medicine, München, 1975.

22) Nanda NC, Gramiak R, Manning J, Mahoney EB, Lipchik EO, and DeWcese JA: *Echocardiographic recognition of the congenital bicuspid aortic valve.*
Circulation 49: 870, 1974.

23) Radford DJ, Bloom KR, Izukawa T, Moes CAF, and Rowe RD: *Echocardiographic assessment of bicuspid aortic valves.*
Circulation 53: 80, 1976.

24) Scovil JA, Nanda NC, Gross CM, Lombardi AC, Gramiak R, Lipchik EO, and Manning JA: *Echocardiographic studies of abnormalities associated with coarction of the aorta.*
Circulation 53: 953, 1976.

25) Dillon JC, Feigenbaum H, Konecke LL, Davis RH, and Chang S: *Echocardiographic manifestations of valvular vegetations.*
Amer. Heart J. 86: 698, 1973.

26) Spangler RD, Johnson ML, Holmes JH, and Blount SG Jr.: *Echocardiographic demonstration of bacterial vegetations in active infective endocarditis.*
J. Clin. Ultrasound 1: 126, 1973.

27) Martinez EC, Burch GE, and Giles TD: *Echocardiographic diagnosis of vegetative aortic bacterial endocarditis.*
Amer. J. Cardiol. 34: 845, 1974.

28) Gottlieb S, Khuddus SA, Balooki H, Dominguez AE, and Myerburg RJ: *Echocardiographic diagnosis of aortic valve vegetations in Candida endocarditis.*
Circulation 50: 826, 1974.

29) De Maria AN, King JF, Salel AF, Caudill CC, Miller RR, and Mason DT: *Echography and phonography of acute aortic regurgitation in bacterial endocarditis.*
Ann. Intern. Med. 82: 329, 1975.

30) Roy P, Tajik AB, Giuliani ER, Schattenberg TT, Gau GT, and Frye RL: *Spectrum of echocardiographic findings in bacterial endocarditis.*
Brit. Heart J. 53: 474, 1976.

38

31) Wray TM: *The variable echocardiographic features in aortic valve endocarditis.*
Circulation 52: 658, 1975.

32) Wray TM: *Echocardiographic manifestations of flail aortic valve leaflets in bacterial endocarditis.*
Circulation 51: 832, 1975.

33) Brown OR, DeMots H, Kloster FE, Roberts A, Menashe VD, and Beals RK: *Aortic root dilatation and mitral valve prolapse in Marfan's syndrome.*
Circulation 52: 651, 1975.

34) Nanda NC, Gramiak R, and Shah PM: *Diagnosis of aortic root dissection by echocardiography.*
Circulation 48: 506, 1973.

35) Moothart RW, Spangler RD, and Blount SG: *Echocardiography in aortic root dissection and dilatation.*
Amer. J. Cardiol. 36: 11, 1975.

36) Brown OR, Popp RL. and Kloster FE: *Echocardiographic criteria for aortic root dissection.*
Amer. J. Cardiol. 36: 17, 1975.

37) Hirschfeld DS, Rodriguez JH, and Schiller NB: *Duplication of aortic wall seen by echocardiography.*
Brit. Heart J. 38: 943, 1976.

Right-sided heart valves

by Graham J. Leech,
Cardiac Department, St. George's Hospital,
London S.W. 1, England.

In normal subjects, the right-sided heart valves are much harder to locate than the left. Although it is possible to direct the ultrasound beam at them, it is difficult to do so in such a way that the reflected echoes return to the transducer. Thus, it is unusual to record the complete motion pattern of either the tricuspid or the pulmonary valve in a normal adult and, indeed, to do so is itself an indication of right-sided abnormality. Nevertheless, some useful information about them can be obtained by M-mode echocardiography.

The anatomic relationship of the valves and chambers of the right side of the heart is shown in fig. 1. The best way to locate the tricuspid valve is to begin with a view of the aortic root from the fourth left intercostal space. The ultrasound beam is then angled medially and quite strongly inferiorly. The large anterior tricuspid leaflet produces an echo trace almost identical to the mitral valve, but much nearer to the chest wall. Continuing inferior beam angulation will detect echoes from the postero-septal leaflet; the moment of tricuspid valve closure can then be determined from the point of apposition of the anterior and posterior leaflets.

The haemodynamic events governing the motion of the tricuspid valve correspond to those for the mitral valve on the left side, and the same nomenclature is used to describe them (fig. 2.) There is an initial rapid opening at the onset of diastole, D-E; followed by partial mid-diastolic closure, E-F, then atrial systolic re-opening, A, and closure at the onset of systole, C. There may be slight posterior displacement of the closed valve during iso-volumic contraction, but then there is steady anterior motion until the valve opens again at the beginning of the next cycle. Rapid filling occurs during the D-E phase, and is probably nearly completed by the E point, which marks the halting of the opening movement and coincides with an opening snap, when present. The A wave peak coincides with a right-sided atrial filling sound, and the C point with the tricuspid component of the first heart sound.

For practical purposes, rheumatic tricuspid stenosis is always secondary to mitral valve disease, and there will usually be aortic involvement as well. Since tricuspid stenosis is relatively rare, and many of the clinical signs are masked by mitral stenosis, routine echocardiographic assessment of a patient with rheumatic heart disease should always include examination of the tricuspid valve. The echocardiographic signs of tricuspid stenosis are the same as for mitral stenosis: thickening or calcification of the leaflets; reduction of diastolic opening excursion; loss of F point,

41

Echocardiology, N. Bom editor, published by Martinus Nijhoff, the Hague 1977.

indicating prolongation of ventricular filling; and reduced, or reversed posterior leaflet motion indicating commissural fusion (fig. 3). Additional evidence can be obtained by demonstrating an opening snap at the left sternal border coincident with the E point on the valve echo.

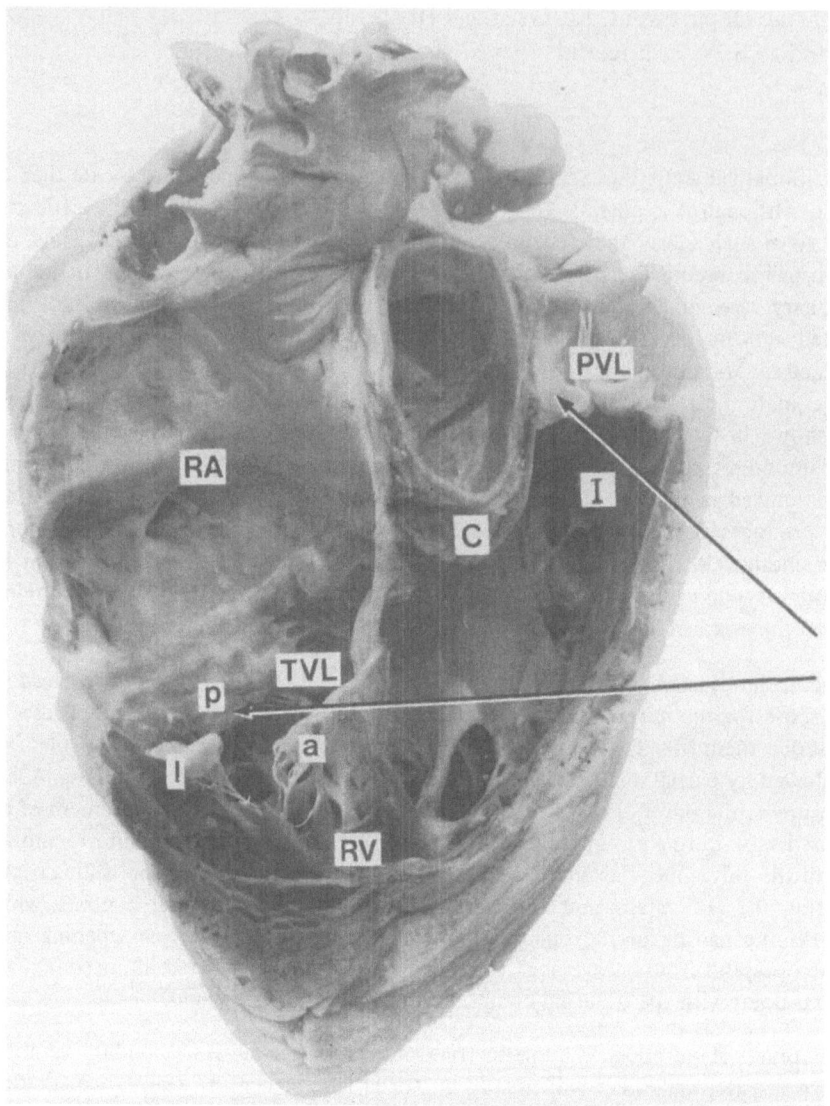

fig. 1. The right side of the heart opened to show the relationship of its structures and the path taken by the ultrasound beam when recording tricuspid and pulmonary valves. Key: RA = Right atrium: TVL = Tricuspid valve leaflets: a = anterior: p = postero-septal: l = lateral: RV = Right ventricle: C = Crista supraventricularis: I = Pulmonary infundibulum: PVL = pulmonary valve leaflets.

Echocardiography is a very sensitive method for detecting tricuspid stenosis, and it is frequently difficult to obtain auscultatory or catheterisation data to confirm the findings. Catheterisation, particularly, is very un-rewarding, even when a double-lumen catheter is used, since a gradient of only 1 - 2 mm Hg represents significant stenosis. Even surgical inspection of the valve not infrequently finds only trivial disease in cases where the echo recordings are clearly abnormal, so care must be taken in equating the echo findings with the presence of disease which is haemo-dynamically severe enough to require surgical treatment.

Tumors of the right side of the heart are very rare, but have been detected by echo-cardiography 1). In our laboratory, twin myxomata attached to the underside of the tricuspid valve were once found during a routine study of a patient presenting with bacterial endocarditis.

The primary echocardiographic sign of tricuspid regurgitation is of right ventricular volume overloading. This is shown by enlargement of the chamber, coupled with reduced, or reversed septal motion, i.e. instead of moving towards the posterior left ventricular wall during systole, the septum moves towards the right ventricle.

However, other conditions which produce right ventricular volume overloading, for example atrial septal defect, anomalous pulmonary venous drainage and pulmonary regurgitation, show the same echocardiographic signs. A very approximate indic-

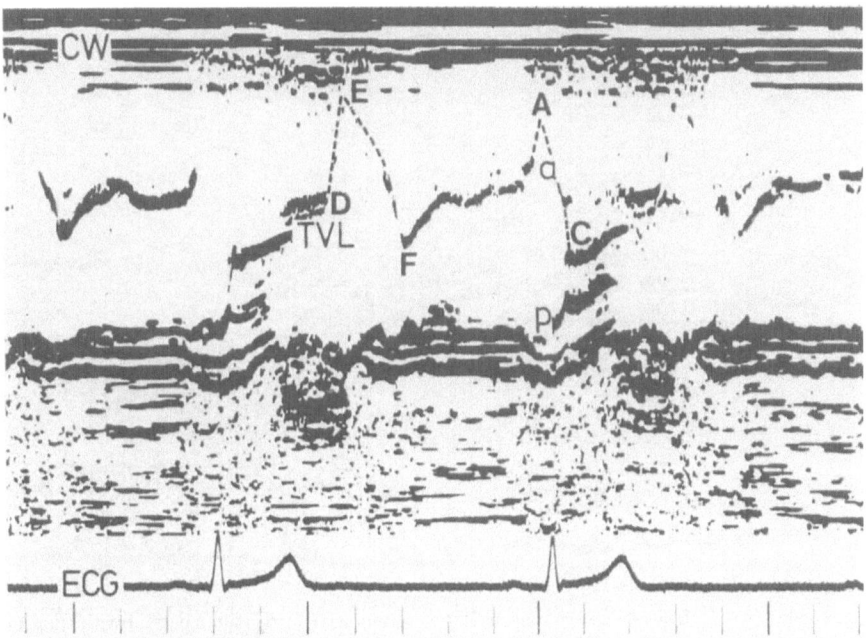

fig. 2. Tricuspid valve recording from a normal adult. The broken line indicates portions of the motion pattern not seen. For nomenclature see fig. 1 and text.

ation of the degree of volume overload can be obtained from the size of the right ventricle, but the geometry of the chamber, and inability to define the ultrasound beam direction across it preclude accurate quantitative assessment.

A posterior "bowing" or "hammock" pattern of the closed tricuspid leaflets, similar to that associated with mitral valve prolapse, is sometimes seen during systole. In so far as this pattern is uncommon, and nearly always accompanied by echo evidence of mitral prolapse, it probably indicates a "floppy" tricuspid valve 2). However, there is normally no associated murmur to indicate tricuspid regurgitation, and so it is probably a benign condition. Vegetations on the tricuspid valve due to infective endocarditis are also relatively uncommon, but have been visualised by echocardiography. However, absence of abnormal echo signs does not preclude infection 3).

In children, recording the tricuspid valve is much easier as the ultrasound beam can penetrate the sternal cartilages and the heart can be approached from the right side of the sternum. In infants, it is usually the most prominent valve, and failure to detect it in a newborn should raise the possibility of abnormal positioning or absence of the valve. Even in adults, congenital disease producing right ventricular enlargement and rotation of the heart makes the tricuspid valve easy to record, and

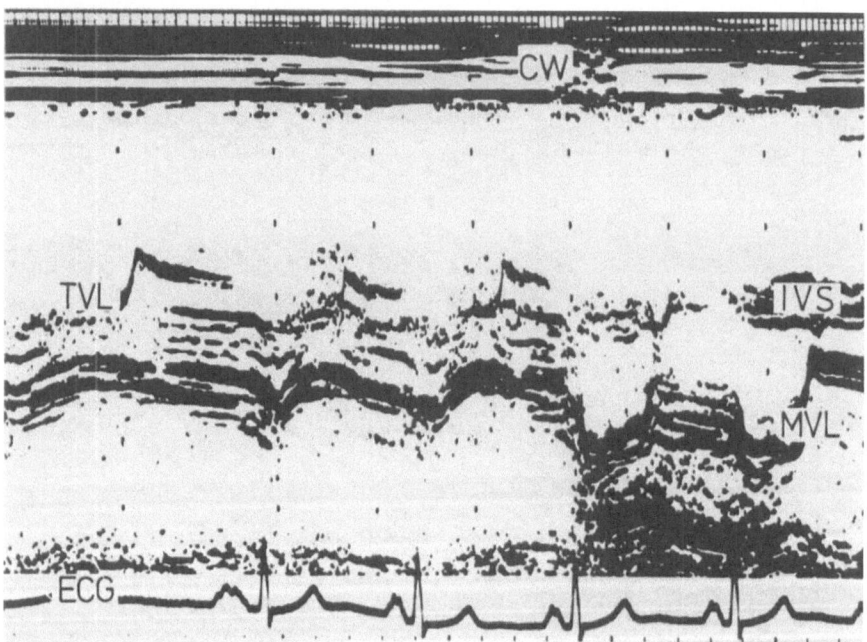

fig. 3. Slow sweep from tricuspid valve at left to mitral valve at right in a patient with tricuspid and mitral stenosis. Note the similarity of the motion patterns. No end-diastolic gradient could be demonstrated across the tricuspid valve at catheterisation, but at surgery it was seen to be diseased and was replaced.

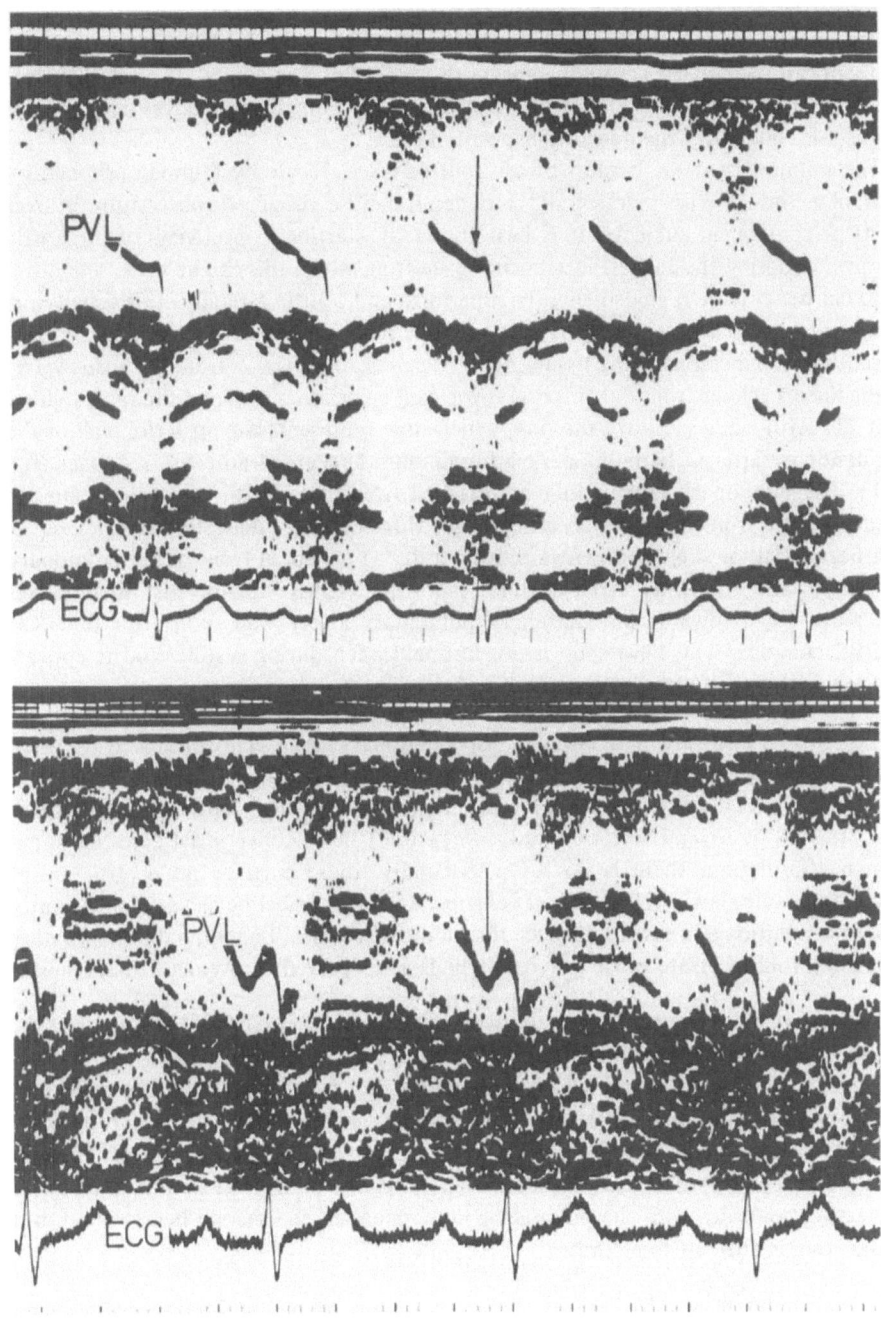

fig. 4. Pulmonary valve recordings from a normal subject (top) and a patient with severe pulmonary stenosis (bottom). The A-dip (arrowed) is much more obvious in the lower recording.

45

allows the complete motion pattern to be seen. The very large tricuspid valve with late closure, which can be shown to coincide with a very loud, late sound on the phonocardiogram, assists in the diagnosis of Ebstein's anomaly. The relative sizes of the anterior and posterior leaflets of the mitral and tricuspid valves may make it possible to identify them in L-transposition 4).

The pulmonary is the hardest of the four valves to locate by M-mode echocardiography, though with practice and patience it can be visualised successfully in over 80 percent of all subjects. It is best found by starting from a view of the aortic valve, choosing the highest intercostal space from which this can be seen. The ultrasound beam is then angled slightly superiorly and a little laterally. It is usually necessary to turn the subject partially onto the left side and have him exhale, to prevent interference from lung tissue. As the beam is angled away from the aortic valve, the line of echoes from the anterior aortic wall ceases to move, and the space behind it fills with echoes. Above the line, which now represents the posterior wall of the pulmonary artery, the pulmonary infundibulum appears as an echo-free space (fig. 1). The pulmonary valve is thus approached from underneath, and echoes are obtained only from the most posterior of the three cusps. In diastole, they are seen as a horizontal, or slightly downward-sloping line, 1 - 2 cm in front of the pulmonary artery wall. Following atrial systole, this dips slightly downwards, then moves rapidly down towards the stationary pulmonary artery wall soon after the ECG QRS complex. The valve echo is not normally seen during systole, and re-appears again during the following diastole (fig. 4).

The small downward deflection of the pulmonary valve echo produced by atrial systole, known as the "A-dip", represents upward displacement of the closed valve cusps caused by inflow of blood into the right ventricle during atrial systole. Its size is affected by several factors. Firstly, there must be effective atrial contraction; in atrial fibrillation, there is no A-dip. Secondly, there must be no obstruction at tricuspid valve level. Thirdly, right ventricular pressure must be elevated sufficiently by the additional inflow to displace the pulmonary cusps. Finally, pulmonary artery end-diastolic pressure must not be so high as to prevent movement of the cusps.

Pulmonary valve opening normally occurs very soon after tricuspid closure, but the exact point is difficult to define when only one cusp is seen. Halting of opening coincides with any pulmonary ejection sound that may be present. The pattern of mid-systolic motion is uncertain. In pulmonary hypertension, the valve partially closes in mid-systole (fig. 5), and it is likely that a similar pattern is present in normal subjects, but it is hard to detect. The moment of valve closure at the end of ejection coincides with the pulmonary component of the second heart sound, but this, too, is difficult to record.

In mild pulmonary valve stenosis, the valve appears normal on echo recordings, and the only useful finding is to confirm the pulmonary origin of the ejection sound by demonstrating its coincidence with maximal valve opening. With development of

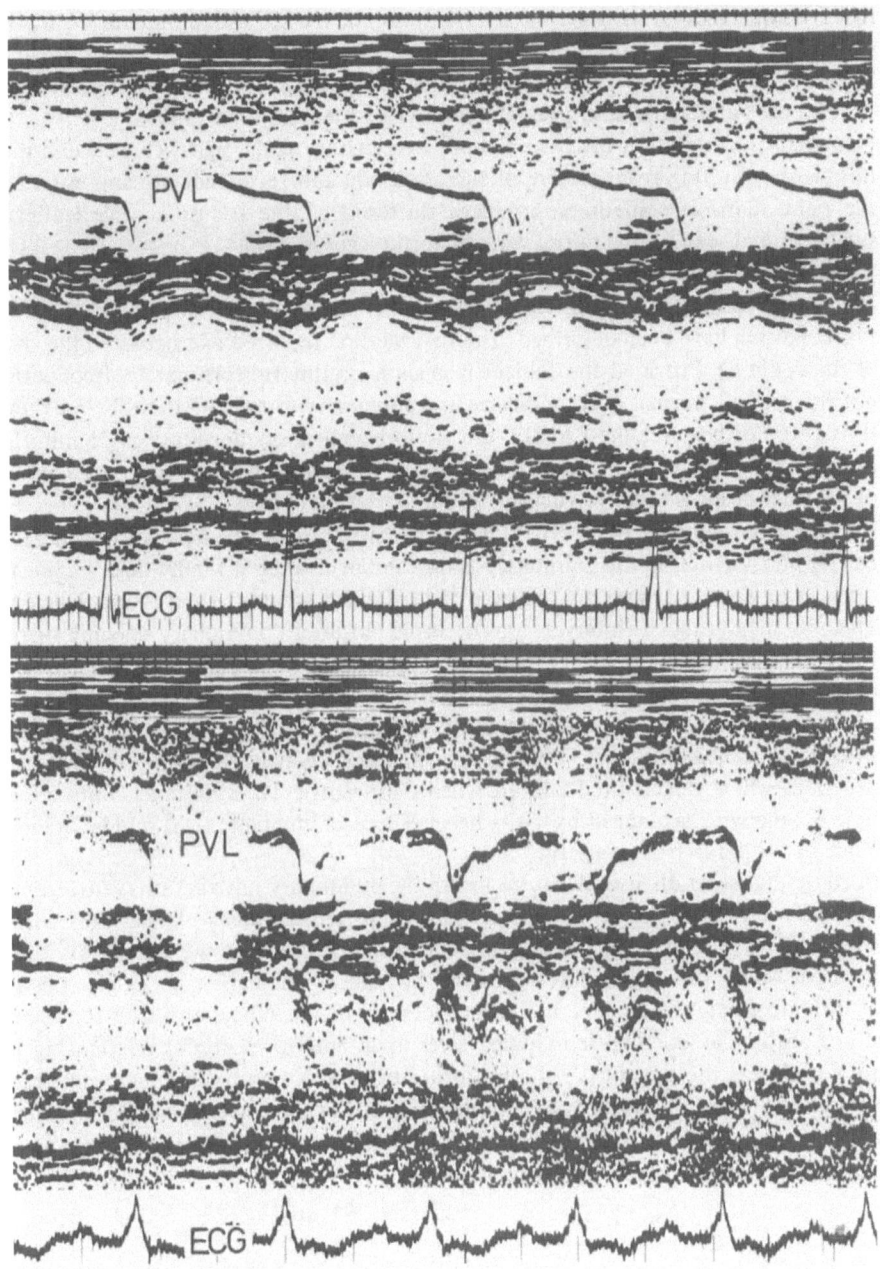

fig. 5. Pulmonary valve recordings from two patients with pulmonary hypertension, both in sinus rhythm. Note the absence of any A-dip, and the mid-systolic partial closure of the valve. In the lower recording from a patient with an Eisenmenger ASD, thickening of the valve cusps is evident.

right ventricular hypertrophy, the ventricle cannot readily accommodate the atrial systolic inflow, and the resulting pressure rise increases the size of the A-dip (fig. 4). With additional inspiratory augmentation of filling, this effect may be great enough to open the pulmonary valve prematurely, before the ECG QRS onset.

Pulmonary regurgitation produces volume overloading of the right ventricle and the turbulence resulting from mixing of the antegrade and retrograde streams entering the right ventricle sometimes produces fluttering of the tricuspid valve leaflets, similar to that seen on the mitral valve in aortic regurgitation.

The clinical implications of pulmonary hypertension make non-invasive detection and quantification very desirable, and a number of features of echo recordings of this condition have been described. The first method reported was based on the size of the A-dip 5). Provided the subject is in sinus rhythm (unfortunately, frequently not the case), a normal A-dip indicates low pulmonary artery end-diastolic pressure (PAEDP). With increasing PAEDP, the A-dip becomes smaller, until at 25 mm Hg or more, it is absent. With severe, long-standing pulmonary hypertension, thickening of the valve cusps is usually evident (fig. 5).

The other consequence of elevated PAEDP is that the right ventricle has to generate greater pressure before the pulmonary valve can open; when it finally does so, opening is more rapid, because the right ventricle dP/dT is greater,6) and is also delayed. Thus, by measuring the interval from tricuspid closure to pulmonary opening (right ventricular isovolumic contraction time), PAEDP can be estimated 7). Since the intervals are quite short, accurate measurement necessitates high speed recordings of the valve motions, but it is possible to estimate PAEDP to within ± 25 percent with 95 percent confidence, even in the presence of atrial fibrillation. The only situations where this method fails are when right ventricular isovolumic contraction time is otherwise prolonged by gross heart failure or complete right bundle branch block of the arborisation variety.

In congenital heart disease, ability to locate the pulmonary valve permits verification of its relationship to the aorta and rules out complete pulmonary atresia. Unlike the left side, there is no echocardiographic continuity between the pulmonary and tricuspid valves, due to the intervening crista superventricularis (fig. 1), but this is of little diagnostic help, since it does not identify the chambers or vessels functionally. Location of the two semi-lunar valves in an anterior-posterior relationship is good evidence, though not proof, of transposition. Where both semilunar valves can be recorded clearly enough to permit measurement of the respective ejection times, the one associated with the pulmonary circulation will have the longer ejection time, except where foetal circulation persists.

References

1) Waxler EB, Kawai N, and Kasparian H: *Right atrial myxoma: echocardiographic, phono-cardiographic and hemodynamic signs.*
Am. Heart J. 83: 251, 1972.

2) Werner JA, Schiller NB, and Prasquier R: *Occurence and significance of echocardiographic-ally demonstrated tricuspid valve prolapse.*
Circulation 53 Supp. II: 232, 1976.

3) Lee C et al: *Detection of tricuspid valve vegetations by echocardiography.*
Chest 66: 432, 1974.

4) Beardshaw J, Gibson DG, Wright JS, Pearson MC, and Anderson RH: *Echocardiographic diagnosis of corrected transposition.*
Brit. Heart J. 38: 878, 1976.

5) Nanda NC, Gramiak R, Robinson TI, and Shah PM: *Echocardiographic evaluation of pul-monary hypertension.*
Circulation 50: 575, 1974.

6) Weyman AE, Dillon JC, Feigenbaum H, and Chang S: *Echocardiographic patterns of pul-monic valve motion with pulmonary hypertension.*
Circulation 50: 905, 1974.

7) Mills PG, Leech GJ, Leatham A, and Ginks WR: *Non-invasive estimation of pulmonary artery end-diastolic pressure.*
Circulation 50 Supp II: 190, 1975.

Cross-sectional echocardiographic evaluation of the Atrioventricular valves in acquired and congenital heart disease

by Walter L. Henry and James M. Griffith,
Cardiology Branch, National Heart, Lung, and Blood Institute
National Institutes of Health, Bethesda, Maryland USA.

The mitral valve was one of the first cardiac structures to be visualized by reflected ultrasound. During his pioneering echocardiographic studies, Edler described the typical motion pattern of the normal mitral valve and also documented that this motion pattern was distinctly different in patients with mitral stenosis 1)-4). Subsequent studies have demonstrated that M-mode echocardiography can be used to diagnose a large number of conditions including mitral valve prolapse 5)-9), hypertrophic obstructive cardiomyopathy (IHSS) 10)-12), aortic regurgitation 13), left atrial myxoma 14), and decreased left ventricular compliance 15), 16). All of these studies describe diagnostic markers that are based on the detection of an abnormal pattern of motion of the mitral valve. However, the technique provides little information about the actual shape of the valve.

Recently devices have been developed that generate a cross-sectional image of the heart at the rate of approximately one complete image every one-thirtieth of a second 17)-19). With these devices, a complete two-dimensional image of the mitral valve can be constructed and its shape determined. These cross-sectional images allow important new information to be derived noninvasively.

Orientation of the imaging device

The two-dimensional imaging systems can be oriented to transect the heart in a variety of planes. In most situations, two views are sufficient to derive diagnostic information. These two views involve orienting the imaging devices either parallel or perpendicular to the long axis of the left ventricle 18). In order to obtain the parallel view, the imaging device is oriented parallel to a line connecting the patient's right shoulder and left hip. Minor adjustments are then made until the optimum image of the mitral valve is obtained. A parallel image of the mitral valve obtained with a mechanical sector-scanner is shown in fig. 1. With this parallel orientation, important information can be obtained in a variety of cardiac abnormalities including mitral stenosis 20), 21), obstructive ASH (IHSS or HOCM) 22), and mitral prolapse 23), 24).

The other view of the mitral valve that we have found to be very useful is obtained with the scanner oriented perpendicular to the long axis of the left ventricle (i.e., with the scanner angling the transducer parallel to a line connecting the patient's left shoulder and right flank) (fig. 2). A drawing of a heart that has been cross-

Echocardiology, N. Bom editor, published by Martinus Nijhoff, the Hague 1977.

sectioned in this manner through the tip of the mitral valve is shown in fig. 3. The specific situations in which perpendicular images of the mitral valve are most useful will be discussed in the next several paragraphs.

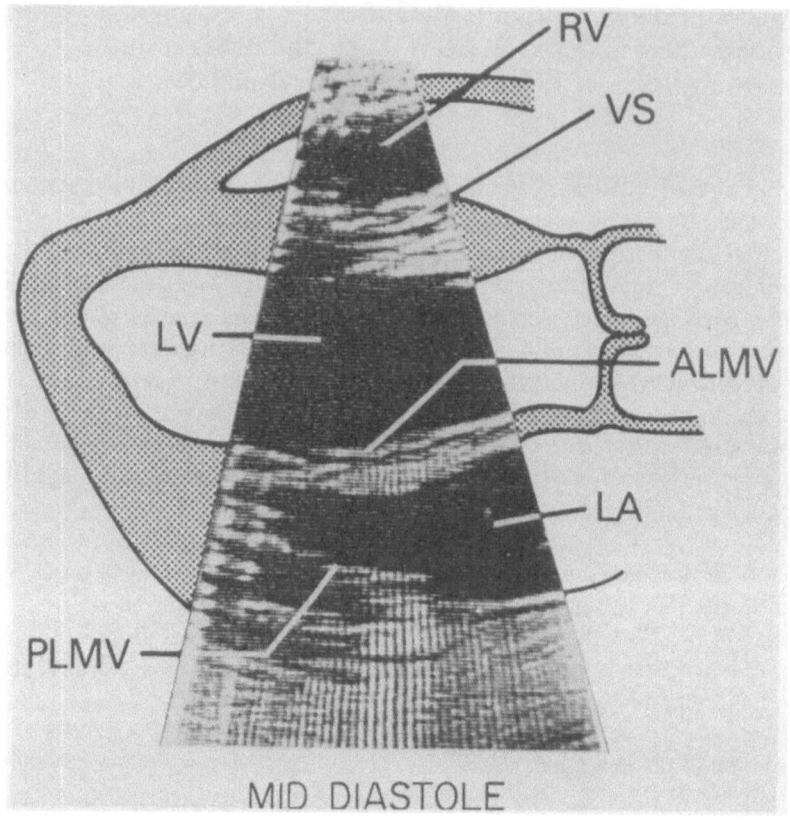

fig. 1. Cross-sectional echocardiogram of a normal subject obtained with a 30° mechanical sector scanner oriented parallel to the long axis of the left ventricle at the tip of the mitral valve (RV = right ventricle, VS = ventricular septum, LA = left atrium, ALMV = anterior leaflet of mitral valve, PLMV = posterior leaflet of mitral valve).

Acquired heart disease

With the cross-sectional imaging device oriented perpendicular to the long axis of the left ventricle, minor angulations are made in a cephalad or caudad direction until the tip of the mitral valve is imaged. In normal subjects, the two leaflets separate widely in early diastole to form a circular structure through which blood rapidly flows from left atrium to left ventricle (fig. 4, left panel). In patients with mitral stenosis, the rheumatic process results in fusion of the commissures between the two mitral leaflets. This fusion results in a much smaller orifice through which blood flows from atrium to ventricle (fig. 4, right panel).

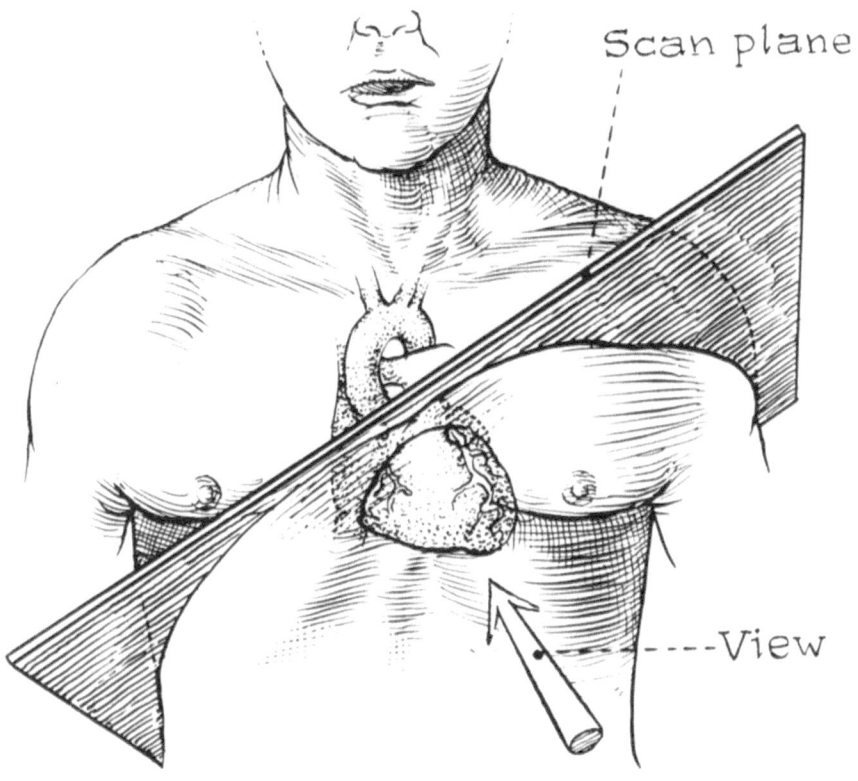

fig. 2. Drawing of the scan plane of a cross-sectional imaging device showing its orientation relative to external landmarks. In the scan plane orientation shown in the drawing, the heart is being transected approximately perpendicular to the long axis of the left ventricle (drawings in fig. 2 and 3 are by Leon Schlossberg of Johns Hopkins University).

Several recent studies have demonstrated that this narrowed orifice can be readily visualized. In addition it has been shown that the cross-sectional area of the mitral orifice can be measured directly from these images. In our initial study, we compared the cross-sectional area obtained by two-dimensional echocardiography with a direct measure of mitral orifice area obtained at operation 20). These two independent measurements were within 0.3 cm^2 of each other in 13 of the 14 patients studied (r = 0.92). This close correlation was attained despite the presence of significant mitral regurgitation in most of the patients in the study. We have recently extended these observations by comparing the mitral orifice area obtained with cross-sectional echocardiography to that calculated with the Gorlin equation during

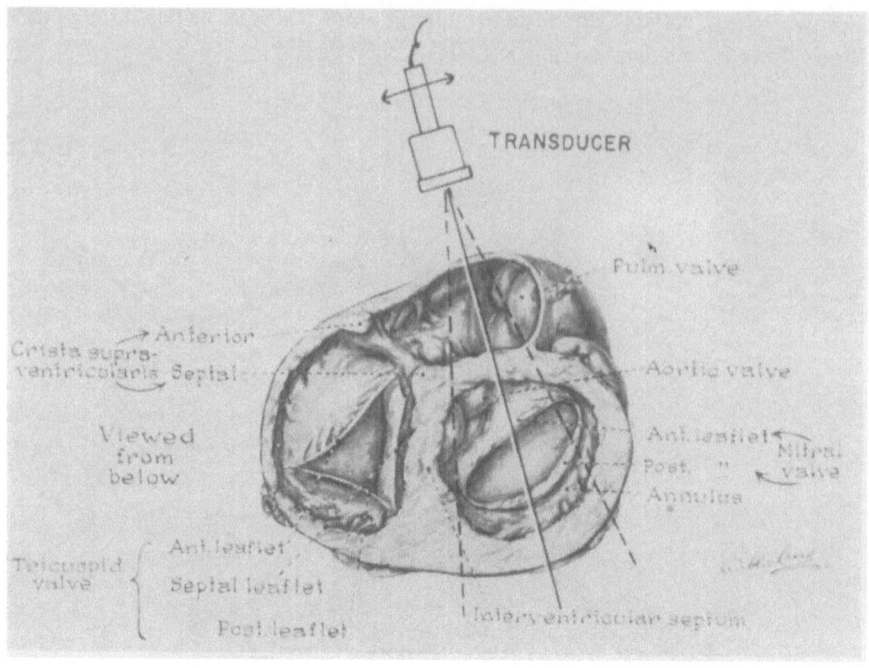

fig. 3. Drawing of a heart cross-sectioned through the tip of the mitral valve and viewed from below (i.e., from the region previously occupied by the apex of the heart).

cardiac catheterization 25). Patients selected for study had little or no mitral regurgitation so that a valid comparison was feasible. The results of this study indicated that the two-dimensional and Gorlin measurements of orifice size were closely related (r = 0.91) by the equation *Cross-sectional Area* = 0.98 *(Gorlin Area)* ±0.3. Nichols et al have published similar data indicating a high correlation between the two-dimensional and Gorlin-derived areas 21).

Thus, cross-sectional echocardiography provides a method for measuring the mitral orifice area directly. Its major advantages are that it is accurate, noninvasive, and not influenced by the presence of coexistent valvular regurgitation.

Congenital heart disease

After evaluating a large number of patients with acquired and congenital heart disease, it became apparent that the mitral valve had a characteristic shape in mid-diastole. The mitral valve consists of two leaflets that are joined medially- and laterally. As a result, it assumes an elliptical (or fish-mouth shape) in mid-diastole after rapid ventricular filling has occurred (fig. 5). Since the mitral valve is always situated in the morphologic left ventricle, it occurred to us that this characteristic elliptical shape might be used as a marker of ventricular situs. Indeed, when we

54

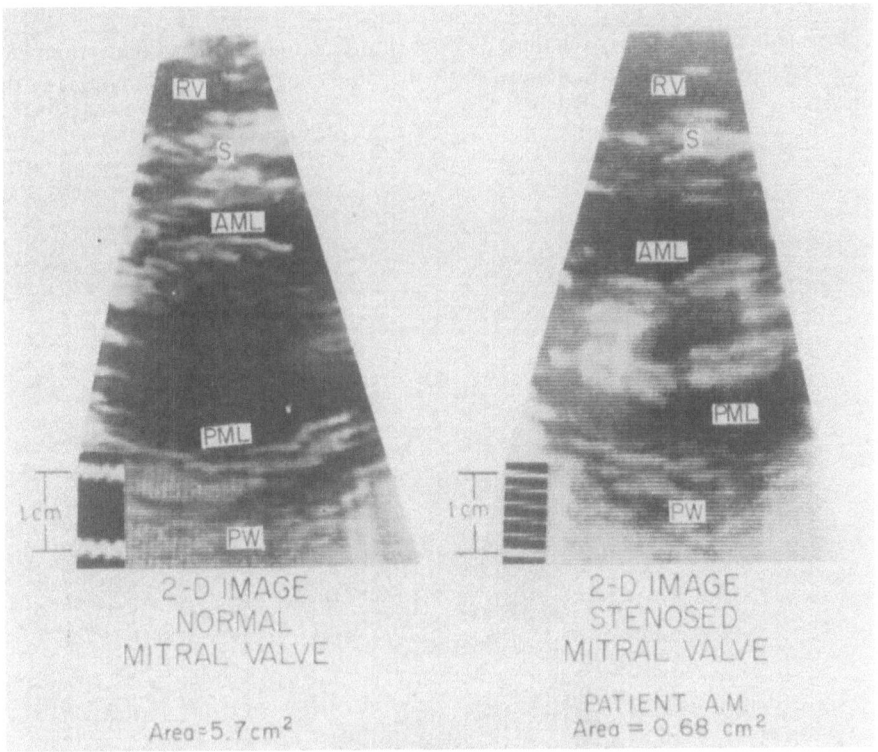

fig. 4. Cross-sectional echocardiograms of the mitral valve orifice in early diastole from a normal subject (left panel) and a patient with mitral stenosis (right panel). One centimeter calibration marks are of similar size in each panel so that the orifice areas can be directly compared to each other.

studied a large number of patients with congenital heart disease (in cooperation with Drs. David Sahn, Stan Goldberg and Hugh Allen of the University of Arizona), we found that an elliptically-shaped atrioventricular valve was able to be visualized to the left of the ventricular septum in every patient with normal ventricular situs 26). Individuals with ventricular inversion did not have an elliptically-shaped valve to the left of the septum but rather had a valve that consisted of three leaflets (i.e., a tricuspid valve) (fig. 6).

Thus if a patient with congenital heart disease is found to have a three-leaflet valve (rather than an elliptically-shaped valve) to the left of the ventricular septum, one can conclude that the ventricle on the left side of the patient contains a tricuspid valve and therefore is a morphologic right ventricle. In our experience, it is possible to reliably determine ventricular situs noninvasively with this method even in complex forms of congenital heart disease. This information, when combined with an

55

assessment of great artery relations 27) and ventricular-great artery connections 28), has extended our ability to noninvasively diagnose congenital malformations of the heart.

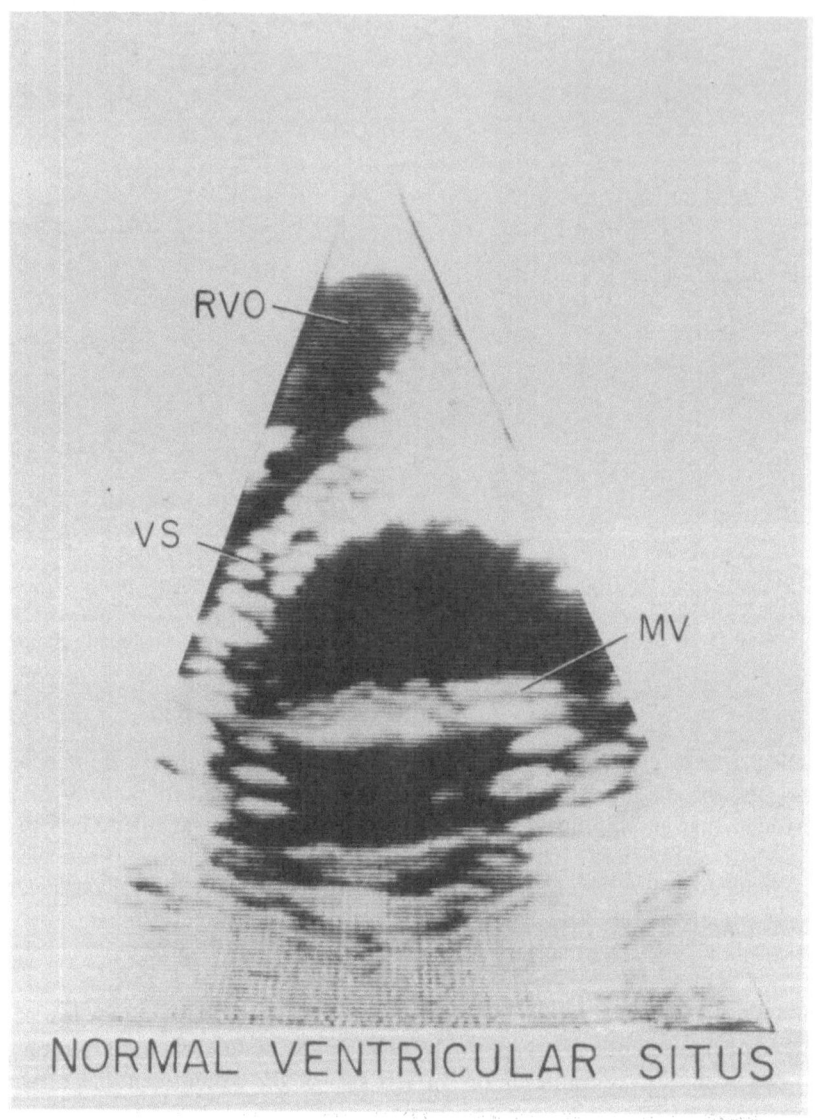

fig. 5. Unretouched stop-frame image of a normal heart obtained in mid-diastole at the level of the tip of the left-sided mitral valve. The valve is identified as a mitral valve by the characteristic elliptical or fish-mouth shape.

56

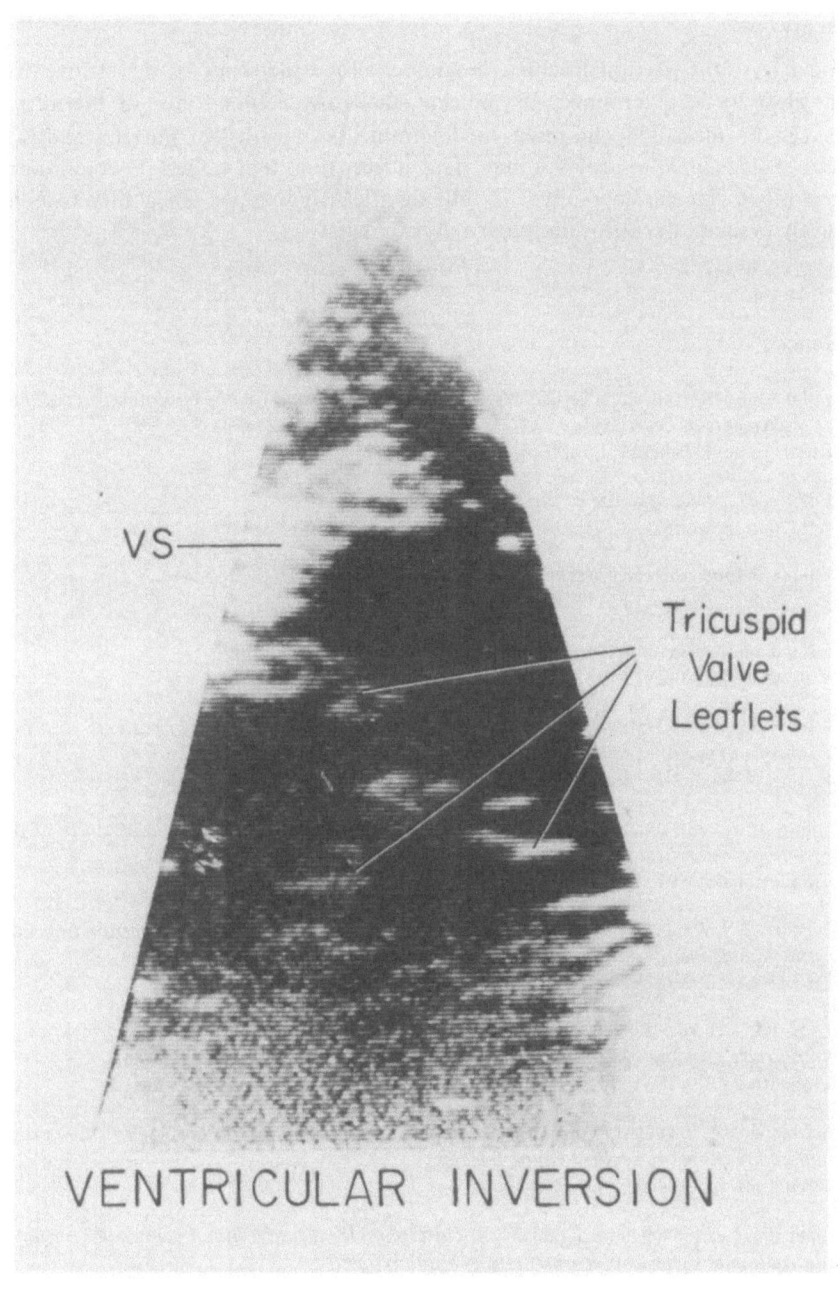

VS———

Tricuspid
Valve
Leaflets

VENTRICULAR INVERSION

fig. 6. Unretouched stop-frame image of a heart with ventricular inversion obtained in mid-diastole at the level of the tip of the left-sided tricuspid valve. The valve to the left of the septum consists of three leaflets and never assumes an elliptical or fish-mouth shape during any portion of the cardiac cycle.

Summary

In summary, cross-sectional echocardiography allows the shape of the atrioventricular valves to be determined. In addition, the cross-sectional area of the mitral valve can be measured and used to determine the severity of mitral stenosis if present. This technique provides important information that cannot be determined with M-mode echocardiography and thus significantly extends our ability to non-invasively evaluate the atrioventricular valves in man.

References

1) Edler I, and Hertz CH: *The use of ultrasonic reflectoscope for the continuous recording of movements of heart wall.*
   Kurgl. Fysiogr. Sallad. i. Lund Forhandl., 24: 5, 1954.

2) Edler I: *The diagnostic use of ultrasound in heart disease.*
   Acta Med. Scandinav. Suppl. 308: 32, 1955.

3) Edler I: *Ultrasound cardiogram in mitral valvular disease.*
   Acta Chir. Scandinav. 111: 230, 1956.

4) Edler I, and Gustafson A: *Ultrasonic cardiogram in mitral stenosis.*
   Acta Med. Scandinav. 159: 85, 1957.

5) Kerber RE, Isaeff DM, and Hancock EW: *Echocardiographic pattern in patients with the syndrome of systolic click and late systolic murmur.*
   N. Engl. J. Med. 283: 691, 1971.

6) Dillon JC, Haine CL, Chang S, and Feigenbaum H: *Use of echocardiography in patients with prolapsed mitral valve.*
   Circulation 43: 503, 1971.

7) DeMaria AN, King JF, Bogren HG, Lies JE, and Mason DT: *The variable spectrum of echocardiographic manifestations of mitral valve prolapse syndrome.*
   Circulation 50: 33, 1974.

8) Popp RL, Brown OR, Silverman JF, and Harrison DC: *Echocardiographic abnormalities in mitral valve prolapse syndrome.*
   Circulation 49: 428, 1974.

9) Markiewicz W, Stoner J, London E, Hunt SA, and Popp RL: *Mitral valve prolapse in one hundred presumably healthy young females.*
   Circulation 53: 464, 1976.

10) Shah PM, Gramiak R, and Kramer DH: *Ultrasound localization of left ventricular outflow obstruction in hypertrophic obstructive cardiomyopathy.*
    Circulation 40: 3, 1969.

11) Popp RL, and Harrison DC: *Ultrasound in the diagnosis and evaluation of therapy of idiopathic hypertrophic subaortic stenosis.*
    Circulation 40: 905, 1969.

12) Henry WL, Clark CE, Glancy DL, and Epstein SE: *Echocardiographic measurement of the left ventricular outflow gradient in idiopathic hypertrophic subaortic stenosis.*
New Engl. J. Med. 288: 989, 1973.

13) Feigenbaum H: *Echocardiography (2nd Edition).*
Philadelphia, Lea and Febiger, 1976.

14) Wolfe SB, Popp RL, and Feigenbaum H: *Diagnosis of atrial tumors by ultrasound.*
Circulation 39: 615, 1969.

15) Quinones MA, Gaasch WH, Waisser E, and Alexander JK: *Reduction in the rate of diastolic descent of the mitral valve echogram in patients with altered left ventricular diastolic pressure-volume relations.*
Circulation 49: 246, 1974.

16) DeMaria A, Miller RR, Amsterdam EA, Markson W, and Mason DT: *Mitral valve early diastolic closing velocity on echogram: relation to sequential diastolic flow and ventricular compliance.*
Amer. J. Cardiol. 37: 693, 1976.

17) Bom N, Lancée CT, Zwieten G van, Kloster FE, and Roelandt J: *Multiscan echocardiography. I. Technical description.*
Circulation 48: 1066, 1973.

18) Griffith JM, and Henry WL: *A sector scanner for real-time two-dimensional echocardiography.*
Circulation 49: 1147, 1974.

19) Vom Ramm OT, and Thurstone FL: *Cardiac imaging using a phased array ultrasound system. I. System design.*
Circulation 53: 258, 1976.

20) Henry WL, Griffith JM, Michaelis LL, McIntosh CL, Morrow AG, and Epstein SE: *Measurement of mitral orifice area in patients with mitral valve disease by real-time, two-dimensional echocardiography.*
Circulation 51: 827, 1975.

21) Nichol PM, Gilbert BW, and Kisslo JA: *Two-dimensional echocardiographic assessment of mitral stenosis.*
Circulation 55: 120, 1977.

22) Henry WL, Clark CE, Griffith JM, and Epstein SE: *Mechanism of left ventricular outflow obstruction in patients with obstructive ASH (IHSS).*
Amer. J. Cardiol. 35: 337, 1975.

23) Sahn DJ, Allen HD, Goldberg SJ, and Friedman WF: *Mitral valve prolapse in children: A problem defined by real-time cross-sectional echocardiography.*
Circulation 53: 651, 1976.

24) Gilbert BW, Schatz RA, Von Ramm OT, Behar VS, and Kisslo JA: *Mitral valve prolapse: Two-dimensional echocardiographic and angiographic correlation.*
Circulation 54: 716, 1976.

25) Kastl DG, Henry WL, McIntosh CL, Michaelis LL, and Morrow AG: *Cross-sectional echo-*

cardiographic studies of the mitral valve before and after mitral commissurotomy: Comparisons of hemodynamic and echocardiographic data.
Circulation: (in press).

26) Henry WL, Sahn DJ, Griffith JM, Goldberg SJ, Maron BJ, McAllister HA, Allen HD, Epstein SE: *Evaluation of atrioventricular valve morphology in congenital heart disease by real-time cross-sectional echocardiography.*
Circulation 52 (Suppl. II): II-120, 1975.

27) Henry WL, Maron BJ, Griffith JM, Redwood DR, and Epstein SE: *The differential diagnosis of anomalies of the great vessels by real-time, two-dimensional echocardiography.*
Circulation 51: 283, 1975.

28) Henry WL, Maron BJ, and Griffith JM: *Cross-sectional echocardiography in the diagnosis of congenital heart disease: Identification of the relation of the ventricles and great arteries.*
Circulation: (in press, July, 1977).

Screening, population and sequential follow-up studies by echocardiography

by Frank E. Kloster
University of Oregon Health Sciences Center
Portland, Oregon 97201, U.S.A.

Echocardiography is very useful for screening or population studies because of several characteristics unique to the technique which meet the requirements for such studies. These include:

1. The noninvasive nature of the technique, with resulting freedom from discomfort or risk to subjects examined.
2. The direct anatomic and physiologic data obtained from ultrasound imaging, providing specific, quantitative cardiovascular information.
3. The relatively low cost of studies compared to other investigations providing comparable information.
4. The high degree of reproducibility of findings by different examiners in the same subject and on repeated studies in the same individual.
5. The availability of reasonably well established criteria for findings in normal individuals and the relatively narrow range of normal values.

Echo studies can be justified in normal or asymptomatic individuals, in patients with disease states not usually requiring invasive laboratory studies and in patients with mild or modest symptoms without the need to demonstrate any direct medical benefit to offset personal risk or pain. Related to the freedom from pain and risk, subjects are less apprehensive and more cooperative about undergoing examination, and as a result more complete data are available regarding patient groups or populations. This is particularly true in family studies, where the most complete data are necessary for valid results but may be unavailable if the study technique is disagreeable, or when investigating those individuals with these disease states not commonly requiring invasive diagnostic tests and hence usually not well studied in the past. Because examinations can be performed on an outpatient basis at relatively low cost, large numbers of subjects can be examined to obtain meaningful population data.

Direct diagnostic information regarding cardiac anatomy and performance is obtained rather than subjective physical findings or the indirect, non-specific information provided by many other noninvasive studies. With these direct, specific cardiac findings it is possible to uncover information and insights previously unavailable and unknown. These factors, in conjunction with the highly reproducible nature of echo data, have made echocardiography particularly attractive for sequential or multiple followup studies.

61

Echocardiology, N. Bom editor, published by Martinus Nijhoff, the Hague 1977.

Some of the areas where echocardiography has been or can be used for such studies are as follows:

Genetic studies.
Echo studies have been extremely useful in evaluating families for the presence of cardiovascular findings suspected or known to be genetically transmitted. The high level of cooperation and availability for examination of virtually all family members was referred to above. Of particular use has been the demonstration of disease markers or findings previously unrecognized and undetectible on physical examination or by other techniques. Classic among these is the recognition of asymmetrical septal hypertrophy (ASH) in the cohorts of patients with idiopathic hypertrophic subaortic stenosis (IHSS) and the recognition that the two are parts of the spectrum of a single genetic disease. From such studies new insights will be gained into modes of genetic transmission of cardiovascular disease, including dominance, sex-linkage, penetrance and expressivity.

Investigation of disease entities.
In some disease states, such as hypertension, direct anatomic and pathophysiologic information has been sparse due to the lack of clinical indications for invasive studies as part of patient evaluation and care. In many others, including valvular and congenital heart diseases, invasive catheter studies are commonly deferred until the patient's symptoms have progressed to the point that operative intervention is indicated, so studies early in the course of the disease or sequentially are uncommon. Echocardiography provides the opportunity to study patients with such disease entities early and repretitively during the natural history of the disease. From such investigations it is possible to define echo criteria, to correlate them with physical and catheterization findings, and to establish the range and severity of cardiovascular abnormalities present.
Sequential studies may be performed during the course of long term follow-up of such patients to determine the natural progression of the disease. Once this has been established, the influence of prophylactic treatment can be evaluated, and both the timing and influence of theraputic interventions, such as valve replacement in rheumatic heart disease or pharmacologic treatment in hypertension, can be determined.

Studies of selected populations.
Populations of individuals without known cardiovascular disease but with specific cardiovascular characteristics in common can be studied for physiologic data never available previously. A group of particular interest has been trained athletes, with subgroups including those primarily in endurance sports (distance runners), in sports involving isometric effort (weight lifting) or those requiring isotonic activity (wrestling). Studies already completed have demonstrated significant differences between athletes involved in sports requiring varying amounts of isometric, isotonic or endurance abilities with regard to cardiac chamber size and wall thickness, and extensions of these initial studies are under way.

Studies of general populations.

Thus far studies of large populations have been directed primarily toward determining the incidence of disease entities, such as prolapsing mitral valve, or determining normal values for individuals without apparent heart disease in different age ranges. An important future application may be the use of echocardiography in screening for clinically unrecognized cardiovascular disease. It is possible that as more specific criteria for heart disease of high prevalence such as coronary disease or hypertension are established, it will be feasible to screen populations in schools, shopping centers, etc.

As with any studies of patient or normal populations, there are potential pitfalls or limitations related to the technique and/or research study design. Some problems that have been recognized in investigations carried out at our institution, with examples from specific research studies, include the following:

Equivocal, false positive or false negative findings.

Incompletely established criteria for abnormality or a "borderline" range can make interpretation and reporting of results difficult. In a familial study of ASH we used the original criterion of a septal/posterior LV wall ratio $\geqslant 1.3$ as diagnostic. Subsequently, there have been supplemental criteria (septum > 15 mm in thickness, ratio $\geqslant 1.5$, absence of any other disease potentially causing right or left ventricular hypertrophy) which may change some "abnormal" interpretations. In our study of Marfan's syndrome, no single criterion for aortic enlargement appeared satisfactory, so three separate criteria (aortic size, aortic size corrected for BSA and left atrial/aortic ratio) were used, with a resulting "equivocal" population of subjects meeting one or two but not all three criteria.

Using improper echo techniques can also produce incorrect results. In a study of normal subjects to determine the incidence of mitral valve prolapse we deliberately made recordings from one interspace above the standard position, and found we could produce "false prolapse" in a significant number.

Such pitfalls can clearly result in misleading or erroneous conclusions. In addition, there can be a serious emotional impact on normal individuals who are falsely interpreted as being abnormal.

Biased populations.

"Normal" populations clearly must be selected carefully to assure they consist of truly normal individuals. Hospital patients without apparent cardiovascular disease are commonly used, but may include a significant number of individuals with unrecognized disease unrelated or related to their primary diagnosis. Even "normal volunteers" who are apparently healthy may be biased inadvertently. In our study of the incidence of mitral prolapse in a population recruited from paid, young adults, we encountered a small but suspicious number of individuals with a history of a heart murmur or palpitations and an unusually strong interest in their echo findings.

Management of asymptomatic or previously unrecognized abnormalities.

Inherent in the remarkable potential for studying asymptomatic, apparently normal individuals is the likelihood that some will be found to have abnormalities. In the case of familial disease, particularly those with serious consequences such as Marfan's syndrome or ASH-IHSS, this can present serious problems in dealing with the individual or the family. We have felt obligated to discuss the finding with the patient (or parents), including some mention of potential therapy (such as prophylactic antibiotics to prevent infective endocarditis), and have referred them to their physicians for further management.

The proper course is even less certain with findings which may be "non-diseases" in some individuals, particularly mitral valve prolapse by echo in otherwise normal young women. When the findings are unequivocal we have discussed them with the person as indicated above. This is with the recognition that there is some risk of creating a cardiac neurosis in a person without significant disease, but the feeling that that possibility is outweighed by the greater risks and consequences of unrecognized heart disease, particularly complicated by endocarditis.

References

Mitral valve prolapse

1) Brown OR, Kloster FE, and DeMots H: *Incidence of mitral valve prolapse in the asymptomatic normal.*
   Circulation 52: II-76, 1975.

2) Markiewicz W, Stoner J, London E, Hunt SA, and Popp RL: *Mitral valve prolapse in one-hundred presumably healthy young females.*
   Circulation 53: 464, 1976.

3) Procacci PM, Savran SV, Schreiter SL, and Bryson AL: *Prevalence of clinical mitral valve prolapse in 1169 young women.*
   N Engl J Med 294: 1086, 1976.

Marfan's syndrome

1) Brown OR, DeMots H, Kloster FE, Roberts A, Menashe VD, and Beals: *Aortic root dilatation and mitral valve prolapse in Marfan's syndrome.*
   Circulation 52: 651, 1975.

Asymmetric Septal Hypertrophy

1) Clark CE, Henry WL, and Epstein CE: *Familial prevalence and genetic transmission of idiopathic hypertrophic subaortic stenosis.*
   N Engl J Med 289: 709, 1973.

2) Van Dorp WG, Ten Cate FJ, Vletter WB, Dohmen H, and Roelandt J: *Familial prevalence of asymmetric septal hypertrophy.*
Europ J Cardiol 413: 349, 1976.

Athletes

1) Morganroth J, Maron BJ, Henry WL, and Epstein SE: *Comparative left ventricular dimensions in trained athletes.*
Ann Intern Med 82: 521, 1975.

2) Roeske WR, O'Rourke RA, Klein A, Leopold G, and Karliner JS: *Noninvasive evaluation of ventricular hypertrophy in professional athletes.*
Circulation 53: 286, 1976.

3) Rost R, Schneider KW, and Stegmann N: *A comparative echocardiographical examination of the hearts of highly trained athletes and untrained persons.*
J Sports Med Phys Fitness 15: 305, 1975.

Echocardiologic Assessment
in Asymmetric Septal Hypertrophy (ASH)

F.J. ten Cate
Department of Clinical Echocardiography
The Thoraxcenter, University Hospital Dijkzigt and
Erasmus University Rotterdam.

The anatomic marker of Idiopathic Hypertrophic Subaortic Stenosis (IHSS) is the disproportionally thickened septum. Because echocardiography allows determination of sizes of ventricular cavities and walls, this method is excellent to confirm or deny the existence of the disease, even in the asymptomatic patient. All features of anatomy and physiology are evident on the echocardiogram (tabel I):

Table I: Characteristic Echocardiographic findings of ASH

Septum	- increased diastolic thickness - systolic thickening decreased ($<$ 20 percent)
AMVL	- systolic anterior motion (SAM) possible - decreased diastolic closure rate
LV	- size normal or decreased - "banana" shape - narrow outflow tract
LV post wall	- normal diastolic thickness - systolic thickening normal or increased

In all cases there is asymmetric hypertrophy of the ventricular septum (ASH), with small or no hypertrophy of the left ventricular posterior wall 1). Septal thickness usually exceeds 15mm and ratio of septal to posterior wall thickness is above 1.5 in classical cases 2). Sometimes a ratio of 1.3 is considered suggestive of ASH when also a thickened septum is present 1).

67

Echocardiology, N. Bom editor, published by Martinus Nijhoff, the Hague 1977.

Furthermore the left ventricular (LV) outflow tract is narrow (less than 20 mm) in all cases. The ventricular septum does not contract well in ASH 3). These features are shown in fig. 1.

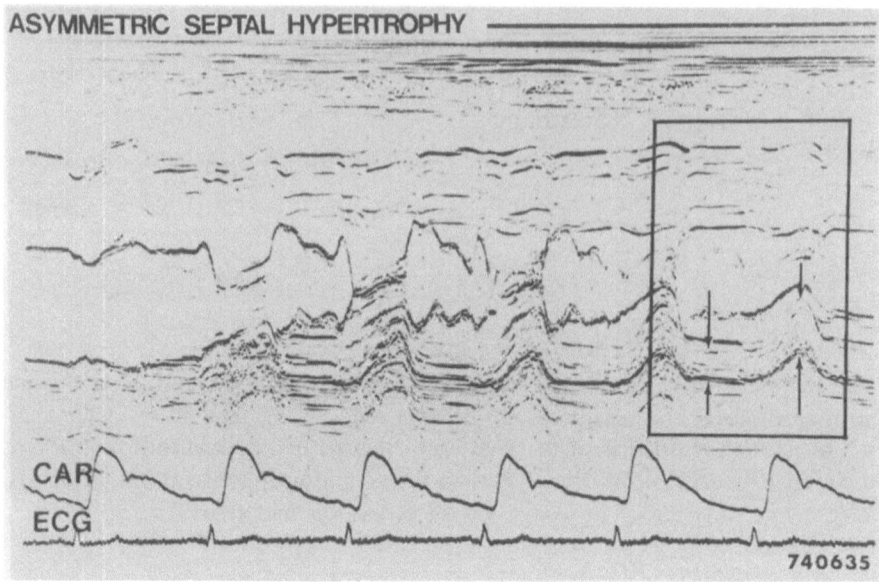

fig. 1. Echocardiogram of a patient with asymmetric septal hypertrophy and no gradient across the left ventricular outflowtract under basal conditions. The disproportionately thickened ventricular septum, which is not contracting, is evident. The posterior wall in contrary is contracting well.

In our laboratory we have studied septal and posterior wall contraction pattern in 19 cases with ASH (11 with and 8 without obstruction to left ventricular outflow). Systolic thickening of the septum in ASH is less than 20 percent (normal ⟩ 40 percent) whereas posterior wall systolic thickening is normal or even augmented 3).

Another feature of the disease is the small left ventricular size. When outflow gradient exists a peculiar systolic anterior motion (SAM) of the anterior mitral valve leaflet (AMVL) is observed (fig. 2).

This motion consists of an abrupt anterior motion of the anterior mitral leaflet just after beginning of systole, reaches its apex in midsystole and returns to its origin in late systole. Measurement of the extent of reduction of the left ventricular outflowtract due to SAM have been used to calculate an obstructionindex which correlates well with the gradient across the left ventricular outflowtract during cardiac catheterization 1). However, this concept should be extended further and confirmed by other echocardiographers in the future, before it could be used in routine echocardiography.

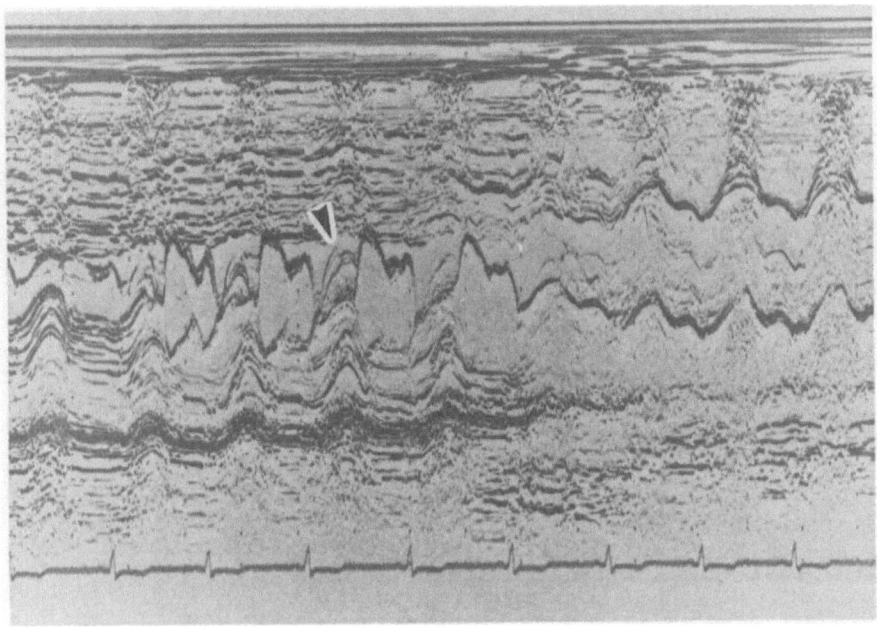

fig. 2. Echocardiogram of a patient with asymmetric septal hypertrophy and a gradient across the left ventricular outflowtract under basal conditions.
Systolic anterior motion (SAM) of the anterior mitral leaflet (see arrow) together with the other characteristic features of the disease are seen (see also text).

The massive hypertrophy and small left ventricular cavity accounts for a stiff left ventricle in this disease; this feature is reflected by a decreased diastolic closure rate of the anterior mitral valve leaflet (table I). The unique possibilities of the multiscan system allows description of functional anatomy in ASH (fig. 3).

The shape of the left ventricle is abnormal and resembles the shape of a ''banana''. The hypertrophied septum is seen extending for its largest portion into the left ventricular outflowtract (LVOT), about 2 - 4 cm beneath the aortic valve cusps. In cases with outflow obstruction the anterior mitral valve leaflet is seen in an abnormal position in the LVOT during systole. The posterior wall is contracting well, whereas the septum does not. LV cavity is small and left atrial cavity sometimes enlarged, when severe mitralinsufficiency is present.

Echocardiographic studies in asymptomatic first degree relatives of symptomatic patients have shown a high familial incidence 1), 4). The disease is genetically transmitted as an autosomal, dominant trait with high degree of penetrance.

Echocardiography, together with other cardiological diagnostic tools, allows careful follow-up of symptomatic cases and their asymptomatic diseased relatives to give further insight into the progression of the disease.

ASYMMETRIC SEPTAL HYPERTROPHY

END DIASTOLE

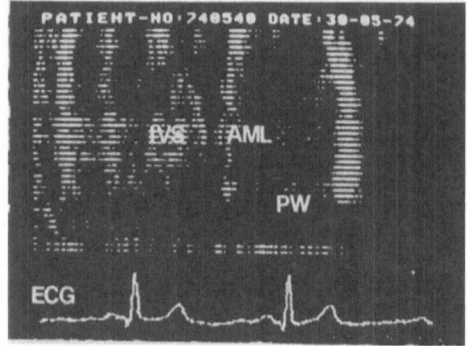 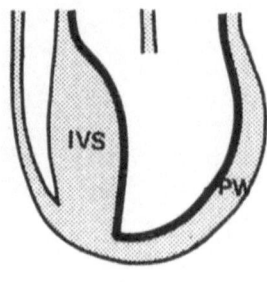

END SYSTOLE

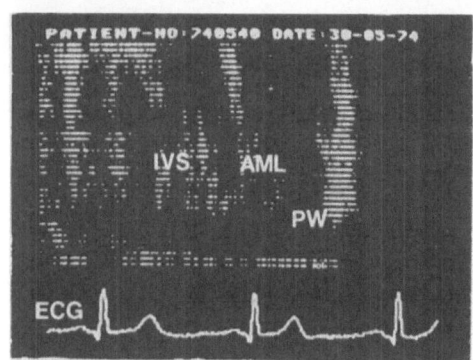 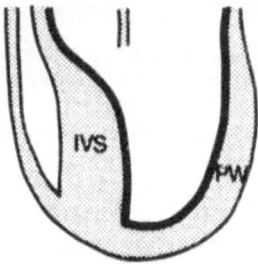

fig. 3. Multiscan echocardiographic enddiastolic and endsystolic frames of the same patient as described in figure 2.
The left ventricle is small and has an abnormal "banana" shape. The hypertrophied ventricular septum is clearly observed with its largest portion extending into the left ventricular outflow tract 2 - 4 cm beneath the aortic cusps. (IVS = inter ventricular septum; PW = posterior wall; AML = anterior mitral leaflet).

Based on echocardiologic observations and clinical experience a classification of the progression of the disease is proposed and given in table II In the evaluation of the disease stage it is known that familial forms have a tendency to show a worse prognosis 5).

Patients with only echocardiographic signs of ASH and no clinical symptoms are classified as preclinical. When slightly symptomatic patients are detected for instance

Table II: Stages of ASH

Degree	Complaints	LV size	SAM	Other findings
preclinical	–	N or ↓	–	–
mild	– or +	N or ↓	– or +	– or +
moderate	+	N or ↓	+	+
severe	+ +	↑ ↑	–	+ +

by screening of 1⁰ relatives these patients are classified as having a mild form of the disease. Symptomatic patients with labile or large gradients are classified to have a moderate form of the disease. When clinical symptoms progress and clinical deterioration is observed, together with LV dilatation, the patients are classified as having a severe form of the disease. However, another severe complication e.g. sudden death seems to occur irrespective of the progression of the disease.

Echocardiology is an excellent technique to observe all hemodynamic and anatomic features of this peculiar disease.

Routine use of this technique in screening of all first degree relatives of symptomatic patients would allow further insight in the natural history of this disease in the future.

References

1) Epstein SE, Henry WL, Clark CE, Roberts WC, Maron BJ, Ferrans VJ, Redwood DR and Morrow AG: *Asymmetric septal hypertrophy*.
Ann Int Med 81 : 650, 1974.

2) Abbassi AS, Mc Alpin RN, Eber LM, Pearce ML: *Echocardiographic diagnosis of idiopathic hypertrophic cardiomyopathy without outflow obstruction*.
Circulation: 46, 897, 1972.

3) ten Cate FJ, van Dorp WG, Vletter WB and Roelandt J: *Ultrasonic analysis of the mechanical behaviour of the left ventricle in Asymmetric septal hypertrophy (ASH)*.
Abstract Book 1, 7th European Congress of Cardiology, Amsterdam, p 218, 1976 (abstract).

4) van Dorp WG, ten Cate FJ, Vletter WB, Dohmen H and Roelandt J: *Familial prevalence of asymmetric septal hypertrophy*.
Europ J of Cardiol 4/3 : 349, 1976.

5) Frank S and Braunwald E: *Idiopathic hypertrophic subaortic stenosis. Clinical analysis with emphasis on the natural history*.
Circulation: 37, 759, 1968.

Mitral valve prolapse

by A. Bloch,
Centre de Cardiologie, Hôpital Cantonal,
Geneva, Switzerland.

The diagnosis of mitral valve prolapse is one of the most important applications of echocardiography. This is due to several reasons:

1. Mitral valve prolapse is a frequent condition.
2. The clinical diagnosis of mitral prolapse may be difficult.
3. The identification of mitral prolapse is useful because this condition, although usually benign, may lead to several complications.
4. Echocardiography is with left ventricular angiography the best technique for the diagnosis of mitral prolapse and represents the only reliable non-invasive method.

Many terms have been used for the syndrome of mitral valve prolapse, such as: Barlow's syndrome, floppy mitral valve, billowing mitral leaflet syndrome, click-murmur syndrome and midsystolic click-late systolic murmur. Mitral valve prolapse is presently the most commonly used term. Patients with the syndrome of mitral valve prolapse usually present 1) atypical chest pain, lightheaddedness, shortness of breath, fatigue and palpitations. The typical auscultatory finding is a nonejection, mid to late systolic click often followed by a late systolic murmur. However, patients with proven mitral valve prolapse may have multiple systolic clicks, an early systolic click, a pansystolic murmur, a late systolic murmur without click or a normal auscultation ("silent prolapse"). The typical electrocardiographic abnormalities consist of inverted T waves in leads II, III and aVF; similar changes can be seen in the precordial leads. Arrhythmias, particularly premature ventricular beats, are frequent.

Although mitral valve prolapse is usually a benign condition, several complications are possible. The most frequent ones are severe arrhythmias and significant mitral regurgitation; isolated cases of bacterial endocarditis and sudden death have also been described. The normal echocardiographic appearance of the mitral valve in systole consists of a gradual upward (or anterior) displacement of the leaflets. The criteria for the echocardiographic diagnosis of mitral valve prolapse include two different patterns of mitral valve motion 2), 6):

1. Early in systole the leaflets are either flat or move in a slightly anterior direction, but in mid or late systole a relatively abrupt posterior displacement of one or both leaflets occurs. This is the late systolic prolapse pattern. (fig. 1 and 2).

Echocardiology, N. Bom editor, published by Martinus Nijhoff, the Hague 1977.

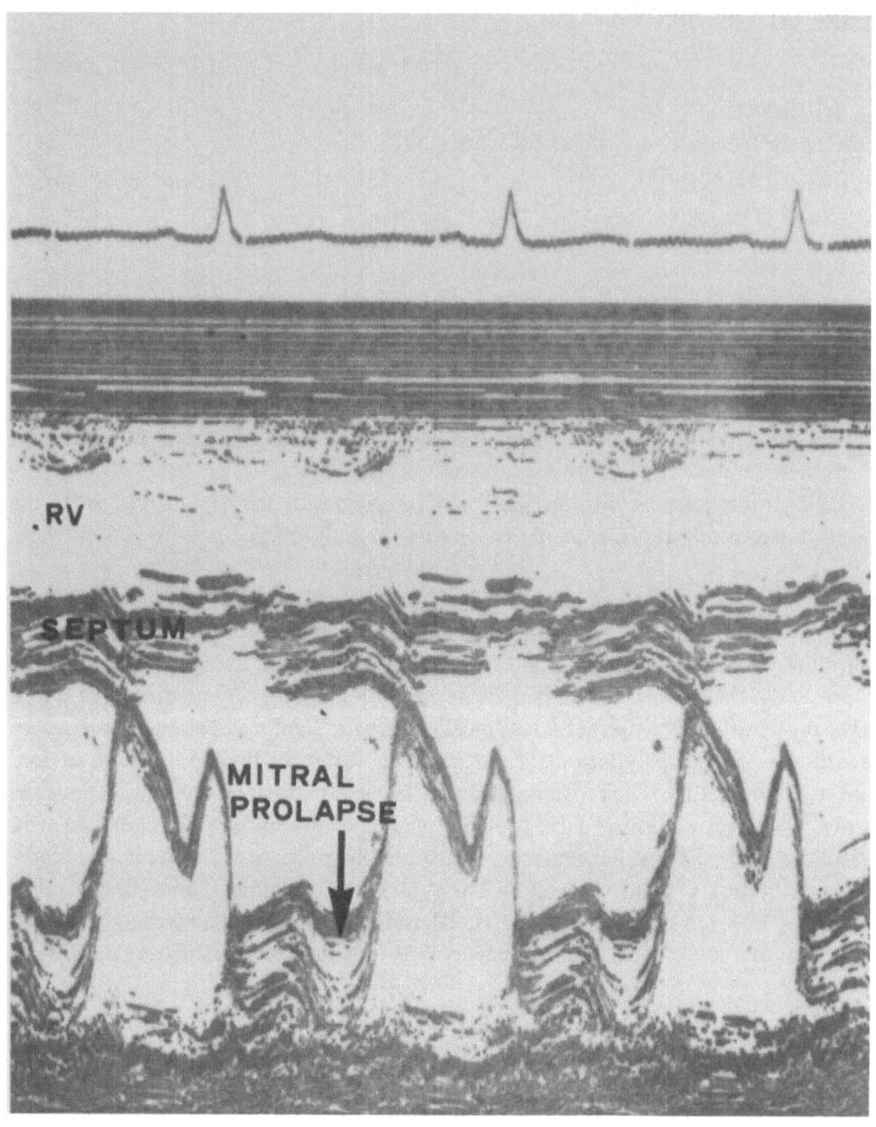

fig. 1. Late systolic mitral valve prolapse in a 22 year old female with systolic click and late systolic murmur.

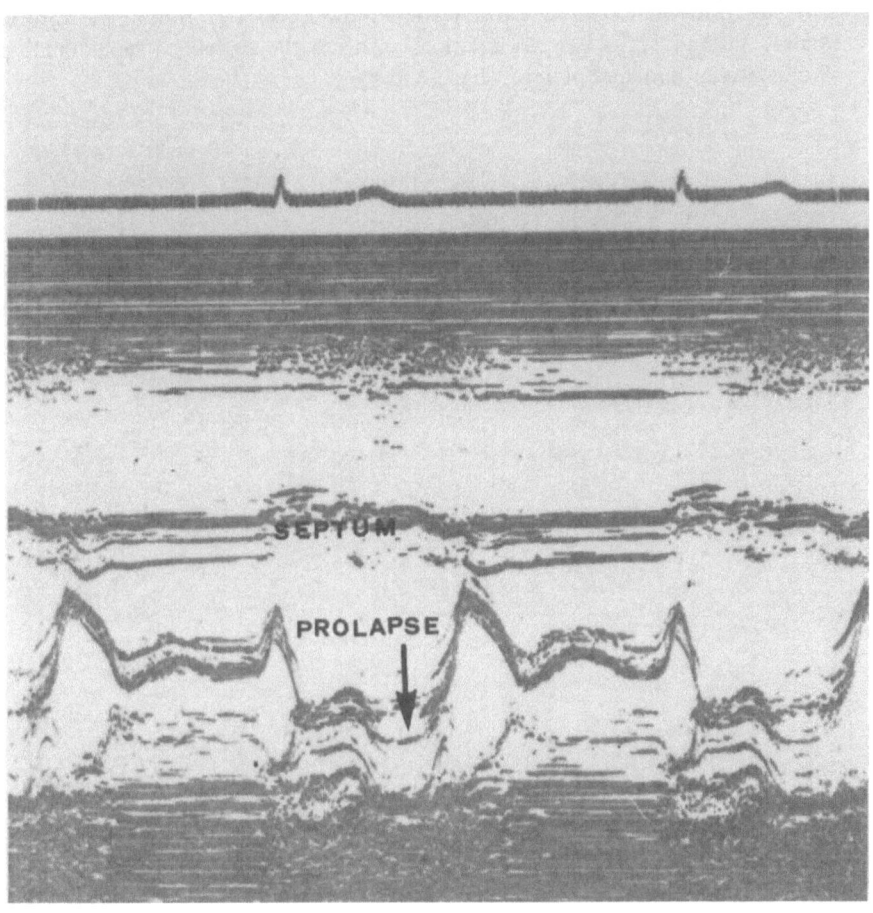

fig. 2. Late systolic mitral valve prolapse in a 60 year old man with a systolic click and late systolic murmur.

2. Early in systole one or both mitral leaflets show a posterior motion and approximately in mid systole move anteriorly. This is the so-called "hammock" or "holosystolic" prolapse pattern. (fig. 3 and 4).

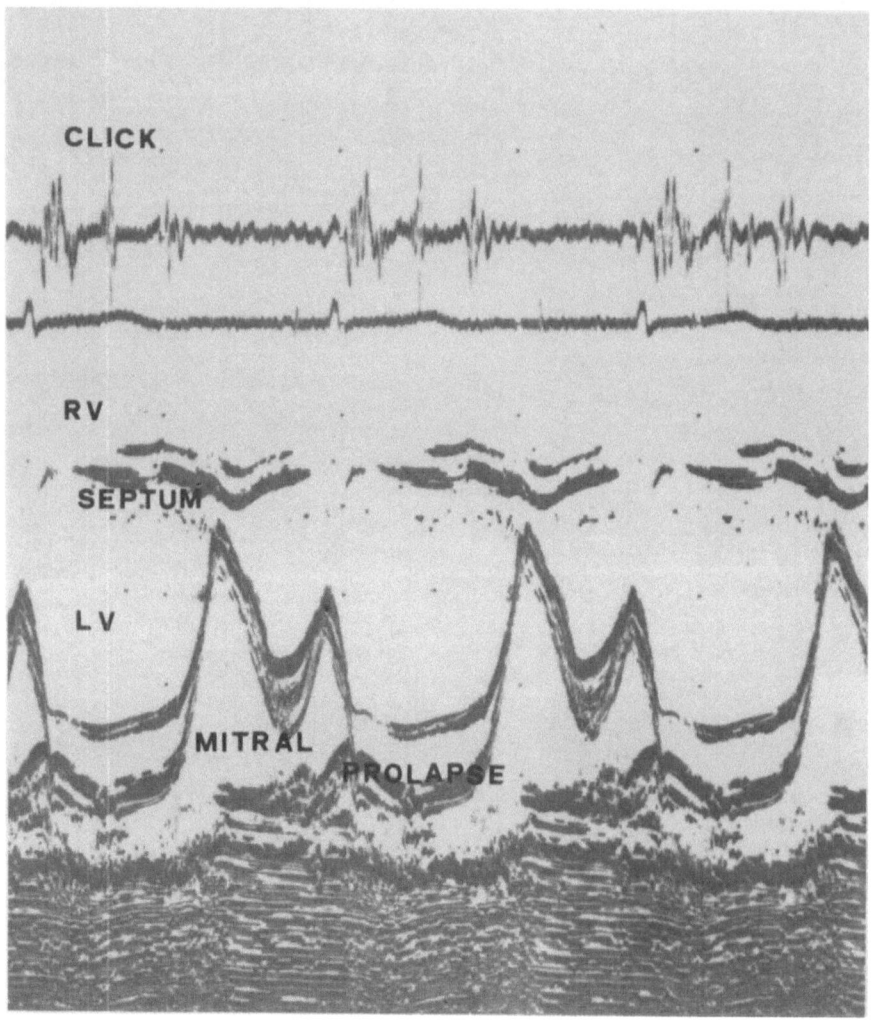

fig. 3. Holosystolic mitral valve prolapse in a 27 year old female. The loudest systolic click is simultaneous with the maximal prolapse of the leaflets.

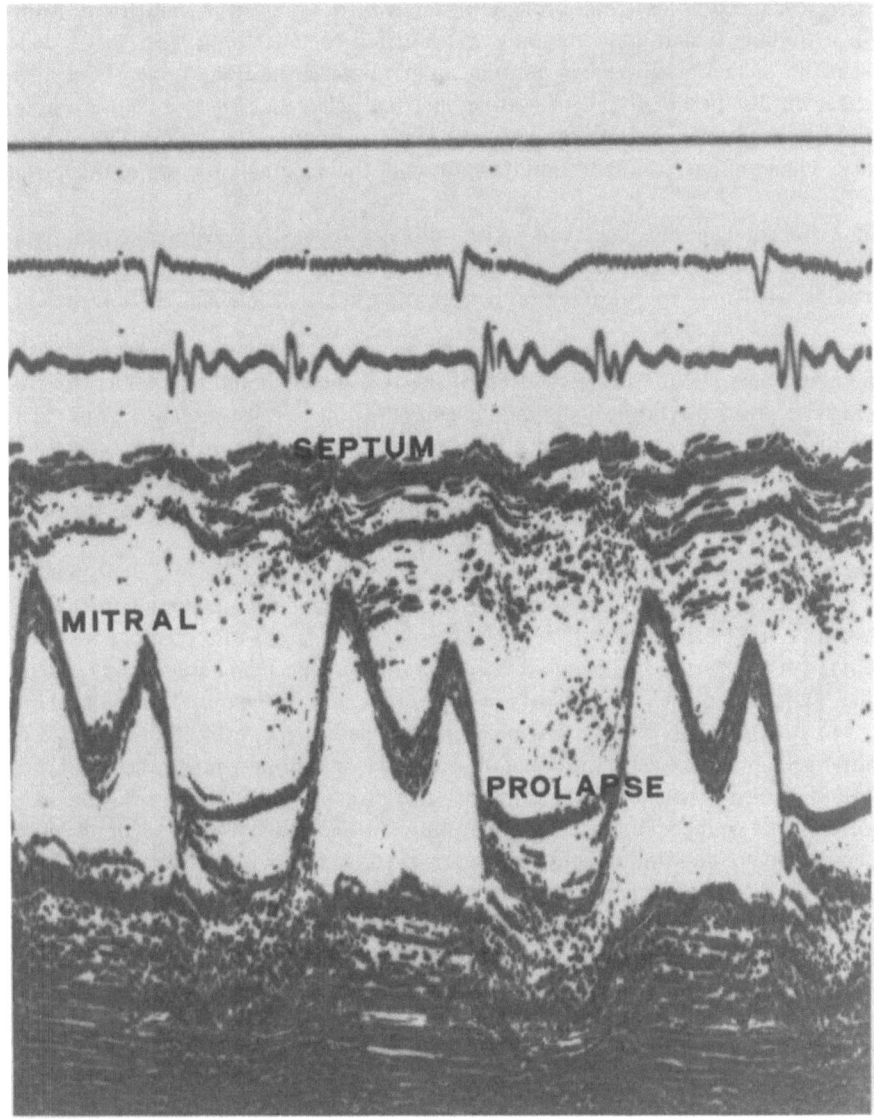

fig. 4. Holosystolic mitral valve prolapse in a 29 year old man with the Marfan syndrome.

These two echocardiographic criteria have been shown to correlate well with prolapse demonstrated by angiography 4), 6), 7). The distinction between these two echocardiographic patterns may be somewhat artificial. When long tracings are recorded with the transducer in several positions and orientations, it is not uncommon to see both patterns in a single individual. Moreover, a late systolic prolapse can be converted into a holosystolic prolapse if amyle nitrite is given to the patient. Additional findings which are commonly seen but not specific to prolapse are: a wide excursion of the mitral valve in diastole, a slight anterior motion of one of the valve echoes during the initial half of systole, and multiple echoes in systole or diastole. Mitral prolapse affects either the posterior leaflet alone or both leaflets. The systolic click, when present, is usually simultaneous with the maximal prolapse of the mitral leaflets.

The echocardiographic diagnosis of mitral prolapse is usually easy but the technique of recording can be at times quite difficult. In some patients the prolapse can be demonstrated only at the junction between the left ventricle and the left atrium.

The maximum prolapsing echo may be faint and thus can be missed if the gain is set too low. Excessive inferior angulation of the transducer should be avoided to prevent false positive echocardiographic diagnosis of mitral valve prolapse. False positive diagnosis of prolapse have also been reported in patients with large pericardial effusions or with hypertrophic subaortic stenosis. In some severe cases of prolapse, the echocardiographic appearance of the mitral valve may be similar to that of a flail valve due to ruptured chordae.

Since echocardiography has provided a non invasive method for the identification of mitral valve prolapse, this condition is being recognized with increasing frequency. Brown et al. 8) have demonstrated mitral prolapse in 31 out of 35 patients (89 percent) with the Marfan syndrome. In a left ventricular cineangiographic study, Betriu et al. 9) have identified prolapse of the posterior leaflet of the mitral valve in 20 out of 54 patients (37 percent) with secundum atrial defect. However, the prevalence of mitral prolapse in the general population is still not well known. Brown et al. 10) have identified echocardiographic mitral valve prolapse in 30 out of 700 (4.3 percent) normal young volunteers. In this group, 23 had systolic clicks and/or murmurs recorded by phonocardiography. However, systolic clicks and/or murmurs at the apex were also recorded from 11 subjects without evidence of prolapse on echocardiographic examination. In a similar study, Markiewicz et al. 11) have reported an unexpected high incidence of 21 percent of echocardiographic mitral valve prolapse in a group of 100 presumable healthy paid female volunteers.

We had the opportunity to perform in Boston an echocardiographic study on normal volunteers 12). The study population was made up of 136 individuals having no clinical evidence of cardiac disease or hypertension; however, subjects were not excluded if they were found to have systolic clicks and/or soft systolic murmurs of doubtful significance. Echocardiograms judged to be satisfactory for interpretation of mitral valve motion were obtained in all cases. All tracings were read independently by two of the investigators. Each tracing which was "suggestive" or "diagnostic" of mitral valve prolapse was then reread separately by each of an additional three experienced echocardiographers. Only when at least four of five independent observers agreed that there was evidence of systolic prolapse of one or both leaflets were the results recorded as such.

Six of the subjects (4.4 percent) had echocardiograms which demonstrated mitral valve prolapse. One reported occasional palpitations, while the remainder was asymptomatic. In all cases were both mitral leaflets involved. The pattern was late systolic in 1 and holosystolic in 5 out of 6. Another subgroup of 18 subjects (13 percent) demonstrated some degree of posterior systolic motion of the mitral valve leaflets which was suggestive but not diagnostic of prolapse. Three of these 18 reported occasional palpitations, while the remaining 15 were asymptomatic. 15 of these 18 subjects had an involvement of both mitral leaflets. A few of these individuals with clearly defined or possible mitral prolapse had a systolic click or an innocent murmur. However, by study design, no subject was included who had the classical "mid systolic click-late systolic murmur" syndrome.

In our study, the tracing was considered "diagnostic" of prolapse when the posterior displacement of the mitral leaflets was greater than or equal to 5 mm (when measured from the C point of the mitral echo). In these cases prolapse could be easily demonstrated from multiple positions of the transducer on the chest wall. The tracing was considered "suggestive" of prolapse when the posterior systolic motion (when measured from the C point) was less than 5 mm. Frequently this minor posterior displacement could only be recorded at a single transducer position and orientation.

Our limit of a 5 mm posterior displacement is quite arbitrary. Markiewicz et al. 11) for example have defined mitral prolapse as a holosystolic or midsystolic posterior motion of the mitral echo of more than 2 mm from a line joining the C and D points. Recently stressed 13), 14) has been the importance of avoiding excessive inferior angulation of the echo transducer to prevent the false positive echocardiographic diagnosis of mitral prolapse. Markiewicz et al. 14) have suggested that the optimal way to analyze mitral valve prolapse is to record both mitral leaflets and left atrium with the transducer either perpendicular to the chest or pointing slightly upward. It is presently not known if a minor posterior displacement of the mitral leaflets in systole is an abnormal finding. There is no correlative study with left ventricular angiography for such cases. Prospective studies will be necessary to know if a slight systolic posterior displacement of the mitral valve has any clinical of functional significance or if it represents a variant of normal mitral valve motion.

We believe that one should be presently cautious not to overdiagnose mitral prolapse echocardiographically.

In summary

Echocardiography has provided an excellent means for the non-invasive detection of mitral valve prolapse. It has revealed that mitral prolapse is a very common condition. In border-line cases, the limit between a normal and an abnormal systolic motion of the mitral valve may be difficult to define; however, in most cases, the echocardiographic diagnosis of mitral valve prolapse is quite easy.

References

1) Jeresaty RM: *Mitral Valve Prolapse - Click Syndrome.*
Progress in Cardiovascular Diseases 15: 623, 1973.

2) Dillon JC, Haine CL, Chang S, and Feigenbaum H: *Use of echocardiography in patients with prolapsed mitral valve.*
Circulation 43: 503, 1971.

3) Kerber RE, Isaeff DM, and Hancock EW: *Echocardiographic patterns in patients with the syndrome of systolic click and late systolic murmur.*
NEJM 284: 691, 1971.

4) Popp RL, Brown OR, Silverman JF, and Harrison DC: *Echocardiographic abnormalities in the mitral valve prolapse syndrome.*
Circulation 49: 428, 1974.

5) Shah PM, and Gramiak R: *Clinical usefulness of echocardiography.*
Progress in Cardiology 3. Edited by PN Yu and JF Goodwin. Philadelphia, Lea and Febiger, 1974 p 293.

6) DeMaria AN, King JF, Bogren HG, Lies JE, and Mason DT: *The variable spectrum of echocardiographic manifestations of the mitral valve prolapse syndrome.*
Circulation 50: 33, 1974.

7) Malcolm AD, Boughner DR, Kostuk WJ, and Ahuja SP: *Clinical features and investigative findings in presence of mitral leaflet prolapse. Study of 85 consecutive patients.*
British Heart Journal 38: 244, 1976.

8) Brown OR, DeMots H, and Kloster FE: *Prevalence of aortic root dilation and mitral valve prolapse in Marfan's syndrome: an echocardiographic study.*
Amer. J. Cardiology 35: 124, 1975.

9) Betriu A, Wigle DE, Felderhod CH, and McLoughlin MJ: *Prolapse of the posterior leaflet of the mitral valve associated with secundum atrial defect.*
Amer. J. Cardiology 35: 363, 1975.

10) Brown OR, Kloster FE, and DeMots H: *Incidence of mitral valve prolapse in the asymptomatic normal.*
Circulation 52, Suppl II: 77, 1975.

11) Markiewicz W, Stoner J, London E, Hunt SA, and Popp RL: *Mitral valve prolapse in one hundred presumably healthy young females.*
Circulation 53: 464, 1976.

12) Bloch A, Vignola PA, Walker H, Kaplan AD, Chiotellis PN, Lees RS, and Myers GS: *Echocardiographic spectrum of posterior systolic motion of the mitral valve in a general population.*
(To be published).

13) Weiss AN, Mimbs JW, Ludbrook PA, and Sobel BE: *Echocardiographic detection of mitral valve prolapse. Exclusion of false positive diagnosis and determination of inheritance.*
Circulation 52: 1091, 1975.

80

14) Markiewicz W, Stoner J, London E, Hunt S, and Popp RL: *Effect of transducer placement on echocardiographic mitral valve systolic motion.*
Europ. J. Cardiology 4: 359, 1976.

A dual M-mode system for simultaneous time motion analyses of cardiac structures and evaluation of cardiac function: initial clinical applications.

by David J. Sahn,
University of Arizona Health Sciences Center, Tucson, Arizona: and
N. Bom, C.T. Lancee, F.C. van Egmond, J. Roelandt,
Thoraxcenter, Erasmus University and Academic Hospital Dijkzigt,
Rotterdam, the Netherlands.

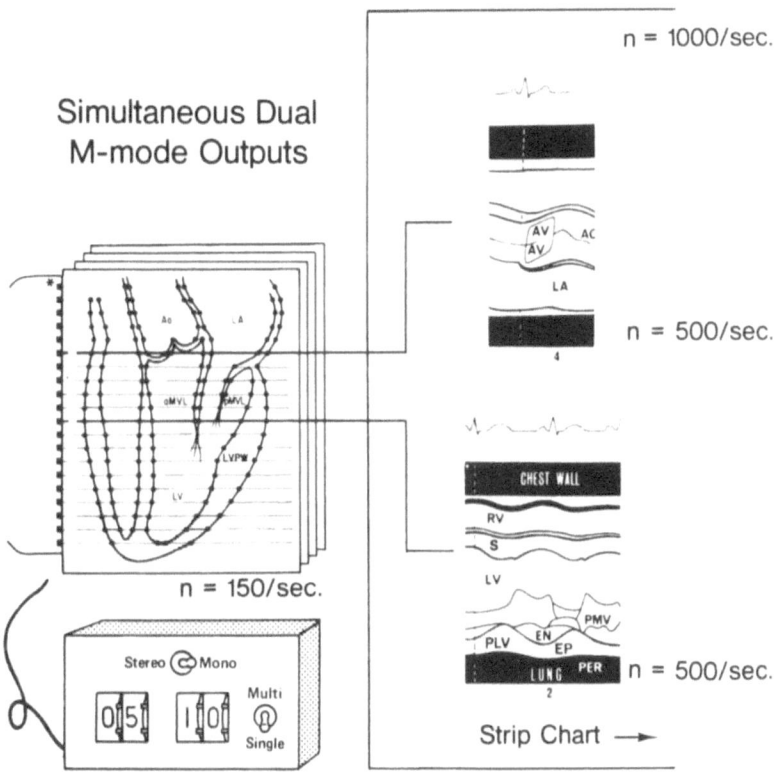

fig. 1. The functioning of the simultaneous dual M-mode system is shown (see text for details). Please note that the diagrammatic traces are not lined up so as to truly be simultaneous. The actual traces in figures 2, 7, 9 and 10 are acquired simultaneously. Abbreviations: n = number of samples per second; Ao = aorta; AV = aortic valve; AC = aortic cusp; LA = left atrium; AMVL = anterior mitral leaflet; PMVL = posterior mitral leaflet; PLV = posterior left ventricular wall; EN = endocardium; EP = epicardium; PER = pericardium; S = septum; RV = right ventricle.

83

Echocardiology, N. Bom editor, published by Martinus Nijhoff, the Hague 1977.

Time motion or M-mode echocardiography has had a major impact in cardiovascular disease because it has allowed rapid noninvasive analysis of the motion of intracardiac structures. The M-mode has provided not only anatomical but also functional or physiological information. For example, analysis of the motion of the aortic valve has provided an accurate measurement of left ventricular systolic time intervals 1) which, when combined with an analysis of left ventricular wall motion has allowed the noninvasive determination of ejection phase parameters of cardiac performance of contractility 2), 3). Likewise, time motion analyses of the motions of the pulmonary valve have been very useful for the evaluation of pulmonary vascular resistance 4). Because simultaneous recording of time motion information from different areas of the heart would increase the sophistication with which echo events could be interpreted for functional as well as for anatomic information, we have, as a collaborative endeavor, designed a dual M-mode registration system to allow the echocardiographic recording of different valves simultaneously on a beat-to-beat basis 5).

The functioning of the system is shown in figure 1.

With the multiple-crystal echocardiographic system as initially designed, M-modes are selectable from individual elements within the array with a sample rate of 1024 Hz by excitation of one single element in the array. The M-mode is selectable at a known location with reference to the heart and provides accurate spatial orientation to assist in the interpretation of dimensional data. As shown in the figure, the dual M-mode system allows independent selection of two lines from known locations within the array, shown here when the control box is switched to the stereo mode.

The cross-sectional image then shows two bright lines. In this example, the first index line at line 5 corresponds to the element in proximity to the aortic root, the second at line 10 corresponds to the element near the free edge of the mitral valve.

Then, when the instrument is placed into the single element recording mode, the two single element M-modes are obtained in alternating fashion at a line rate of 512 Hz with simultaneous recording of the electrocardiogram on a strip chart recorder. As shown in figure 2, the M-mode echocardiograms are adequate for the measurement of systolic time intervals and calculation of indices of ventricular contractility. The addition of an independent Honeywell time line generator to this system (as shown in figure 9) has increased the accuracy with which these timing measurements can be made.

Our initial experiences with this technique suggest that simultaneous mitral and aortic valve traces of adequate quality for timing can be obtained in 75 percent of children and approximately 40 percent of adults. The utility of these traces can be illustrated in figure 2. The aortic ejection time can be calculated from the upper trace and combined with the simultaneously derived left ventricular diastolic and systolic dimensions for the calculation of mean velocity of circumferential fiber

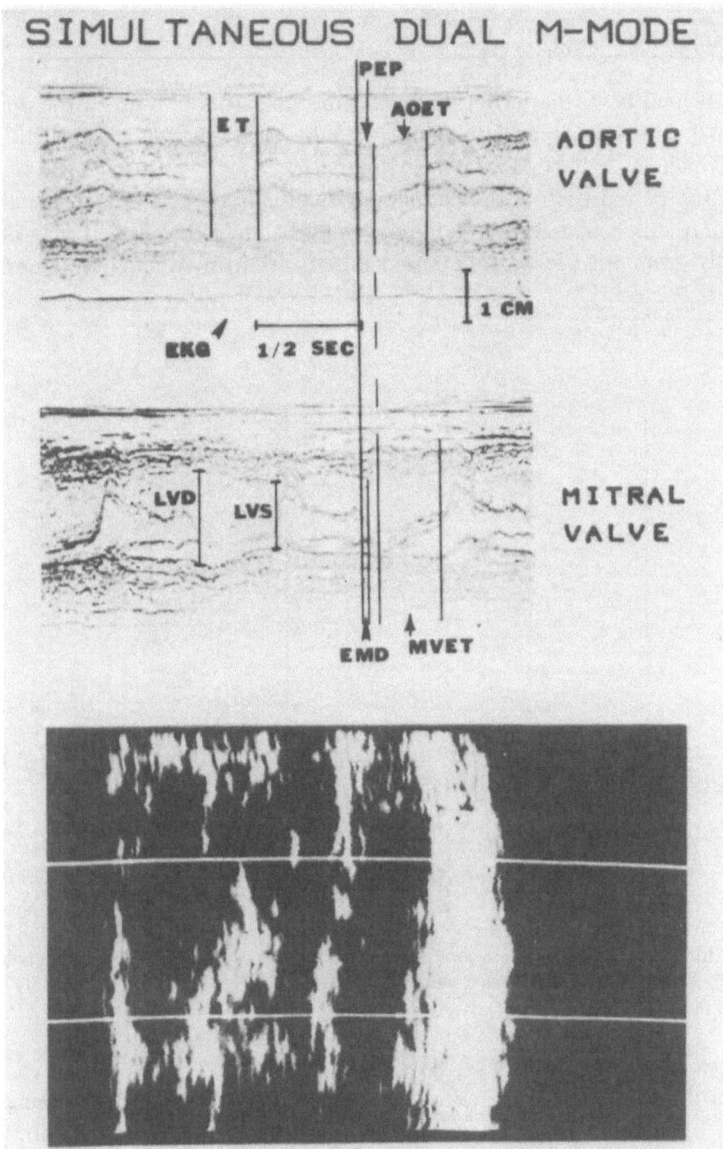

fig. 2. The simultaneous dual M-modes from the mitral and aortic valves and echocardiographic cross-sectional still frame showing the index lines used to derive them are shown. The top line corresponds to the tracing of the aorta and aortic valve seen on the top trace. The bottom line corresponds to the trace through the septum, mitral valve and left ventricular posterior wall shown in the bottom of the simultaneously derived traces. ET = ejection time; AoET = aortic ejection time; PEP = pre-ejection period; EKG = electrocardiogram; EMD = electromechanical delay; MVET = mitral valve ejection time; LVD = left ventricular diastolic dimension; LVS = left ventricular systolic dimension. See text for details.

shortening $V_{cf} = \dfrac{LVD - LVS}{LVD \times ET}$, an index of contractility which is normal in this patient.

On the second beat, the mitral valve ejection time from closure to the opening of the mitral valve is compared to the aortic valve ejection time and is slightly longer since it includes a portion of the isovolumic contraction period. The isovolumic contraction period itself is the period between the onset of mechanical contraction of the left ventricular wall and the opening of the aortic valve. It may differ significantly from the pre-ejection period in patients with conduction abnormalities.

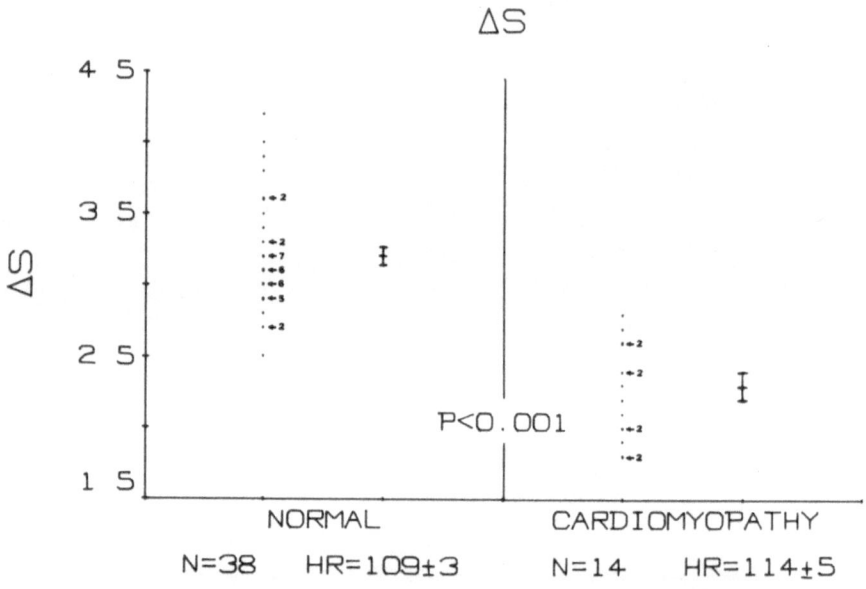

fig. 3. Individual patient values, group means and standard errors are shown for the left ventricular fractional shortening of the minor axis (Δ S) expressed in percent and compared between normal (left) and children with cardiomyopathy (right). The groups were statistically separable as shown by the p <0.01.

The isovolumic contraction period can be calculated from the simultaneous dual outputs by determining the electromechanical delay (EMD), the period starting from the Q wave (the onset of electrical ventricular depolarization) and ending with the first rapid closing movement of the mitral valve complex. The EMD is then subtracted from the pre-ejection period to determine the isovolumic contraction time which is .04 seconds on the second beat in figure 2.

We have recently investigated the percent of left ventricular fractional shortening $\dfrac{(LVD - LVS) \times 100}{LVD} = \Delta S$ and mean velocity of circumferential fiber shortening in a group of 38 (age-matched normal) children and compared our results to those ob-

86

tained in 14 children with documented acute myocarditis or chronic cardiomy-
pathy. The children in both groups had a mean age of 5.4 ± .07 yrs. The fractional
shortening ΔS in the cardiomyopathy children (22 ± 2 percent (SE)) (figure 3) was
significantly depressed when compared to the normal group (32 ± 6 percent) despite
digitalis maintenance in all children with myocarditis. The ΔS index allowed good
separability of the groups.

Further, fractional shortening was relatively independent of heart rate, as shown in
figure 4. In contrast, mean velocity of circumferential fiber shortening determined
with aortic valve ejection time correlated well with heart rate in the normal group
($r = .74$) (figure 5). This result was as expected because of the known variation of
left ventricular ejection time with heart rate.

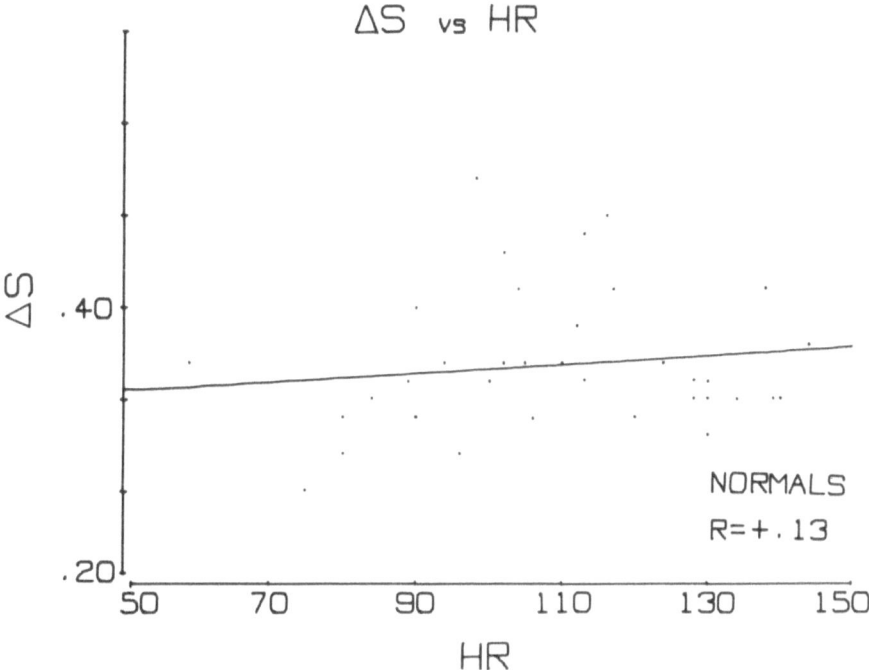

fig. 4. The relationship of ΔS here expressed as a fraction on the ordinate with heart rate shown
on the abscissa is illustrated for our normal children. The index appeared relatively independent
of heart rate.

Finally, Vcf could be regressed for heart rate using the regression formula and expressed as an actual-to-expected ratio in both groups. The mean A:E ratio in the
normal group was 1.01 ± .02 vs. 0.68 ± .05 ($p < 0.001$) in the children with cardiomyopathy (figure 6). As such, the indices derived from double-crystal M-modes
allowed the detection of children with depressed cardiac contractility.

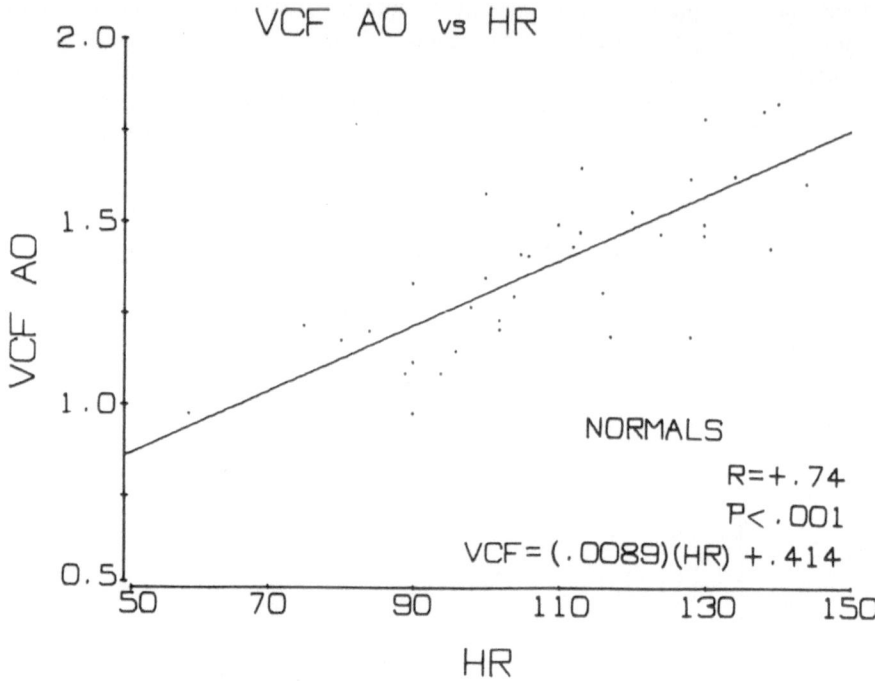

fig. 5. The mean velocity of left ventricular circumferential fiber shortening (Vcf expressed with circumferences/second) determined from simultaneous left ventricular and aortic valve dual M-mode outputs on the ordinate is related to heart rate in our normal children. The correlation coefficient and regression equation for heart rate correction are shown.

As described above, the dual M-mode approach allows determination of the iso-volumic contraction time (ICT) on a beat-to-beat basis. In normal children, ICT showed a mean of 0.052 ± .03, and it was independent of heart rate. Nevertheless, in our small group of cardiomyopathy infants and children, the isovolumic contraction time was somewhat longer but not statistically different from normal children. Another utility of this technique is that it allows the evaluation of diastolic function by calculation of the isovolumic relaxation period from aortic valve closure to the opening of the mitral valve, as shown in figure 7.

This index has reportedly been prolonged in patients with cardiac muscle disease and significantly shortened in patients with mitral stenosis 6). In our normal group, the mean as shown in figure 8 for the isovolumic relaxation period was 0.057 ±.024 and the index was relatively independent of heart rate. In figure 9, we can see an example of a patient with moderately severe mitral stenosis in whom the isovolumic relaxation period is quite short secondary to the elevation of left atrial pressure.

The dual M-mode technique also allows simultaneous comparison of left and right ventricular systolic time intervals using the pre-ejection period and ejection times

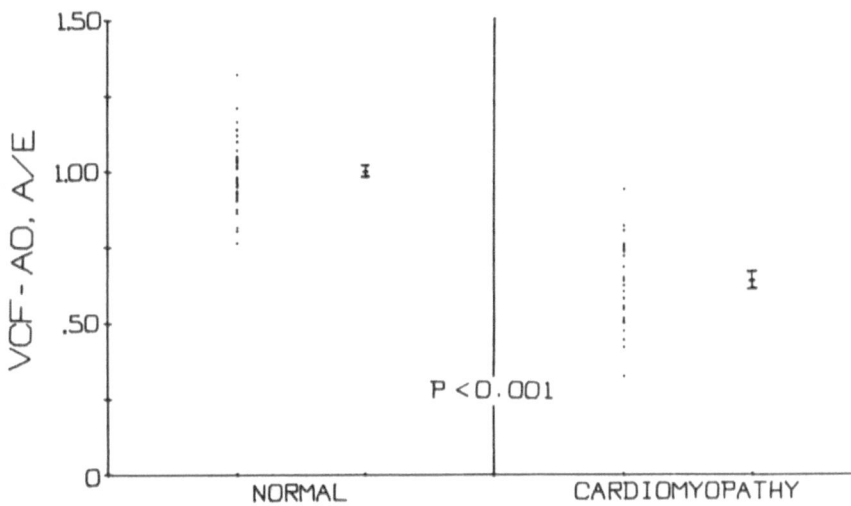

fig. 6. Aortic valve Vcf determined from simultaneous dual M-mode traces and expressed as an actual-to-expected ratio is shown. Expected values were derived after correction for heart rate from the heart rate regression formula for normal children. The cardiomyopathy group was statistically separable with a $p < 0.001$. The individual patient values are at left while the bars for group means and standard errors are shown at right in each panel.

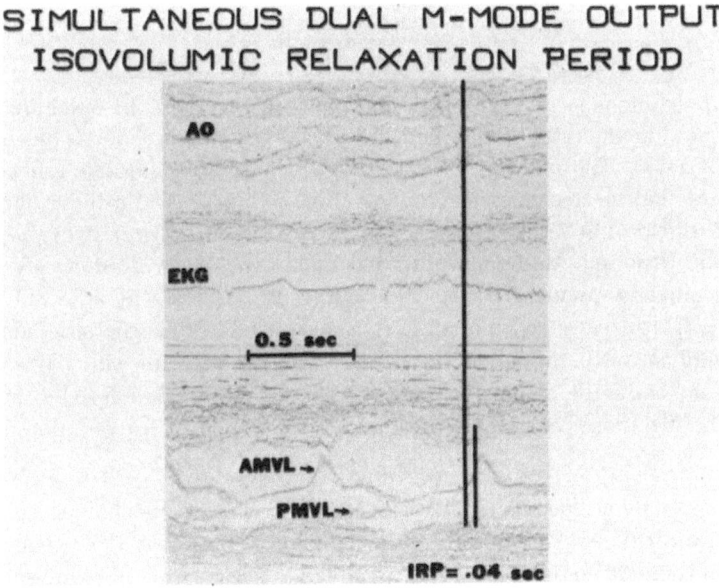

fig. 7. Simultaneous dual M-modes show the calculation of isovolumic relaxation period here .04 seconds from the closure of the aortic valve to the onset of the rapid opening motion of the mitral valve. (Abbreviations as in figure 1.).

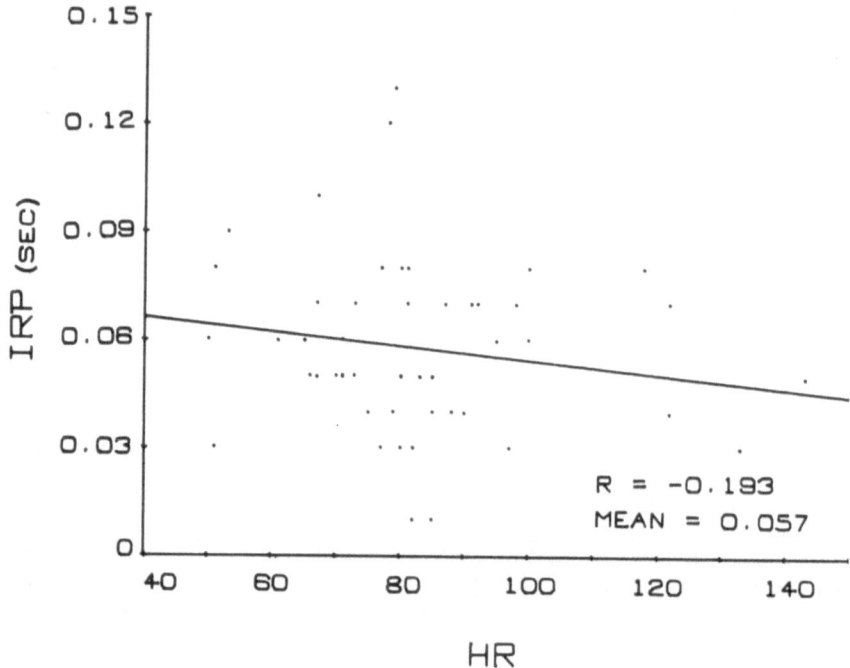

fig. 8. Isovolumic relaxation period (IRP) (ordinate) is related to heart rate (abscissa) in our normal population. The correlation was poor. The mean IRP for the normal group is shown.

calculated simultaneously from aortic and pulmonary valves. In our initial experiences, such tracings could be obtained from 60 percent of children but only 30 percent of adults. The addition to the system of a facility for separate gain controls for each of the selected lines may improve our ability to obtain these tracings in adults. Hirshfeld et al 7) have shown a direct correlation between right ventricular pre-ejection period/ejection time ratio and pulmonary artery diastolic pressure as well as pulmonary vascular resistance. In their study, patients with a RVPEP/RVET ratio > 0.32 had elevated pulmonary resistance. Obtaining aortic and pulmonary traces simultaneously should increase the sophistication with which this data is acquired and allow the parameters on both sides of the circulation to be compared without having to correct each separately for respiration or for variation in heart rate.

We have encountered specific additional instances in which this technique has proven quite useful for the evaluation of cardiac anatomy or physiology. The combined recording of tricuspid and pulmonary valves allows the calculation of right ventricular isovolumic contraction time from tricuspid closure to pulmonary valve opening (fig. 10).

Simultaneous acquisition of this data is even more crucial because of the wide res-

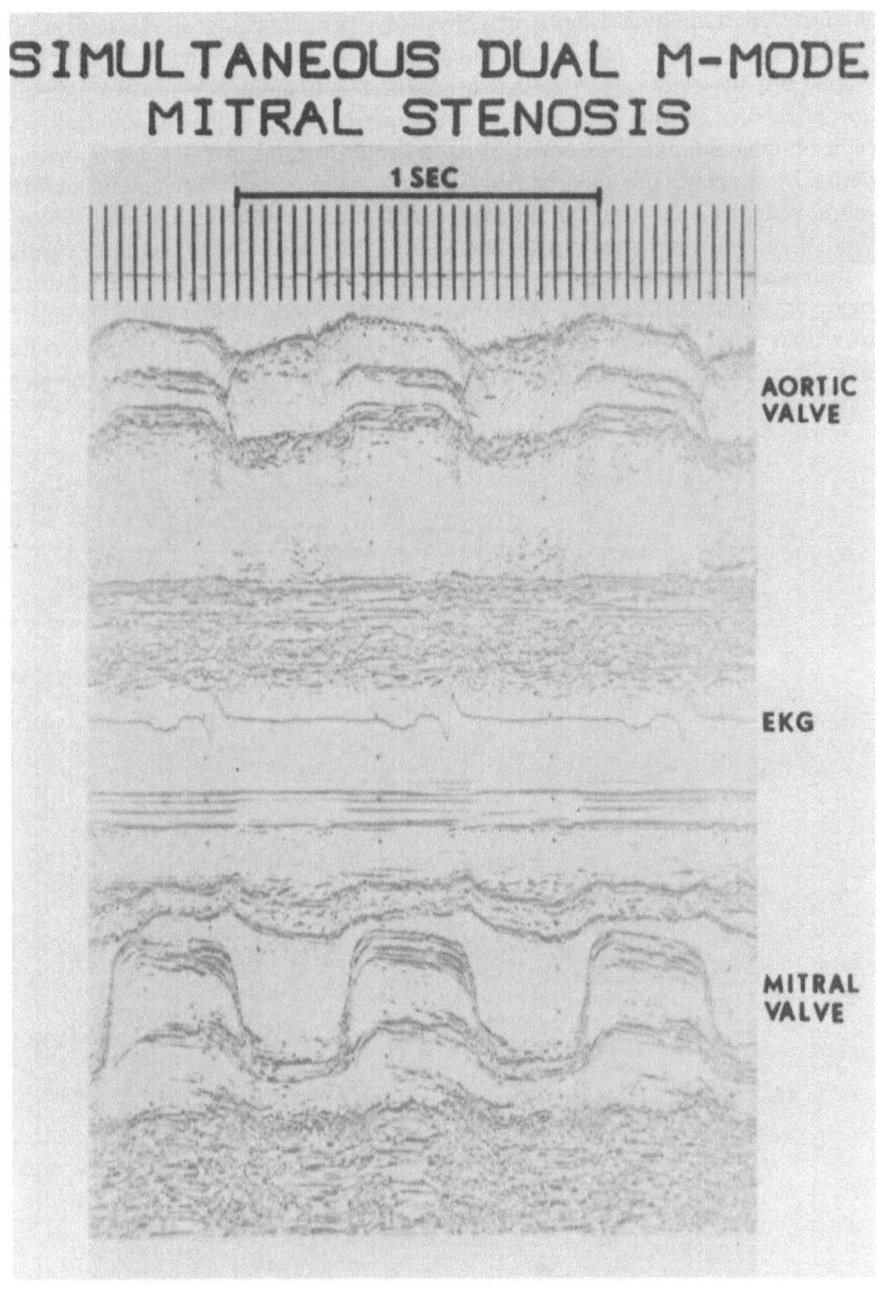

SIMULTANEOUS DUAL M-MODE
MITRAL STENOSIS

1 SEC

AORTIC
VALVE

EKG

MITRAL
VALVE

fig. 9. The simultaneous dual M-mode output derived from a patient with moderate mitral stenosis is shown. Aortic valve closure on the upper trace occurs almost simultaneous with mitral valve opening and the isovolumic relaxation period is therefore quite short.

piratory variations in right ventricular physiology. Simultaneous recording of systolic anterior motion of the mitral valve along with premature closure of the aortic valve graphically illustrates the physiology of obstruction in idiopathic hypertrophic sub-aortic stenosis. Further, we have recently applied the technique to graphically exhibit on dual M-mode the descent of a left atrial myxoma into the left ventricular cavity by watching it disappear from the left atrium while appearing behind the mitral valve. This time motion display in conjunction with the cross-sectional echo display allowed the patient to undergo open heart surgery without prior cardiac catheterization. Simultaneous visualization of left and right ventricles as well as the right ventricular outflow tract and aorta on dual M-modes during the performance of venous saline contrast techniques for the detection of the sites of intracardiac shunting in newborns has decreased the number of injections required to complete

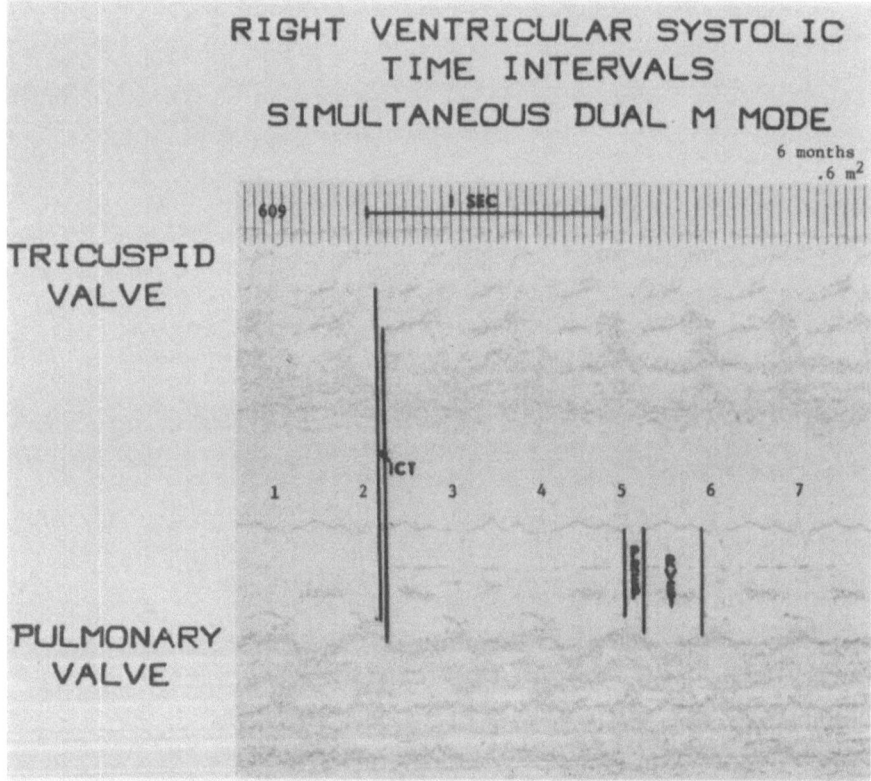

fig. 10. The derivation of right ventricular systolic time intervals is shown from simultaneous tricuspid and pulmonary valve traces in a 6-month-old infant. Right ventricular pre-ejection period (PREP) and ejection time are shown on beat 5 for the pulmonary valve trace. On beat 2, the period between tricuspid valve closure and rapid pulmonary valve opening motion is calculated as the right ventricular isovolumic contraction period (ICT), here .03 seconds.

92

these evaluations as well as allowing the comparisons of the timing of contrast arrival in the different areas of the heart on a beat-to-beat basis.

As such, we believe that the development of this new system will therefore allow a more sophisticated analysis of the right and left ventricular systolic time intervals as well as of the ejection phase parameters of cardiac contractility in systole and of the isovolumic relaxation period in diastole. The system will be useful as an adjunct to both single-crystal and cross-sectional echocardiography. With further refinements of signal to noise ratio and the possible addition to the system of a facility of a separate time gain control for the two selected elements, this system should represent a further advance in diagnostic ultrasound.

References

1) Vredevoe LA, Creekmore SP, and Schiller NB: *The measurement of systolic time intervals by echocardiography.*
   J Clin Ultrasound 2: 99, 1974.

2) Sahn DJ, Deely WJ, Hagan AD, and Friedman WF: *Echocardiographic assessment of left ventricular performance in normal newborns.*
   Circulation 49: 232, 1974.

3) Sahn DJ, Vaucher Y, Williams DE, Allen HD, Goldberg SJ, and Friedman WF: *Echocardiographic detection of large left-to-right shunts and cardiomyopathies in infants and children.*
   Am J Cardiol 38: 73, 1976.

4) Hirschfeld S, Meyer R, Schwartz DC, Korfhagen J, and Kaplan S: *Measurement of right and left ventricular systolic time intervals by echocardiography.*
   Circulation 51: 304, 1975.

5) Sahn DJ, Bom N, Allen HD, Von Egmond F, Goldberg SJ, Lancee CT, and Roelandt J: *A dual M-mode system for simultaneous time motion analyses of cardiac structures: Development and initial clinical results.*
   Proceedings of First World Federation for Ultrasound in Medicine and Biology - Abstract 114, presented WFUMB 8/5/76, San Francisco, California.

6) Kumar S, and Spodick DH: *Study of the mechanical events of the left ventricle by atraumatic techniques: Comparison of methods of measurement and their significance.*
   Am Heart J 80: 401, 1970.

7) Hirschfeld S, Meyer R, Schwartz DC, Korfhagen J, and Kaplan S: *The echocardiographic assessment of pulmonary artery pressure and pulmonary vascular resistance.*
   Circulation 52: 642, 1975.

Advantages of combined hemodynamic
and ultrasonic studies in man

by Jos Roelandt, Warren Walsh, and Paul G. Hugenholtz,
From the Division of Cardiology,
University of Oregon Health Sciences Center, Portland, Oregon and
the Thoraxcenter, Erasmus University and University Hospital,
Dijkzigt, Rotterdam.

A long sought goal in clinical cardiology has been the quantitative description of left ventricular performance in man. Until recently, this has exclusively involved the use of a combined hemodynamic-angiographic method for the derivation of a number of functional indices for both the systolic and diastolic phases of the cardiac cycle. Some of the difficulties which are encountered with the combined hemodynamic-angiographic methods are as follows:

1. Injection of 30 - 50 cc of viscous contrast media into the left ventricle (LV) containing 80 - 100 cc of blood may alter LV shape, volume and wall stress.
2. Contrast media have a direct myocardial depressant effect leading to an increase in end-diastolic and end-systolic LV volume and a fall in ejection fraction and systemic blood pressure.
3. Serial measurements require multiple angiograms with consequent increased risk to the patient and increased radiation hazard to both patient and laboratory personnel.
4. Angiographic measurements are limited to a few cycles only and these are often invalidated by the occurrence of premature ventricular contractions during the injection of contrast media.
5. LV pressure and volume/mass measurements are usually made sequentially rather than simultaneously; hence, slight alterations in cycle length, ejection time and LV pressures may alter the measurements.
6. Accurate determination of LV volume and mass data requires tedious frame by frame analysis of the LV angiogram.

Many of the limitations associated with the combined hemodynamic-angiographic method for assessment of LV performance are largely eliminated by using a combined hemodynamic-ultrasonic method (HUM), since LV minor axis dimensions and wall thickness can be readily obtained from the standard LV echocardiogram. The resolution in time of the ultrasonic technique is excellent and data is available without altering the native hemodynamics. The validity and accuracy of the ultrasonic measurements of cavity dimensions and wall thickness have been confirmed by several investigators 1)-4).

95

Echocardiology, N. Bom editor, published by Martinus Nijhoff, the Hague 1977.

If the ultrasonic technique is combined with the simultaneous use of a catheter tip manometer to obtain high fidelity left ventricular pressure, continuous recordings of LV pressure, dimension and wall thickness throughout each cardiac cycle are produced for as many beats as required. From these, LV functional indices which are dependent on the accurate simultaneous measurement of LV pressure, its diameter and wall thickness (such as LV work, compliance and wall stress) are readily computed and their instantaneous changes can be plotted for systole or diastole during many cardiac cycles. The method permits frequent observations to be per-

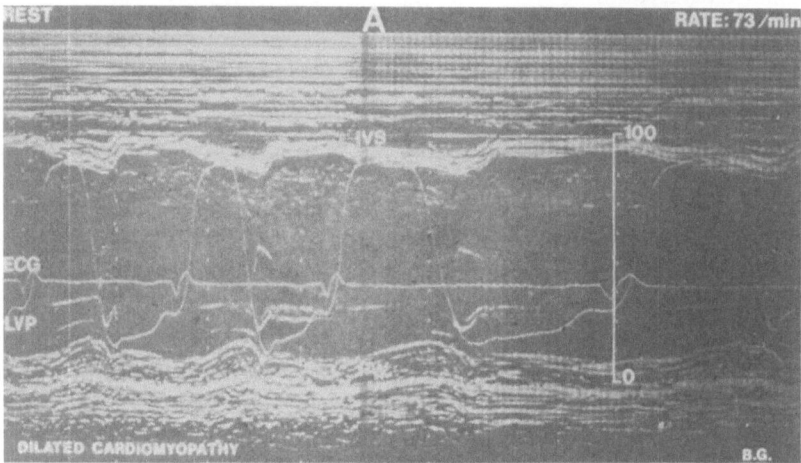

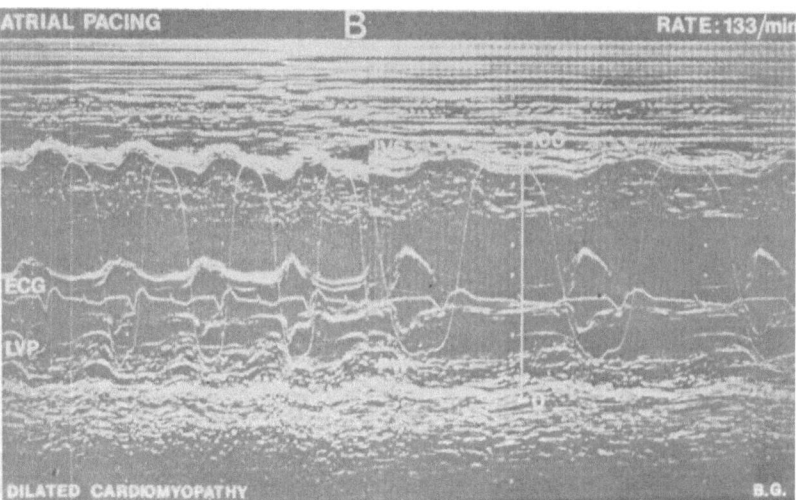

fig. 1. Left ventricular standard echogram recorded simultaneously with left ventricular pressure (LVP) from a patient with dilated cardiomyopathy at rest (panel A) and during atrial pacing (panel B). The right part of the tracing is recorded at a paper speed of 100 mm/sec. IVS: interventricular septum, PW: left ventricular posterior wall.

formed in a single patient, which is of particular value during acute intervention studies as with drugs or atrial pacing stress tests. Examples of simultaneous recordings of the LV pressure and the echocardiogram from a patient with a dilated cardiomyopathy at rest and during atrial pacing are shown in figures 1 A and B.

Left ventricular pressure-dimension loops

The advantages of HUM in producing pressure-dimension loops of the cardiac cycle have been pointed out by Gibson and Brown 5) and McLaurin et al 6). These authors were able to show characteristic changes in pressure-dimension relations in patients with stenotic or regurgitant valvular lesions similar to the previously published pressure-volume loops described by investigators using the more complicated angiographic method 7), 8). In addition, by integrating the area enclosed by the loop, left ventricular stroke work can be calculated. Superimposed pressure-dimension loops at rest (heart rate 73 beats/min) and during atrial pacing at 133 beats/min of the patient whose recordings are shown in fig. 1 are presented in fig. 2.

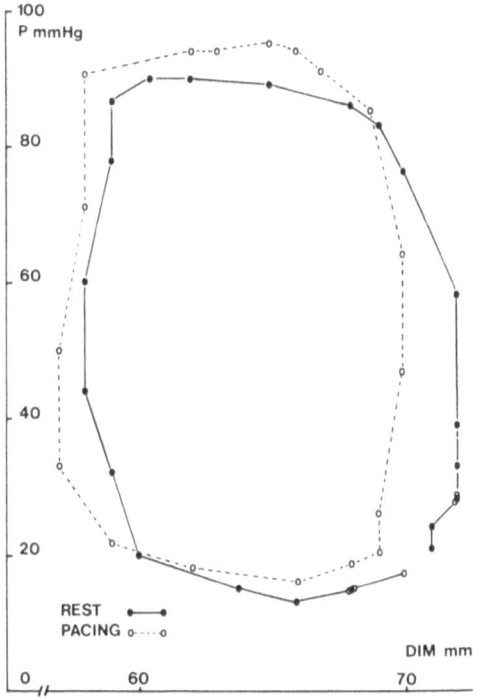

fig. 2. Superimposed pressure (P in mmHg) - dimension (DIM in mm) loops at rest and during atrial pacing of the patient whose left ventricular echocardiographic and pressure recordings are shown in fig. 1. The surface area enclosed by the pressure-dimension loops represents the left ventricular stroke work and is not different for rest and pacing stress. Dots represent intervals of 25 msec.

Although pressure-dimension and pressure-volume loops are usually comparable in the absence of ventricular dyskinesia, it must be remembered that HUM represents the behaviour of only a small region of the LV cavity and is therefore, potentially affected by shape changes occurring during isovolumic contraction and/or relaxation. Gibson and Brown 5) have shown that in patients with valvular heart disease, deformation of pressure-dimension loops may result from incoordinate contraction in the isovolumic periods attributable to left ventricular dysfunction. This situation could lead to a discrepancy between pressure-dimension and pressure-volume loops.

Left ventricular compliance and stiffness
With the development of HUM, interest has again been focussed on the diastolic pressure-dimension relations, with the aim of obtaining a better understanding of LV chamber compliance (dV/dP) or stiffness (dp/dv) in man. Previous studies of diastolic performance have been limited, mainly because of technical difficulties associated with the angiographic analysis. Grossman et al 9)-12) initiated the use of HUM to assess diastolic LV chamber properties in patients with valvular heart disease. These authors proposed as the index of LV chamber stiffness the ratio between the increment of LV pressure to the increment of LV dimension associated with atrial contraction, normalized to the average LV pressure during the interval of measurement. They showed that the highest values for late diastolic stiffness were associated with pressure overloaded ventricles and/or electrocardiographic or echocardiographic evidence of left ventricular hypertrophy. In contrast, patients with mitral stenosis had the lowest, while those with mitral and aortic regurgitation had intermediate values for late diastolic stiffness. Thus, by confirming and extending the findings obtained with the earlier but tedious and complex angiographic methods, Grossman et al demonstrated the validity of HUM for the study of chamber stiffness or complicance in man.

The effects on LV compliance of altering the loading state, of administering various inotropic drugs or of inducing myocardial ischemia have been studied in animals and man using a variety of techniques but the results have been conflicting, mainly due to technical difficulties mentioned earlier. HUM is particularly appropriate for the investigation and the answering of these questions because of the ease of performing serial quantitative studies. The effect of increasing heart rate by atrial pacing from 73 to 133 beats/min on LV diastolic pressure-volume relations of the patient whose recordings are shown in fig. 1 is presented in fig. 3.

McCarns and Parker 13) have examined diastolic pressure-dimension relations during pacing induced myocardial ischemia in man. They demonstrated an increase in LV end-diastolic dimensions but no significant change in late diastolic compliance in their patients. Although most studies of diastolic properties using this new technique have been limited to patients in whom LV wall motion abnormalities are unlikely, it is conceivable that it may be equally applicable to patients with wall motion abnormalities since these are largely systolic events with little effect on late diastolic geometry.

98

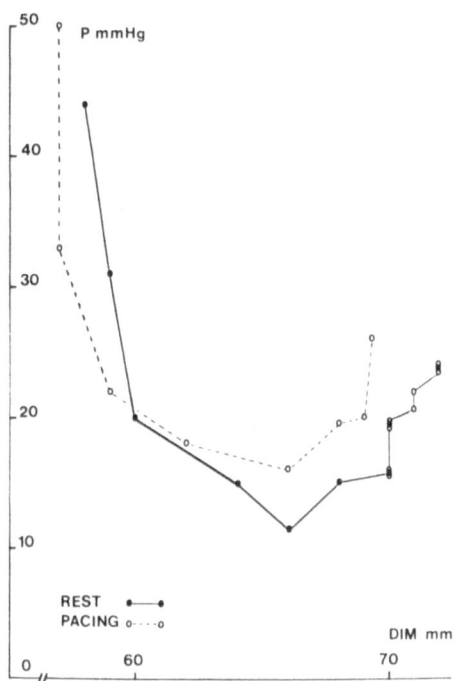

fig. 3. Diastolic left ventricular pressure (P in mmHg) - dimension (DIM in mm) curves at rest and during atrial pacing of the patient whose recordings are shown in fig. 1. Dots represent intervals of 25 msec.

Left ventricular wall stress

HUM provides a much simpler method for the estimation of LV myocardial wall stress, a major determinant of myocardial oxygen consumption and hypertrophy. From simultaneous and continuous measurements of LV minor axis diameter, wall thickness and pressure, the instantaneous meridional and circumferential wall stresses in the LV equatorial plane can be readily computed 14)-17).

Fig. 4 shows the time course of LV meridional wall stress at rest and during atrial pacing of the patient whose recordings are shown in fig. 1. Calculation of circumferential wall stress requires knowledge of the LV long axis diameter 14). This variable can be estimated assuming the LV to be a prolate ellipsoidal model with a 2:1 long to minor axis ratio 16) or it can be calculated from known regression equations 17).

The validity of HUM for the measurement of meridional and circumferential wall stress has been verified by comparison with the standard angiographic method.
Brodie et al 14) compared measurements for meridional wall stress in 9 patients by the two techniques. They found an excellent agreement for calculated meridional

99

stress values throughout the cardiac cycle with correlation coefficients ranging from .91 to .99. Ratshin et al 16) looked at the correlation between the two techniques for the measurement of circumferential wall stress. They measured stress at end-diastole and end-isovolumic systole in 48 patients and obtained correlation coefficients of 0.98 and 0.86 respectively. There are several studies which suggest meridional rather than circumferential wall stress is a more sensitive indicator of myocardial function 15), 17).

Grossman et al 15) used HUM to determine meridional wall stress in patients with volume and pressure overloaded ventricles. They found that in patients with volume overloaded ventricles peak systolic wall stress was not significantly different from control but that end-diastolic stress was consistently higher. Patients with pressure overloaded ventricles however, had values for peak systolic and end-diastolic stresses which were within the normal range. These findings suggest that LV hypertrophy develops to normalize systolic but not diastolic wall stress.

Gibson and Brown 18) have pointed out that in order to measure compliance or stiffness of the ventricular muscle, rather than of the whole LV chamber as previously described, it is necessary to measure stress and strain within the ventricular wall. They defined myocardial stiffness as the slope of the calculated stress-strain curve and obtained instantaneous values for LV circumferential stress and strain (LV minor axis circumference) throughout the cardiac cycle using a digitizing technique. Since this method of assessing myocardial stiffness is partly dependent on wall thickness, they were able to show differences between diastolic stress-strain

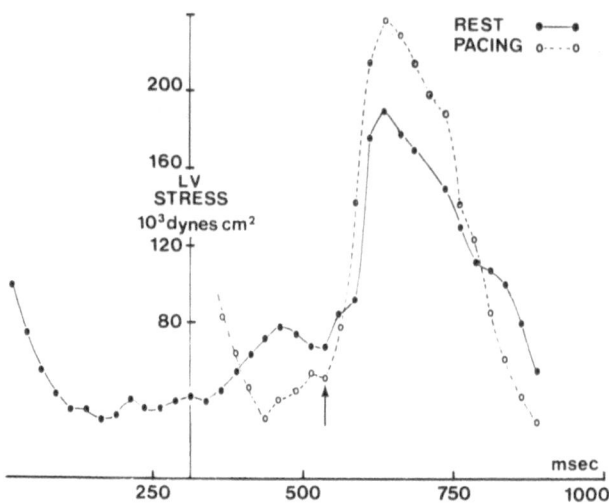

fig. 4. Time course of left ventricular meridional wall stress throughout the cardiac cycles at rest and during atrial pacing from the patient whose recordings are shown in fig. 1. The arrow indicates end-diastole.

curves and pressure-dimension curves, although the slope of both curves did show an increase in wall and chamber stiffness in late diastole, especially in patients with evidence of LV hypertrophy.

Left ventricular force-velocity relationships
An additional application of wall stress determinations with HUM is the relative ease with which force-velocity can be examined in man. Quinones et al 19) have used this technique to study the time course of LV circumferential wall stress and the velocity of LV dimensional shortening (V$_{CF}$) allowing instantaneous force-velocity relationships to be obtained. A stress-V$_{CF}$ plot of the patient whose recordings are shown in fig. 1 is presented in fig. 5.

Quinones et al 19) found that measurement of V$_{CF}$ at peak wall stress was able to separate patients with normal from those with abnormal ventricles. Although these findings confirmed data already available from angiographic studies, the major advantage of HUM is the ability to study the effects of interventions on the force-velocity relation in man on a beat to beat basis. Quinones et al 19) also evaluated the effect of increasing afterload in 7 patients by infusing angiotensin on the force-velocity curve and showed that patients with myocardial disease had much flatter curves than normals. However, force-velocity relations in man using this technique have only just begun to be explored and much further work needs to be done to assess the potential clinical value of measuring those parameters for defining LV performance.

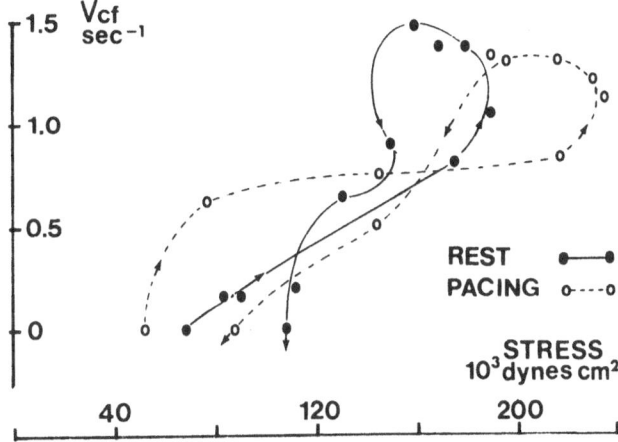

fig. 5. Plot of left ventricular meridional wall stress versus velocity of dimensional shortening (V$_{CF}$) at rest and during atrial pacing from the patient whose recordings are shown in fig. 1. Dots represent intervals of 25 msec. Note that V$_{CF}$ at peak stress during pacing is not significantly different from the resting value.

101

Conclusion

It is concluded that the combined use of LV hemodynamic and ultrasonic data provides a relatively simple method to perform serial studies of ventricular function in man, especially for the assessment of pressure-dimension relations, changes in compliance, wall stress and force-velocity relationships during physiological events and pharmacological or other interventions. Clearly, a computer-aided analysis greatly facilitates extraction of these data.

Acknowledgement
We are most grateful to Lawrence Lima for technical assistance and Shanna Erickson for her secretarial help.

References

1) Gibson DG: *Estimation of left ventricular size by echocardiography.*
   British Heart J 35: 128-134, 1973.

2) Roelandt J: *Practical Echocardiology.*
   Forest Grove, Research Studies Press, 1977 (chapter 8).

3) Sjogren AL, Hytonen I, and Frick MH: *Ultrasonic measurements of left ventricular wall thickness.*
   Chest 57: 37-40, 1970.

4) Troy BL, Pombo J, and Rackley: *Measurement of left ventricular wall thickness and mass by echocardiography.*
   Circulation 45: 602-611, 1972.

5) Gibson DG, and Grown DJ: *Assessment of left ventricular systolic function in man from simultaneous echocardiographic and pressure measurements.*
   British Heart J 38: 8-17, 1976.

6) McLaurin LP, Grossman W, Stefadouros MA, Rolett EL and Young DT: *A new technique for the study of left ventricular pressure-volume relations in man.*
Circulation 48: 56-64, 1973.

7) Bunnell JL, Grant C, and Green DG: *Left ventricular function derived from the pressure-volume diagram.*
Am J Med 39: 881-894, 1965.

8) Dodge HT, and Banley WA: *Left ventricular volume and mass and their significance in heart disease.*
Amer J Cardiol 23: 528-537, 1969.

9) Grossman W, Stefadouros MA, McLaurin LP, Rolett EL, and Young DT: *The quantitative assessment of left ventricular stiffness in man.*
Circulation 45: 567-573, 1973.

10) Grossman W, McLaurin LP, Moos SP, Stefadouros M, and Young DT: *Wall thickness and diastolic properties of the left ventricle.*
Circulation 49: 129-135, 1974.

11) Grossman, McLaurin LP, and Stefadouros MA: *Ventricular stiffness associated with chronic pressure and volume overloads in man.*
Circ Res 35: 793-799, 1974.

12) Grossman W, and McLaurin LP: *Diastolic properties of the left ventricle.*
Ann Int Med 84: 316-326, 1976.

13) McCans JL, and Parker JO: *Left ventricular pressure-volume relationships during myocardial ischemia in man.*
Circulation 48: 775-785, 1973.

14) Brodie BR, McLaurin LP, and Grossman W: *Combined hemodynamic-ultrasound method for studying left ventricular wall stress.*
Am J Cardiol 37: 864-870, 1976.

15) Grossman W, Jones D, and McLaurin LP: *Wall stress and pattern of hypertrophy in the human left ventricle.*
J Clin Invest 56: 56-64, 1975.

16) Ratshin RA, Rackley CE, and Russell RO: *Determination of left ventricular preload and afterload by quantitative echocardiography in man.*
Circ Res 34: 711-718, 1974.

17) Gould KL, Lipscomb K, Hamilton GW, and Kennedy JW: *Relation of left ventricular shape, function and wall stress.*
Amer J Cardiol 34: 627-634, 1974.

18) Gibson DC, and Brown DJ: *Relation between diastolic left ventricular wall stress and strain in man.*
Br Heart J 36: 1066-1077, 1974.

19) Quinones MA, Gaasch WH, Cole JS, and Alexander JK: *Echocardiographic determination of left ventricular stress-velocity relations in man.*
Circulation 57: 689-700, 1975.

Detection of incoordinate left ventricular contraction by echocardiography.

D.G. Gibson, Brompton Hospital, London.

The uses of echocardiography in measuring left ventricular cavity size and rates of wall movement are now well documented. In order to extrapolate these results to the left ventricular cavity as a whole, it is necessary to assume that contraction and relaxation are uniform. This need not be evident from an echocardiogram of the left ventricular cavity considered in isolation. Ways of detecting incoordinate contraction by M-mode echocardiography are discussed.

The first use of echocardiography in studying left ventricular function was to measure the cavity size 1), 2), and there is a considerable body of evidence to suggest that reliable estimates of a minor diameter can be made using the method. More recently, a second index of left ventricular function, the rate of change of dimension has been studied and taken to indicate the myocardial fibre shortening rate 3), 4). Measurements can be made in absolute terms expressed in cm/sec, or normalized to refer to unit length of dimension, when they are often referred to as Vcf or velocity of circumferential fibre shortening. Mean or peak values of shortening rate have been estimated and shown to correlate with corresponding values from angiograms in the same patients 5).

It is a limitation of standard M-mode echocardiography, however, that only a small part of the left ventricular cavity can be studied, so that if attempts are made to extrapolate values obtained by this method to the cavity as a whole, serious errors may result if incoordinate left ventricular function is present. It has been widely assumed, therefore, that M-mode methods are of little value in assessing contraction or relaxation patterns unless overall function is known to be uniform, an assurance that may be difficult to supply under many clinical conditions. It is the purpose of this chapter to describe methods whereby the scope of M-mode echocardiography can be extended to detect incoordinate left ventricular function. It also seems possible that these methods may give information about some of the disturbances that can interfere with the highly organized process constituting normal contraction and relaxation.

Echocardiology, N. Bom editor, published by Martinus Nijhoff, the Hague 1977.

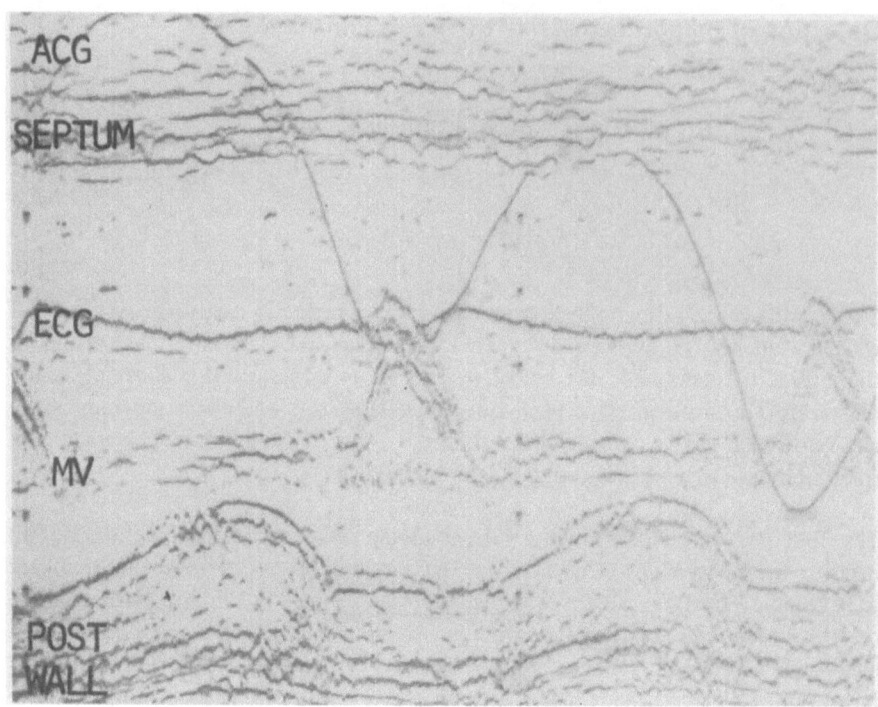

fig. 1. Echocardiogram from a patient who developed a low output state post-operatively. Outward wall movement is almost complete before the start of mitral valve opening.

One possible approach is illustrated in figure 1, which shows simultaneous echoes from the septum, posterior wall and mitral valve of a patient who developed a low output state after open heart surgery.

At first sight, left ventricular function appears good, with a satisfactory amplitude of posterior wall movement, the small degree of reversed septal movement being common after cardiopulmonary bypass. However, on closer inspection, it is apparent that, during diastole, almost all posterior wall movement occurs before the start of mitral valve opening and thus before the start of ventricular filling, so that the apparently normal increase in diastolic left ventricular dimension represents no more than a change in cavity shape during the period of isovolumic relaxation.

Observations such as this, suggested that it might be fruitful to study the relation between mitral valve and left ventricular dimension in normal subjects. Although some information can be gained by direct inspection of the original echocardiograms, the technique can be made more sensitive by digitizing the various echoes using a simple computing technique 6).

The results from a normal subject are shown in figure 2.

The lowest panel represents the original digitized echoes, and the trace above shows the left ventricular dimension, representing the distance between septum and posterior wall. It will be seen that the onset of mitral valve opening corresponds with the start of the dimension increase. However, comparison between the two is made much more sensitive if the relation between the rates of change of dimension and mitral valve position are studied rather than the original echoes themselves. These two rates of change are shown in the top two traces, and it is immediately clear how intimate is the relation between the two.

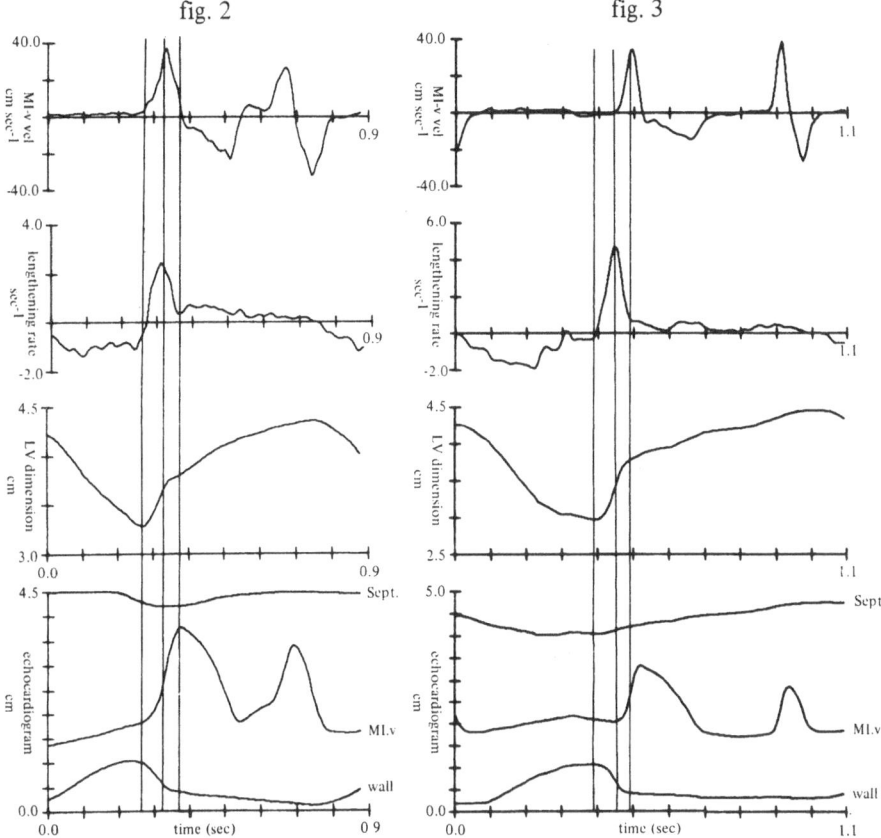

fig. 2. Computer output of digitized mitral valve and left ventricular cavity echoes, showing from below, direct printout of echoes, left ventricular dimension, rate of change of dimension, normalised rate of change of dimension and (top) instantaneous mitral leaflet velocity. Vertical lines demonstrate:
1. Onset of outward wall movement.
2. Peak rate of wall movement.
3. Discontinuity in wall movement at the end of rapid filling.
There is close correlation with the corresponding events of anterior leaflet movement.

fig. 3. Computer output of digitized mitral valve and left ventricular cavity echoes from a patient with ischaemic heart disease and an abnormal left ventriculogram. Layout as for fig. 2.

The onset of left ventricular dimension and mitral valve movements are synchronous: the peak rate of change of dimension occurs at the same time as the peak rate of mitral valve opening, and finally, both traces show a discontinuity at the same time representing the end of the rapid phase of ventricular filling. This picture is seen in all normal subjects and also in patients with ischaemic heart disease and normal left ventricular angiograms. When segmental abnormalities of contraction are present (figure 3), however, a characteristic disturbance is present with the onset of outward wall movement preceding the start of mitral valve opening 7).

This amounts to a mean of 60 msec, when septal movement is normal on the echocardiogram, and to over 100 msec when septal movement is reversed. It is not simply due to impaired left ventricular function, since the normal relation between dimension and mitral valve movement occurs when the cavity is dilated with uniform impairment of contraction. This delay in mitral valve opening, therefore, seems to be the results of segmental abnormalities of contraction. In more general terms, it has been possible to detect non-uniform left ventricular function because the left ventricular dimension has not been studied in isolation, but has been correlated with an index of general function, represented here by the start of filling.

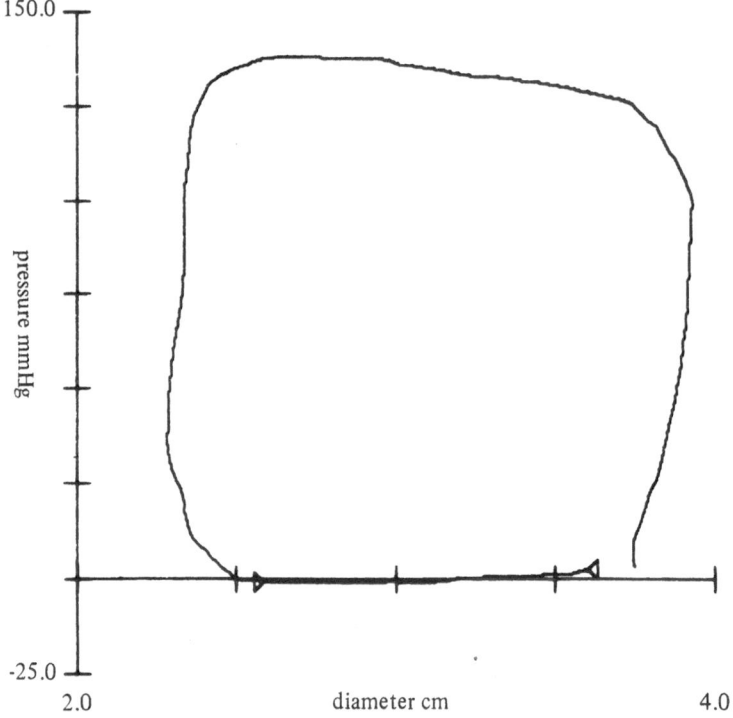

fig. 4. Pressure-Dimension loop from a patient with normal left ventricular function.

Clearly, if left ventricular behaviour is uniform, local and overall function will be in phase with one another, but this close time relation may be lost when non-uniformities are present.

These considerations suggest that the start of left ventricular filling may not be the best index of overall function to choose as a reference for the tracing of local behaviour, since it is applicable for only a short period in the cardiac cycle. In spite of this, however, it is surprisingly informative. An obvious alternative is to use the high fidelity left ventricular pressure trace and to plot the relation between pressure and dimension in the form of a pressure-dimension loop, as suggested by Rushmer 8).

In normal subjects, the shape of the loop is characteristic and approximates to a rectangle (figure 4). Four phases can be recorgnized: isovolumic contraction, when pressure rises at constant dimension, ejection, when the dimension decreases at approximately constant pressure, isovolumic relaxation, when pressure falls, again at constant dimension, and finally filling 9). This rectangular configuration has functional significance in that the area of the loop represents the stroke work per unit area of endocardium performed by that region of myocardium studied with the echo beam: the maximum work that could have been done on the circulation by the myocardium working over the same range of pressure and dimension is given by the product of the two, i.e. by the area of the rectangle that just encloses the loop. A rectangular loop thus represents the condition of efficient energy transfer from the myocardium to the circulation and distortion of the loop represents loss of mechanical efficiency of this process.

Unfortunately, measurement of left ventricular pressure directly requires cardiac catheterisation, but the timing of the upstroke and downstroke of the pressure pulse can be derived, with minor delay, from the corresponding regions of the apexcardiogram 10), (Venco, Gibson and Brown, unpublished, 1976). This is fortunate, since in clinical left ventricular disease, abnormalities of the loop appear to occur most frequently during the periods of isovolumic contraction and early relaxation.

We have therefore examined the use of simultaneous apex and echocardiogram to detect incoordinate contraction. As with pressure, the results are presented in the form of an echo dimension-apexcardiogram loop, which has proved to be rectangular in more than 50 normal subjects. Mitral regurgitation is associated with inward movement of the dimension during the upstroke of the apexcardiogram. When left ventricular function was normal, these effects were small in spite of regurgitation. (figure 5). Aortic regurgitation is associated with an increase in dimension in the early relaxation phase.

The configuration of the loop has been abnormal in approximately 90 percent of patients with ischaemic heart disease and typical examples are shown in figures 6 and 7. Inward or outward movement during the upstroke, in the absence of valvular regurgitation, represents abnormalities of isovolumic contraction, while corresponding abnormalities during the downstroke represent disturbances of early relaxation.

The latter are closely related in individual patients to outward wall movement before mitral valve opening described above. This type of display has also been of value in detecting incoordinate contraction in the presence of valvular heart disease, which may be related, for example, to coronary embolism. It is also useful in following up patients after saphenous bypass grafting, when successful surgery may be associated with a return of the configuration of the loop towards normal (Traill T, unpublished). In addition, the technique is of value is assessing post-operative left ventricular function.

Using methods of angiographic analysis described elsewhere 11) therefore, exactly similar disturbances to those detected by echocardiography can be documented, although naturally their spatial distribution can be described in greater detail.

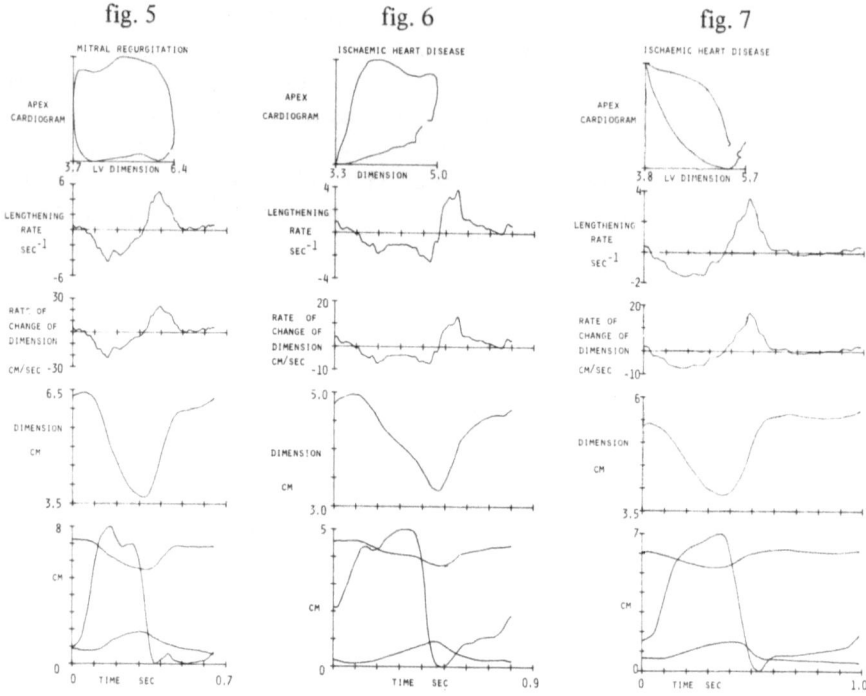

fig. 5. Computer output of digitized echo and apex cardiogram from a subject showing, from below, echoes from septum, posterior wall and apex; above are changes in dimension (D), rate of change of dimension (1/D.dD/dt), and the echo dimension-apex cardiogram loop, which is approximately rectangular.

fig. 6. Echo and apex cardiogram from a patient with ischaemic heart disease and an interior aneurysm. There is significant outward movement during the upstroke of the apexcardiogram, and inward movement during the downstroke.

fig. 7. Echo and apexcardiogram from a patient with ischaemic heart disease. There is abnormal inward movement during the upstroke and outward wall movement during the downstroke of the apexcardiogram.

110

Nevertheless, both methods allow asynchronous onset of contraction, abnormal shape changes during isovolumic relaxation and disturbed filling patterns to be detected and quantified.

M-mode echocardiography can thus be used to give a very full account of the pattern of left ventricular contraction. The size of the cavity along one of its minor axes can be accurately measured, and peak rates of wall movement estimated. In addition, incoordinate contraction, relaxation and filling can be detected. These aspects of left ventricular function are all separate from one another, and studies such as these suggest that left ventricular disease in clinical practice is not a homogeneous process, but that a number of separate disturbances exist which can be present to different degrees in individual patients. Use of the methods described here allows these to be detected and an analysis made of the extent to which one or more are present to account for impairment of overall left ventricular performance.

References

1) Fortuin NJ, Sherman ME, Hood WP Jr., and Craige E: *Evaluation of left ventricular function by echocardiography.*
   Circulation 42 Suppl 3: 120, 1970.

2) Feigenbaum H, Popp RL, Wolfe SB, Troy BL, Pombo JF, Haine CL, and Dodge HT: *Ultrasound measurements of the left ventricle: a correlative study with angiography.*
   Archives of the Internal Medicine 129: 641, 1972.

3) Paraskos JA, Grossman W, Soltz S, Dalen JE, and Dexter L: *A Non-invasive technique for the determination of the velocity of circumferential fibre shortening in man.*
   Circulation Research 29: 610, 1971.

4) Cooper R, Karliner JS, O'Rourke RA, Peterson KL, and Leopold G: *Ultrasound determination of mean fibre-shortening rate in man.*
   Amer. J. Cardiology 29: 257, 1972.

5) Gibson DG, and Brown DJ: *Measurement of peak rates of left ventricular wall movement in man.*
   British Heart Journal 37: 677, 1975.

6) Upton MT, Gibson DG, and Brown DJ: *Instantaneous mitral valve leaflet velocity and its relation to left ventricular wall movement in normal subjects.*
   British Heart Journal 38: 51, 1976.

7) Upton MT, Gibson DG, and Brown DJ: *Echocardiographic Assessment of abnormal left ventricular relaxation in man.*
   British Heart Journal 38: 1001, 1976.

8) Rushmer RF: *Pressure-circumference relations of the left ventricle.*
   Amer. J. Physiology 186: 115, 1956.

9) Gibson DG, and Brown DJ: *Assessment of left ventricular systolic function in man from simultaneous echocardiographic and pressure measurements.*
British Heart Journal 38: 8, 1976.

10) Manolas J, Ruitshauser W, Wirz P, and Arbenz U: *Time relation between apexcardiogram and left ventricular events using simultaneous high-fidelity tracings in man.*
British Heart Journal 37: 1263, 1976.

11) Gibson DG, Prewitt TA, and Brown DJ: *Analysis of left ventricular wall movement during isovolumic relaxation and its relation to coronary artery disease.*
British Heart Journal 38: 1010, 1976.

Cardiac anatomy in congenital heart disease

by Anton E. Becker, Michael J. Tynan and Robert H. Anderson.
From the Department of Pathology, Wilhelmina Gasthuis, Amsterdam,
The Netherlands, the Department of Paediatrics, Guy's Hospital,
Medical School, London and the Department of Paediatrics,
Cardiothoracic Institute, Bromptom Hospital, London, England.

It is common practice to classify congenitally malformed hearts according to pre-
fixed entities. Over the past decade, however, a more systematic approach has led
to a better understanding of these malformations and as a consequence it has been
demonstrated that transitional forms occur between congenital malformations
which were previously considered to be separate entities. At the same time the need
for precise description and classification has become urgent because increasing surgical expertise has made possible the correction of complex cardiac malformations.
The problem with existing classifications of congenital heart disease is their lack of
sufficient flexibility to accurately describe the whole spectrum of complex malformations. Dissatisfaction with these classifications has recently culminated in a pro-
posal for a descriptive nomenclature, using a segmental approach as its framework
1). The principles involved are as follows: firstly, the basic route of circulation
through the heart is described by defining the *connections* of the cardiac segments;
secondly, the *relations* of the segments one to another are described when they are
abnormal; thirdly, other malformations, e.g. septal defects or stenoses, are catalogued; and finally, any morphological interpretation can be added, if so desired.

Segmental approaches to congenital heart disease have already proved their clinical
value 2-4). The nomenclature and classification proposed here is, we believe, the
natural development of these approaches. It is, in our opinion, an improvement
because it is purely descriptive, thereby making the nomenclature independent of
morphogenetic controversy, and because it is extremely flexible.

Segmental Approach

The scope of this paper does not allow us to describe the whole classification in
detail. However, a brief description of its application is unavoidable. As an illustration, the normal heart can be classified as follows (fig. 1A). As a first step the
atrial situs is established, the normal situation being termed situs solitus. The next
step is to describe the connection of the atria to the ventricles. In the case of the
normal heart, the right atrium connects to the morphologically right ventricle and
the left atrium to the morphologically left ventricle. This connection is termed
"concordant". Both atrioventricular valves are perforate in the normal heart, so the

113

Echocardiology, N. Bom editor, published by Martinus Nijhoff, the Hague 1977.

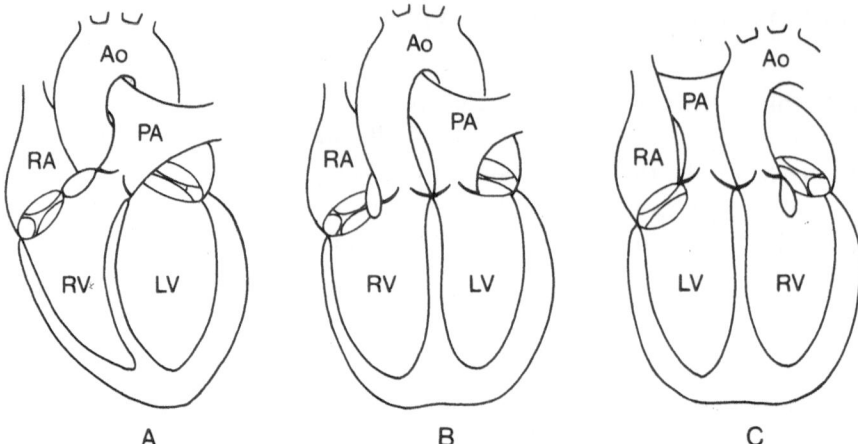

fig. 1. Diagrams of hearts to illustrate the basic principle of the segmental approach by defining the connections between the cardiac segments. Fig. 1A normal heart with the atria in a situs solitus position, i.e. the right atrium is to the right and the left atrium to the left. The atrioventricular connections are concordant, since the right atrium connects to the right ventricle and the left atrium to the left ventricle. The ventriculo-arterial connections are also concordant since the right ventricle connects to the pulmonary artery and the left ventricle connects to the aorta. Fig. 1B shows a diagram of complete transposition of the great arteries. This heart can accurately be described as "situs solitus atria, concordant atrioventricular connections and *dis*cordant (because the aorta arises from the morphologic right ventricle) ventriculo-arterial connections". Fig. 1C shows a diagram of a heart with corrected transposition of the great artery, described as situs solitus atria, *dis*cordant (because the right atrium connects to the morphologic left ventricle) atrioventricular connections, *dis*cordant ventriculo-arterial connections".

classification reads "solitus atria, atrio-ventricular concordance with two perforate atrioventricular valves". Finally, the connection of the ventricles to the great arteries is established. In case of the normal, the connection is described as "concordant", since the morphologically right ventricle connects to the pulmonary trunk and the morphologically left ventricle to the aorta.

In summary, therefore, the normal heart can be accurately described as "situs solitus atria, concordant atrio-ventricular connections with two perforate atrioventricular valves and concordant ventriculo-arterial connections". For the normal heart this seems cumbrous, but for complicated malformations the method will enable an accurate description, which anyone involved in congenital heart disease can understand. As an example, the descriptive analysis of a malformation such as complete transposition of the great arteries would read: "situs solitus atria, concordant atrio-ventricular connections with two perforate atrioventricular valves and *dis*cordant ventriculo-arterial connections (because the aorta arises from the morphologic right ventricle) and the pulmonary trunk from the morphologic left ventricle (fig. 1B). In contrast, in corrected transposition the description would read:

114

"situs solitus atria, *dis*cordant atrio-ventricular connections (because the right atrium connects to the morphologic left ventricle) and *dis*cordant ventriculo-arterial connections (fig. 1C).

For the complete characterization of these malformations, abnormal relationships are then described in full, since with complete or corrected transposition the aorta can be anterior, posterior, right or left in relation to the pulmonary valve. Additional malformations are then catalogued. In the latter condition, for instance, it could be added: "aorta anteriorly and to the left with ventricular septal defect and subpulmonic stenosis".

Segmental Anatomy of Relevance to the Echocardiographer

Plain echocardiography has its limitations for the diagnosis of congenital heart disease because it cannot in all cases identify the morphology of the structures which are detected. This is particularly true with complex congenital malformations of the heart. The absolute determination of the morphology will usually depend upon other procedures, such as angiography.

The real strength of echocardiography is that it does identify atrioventricular valves, semilunar valves and the ventricular septum and from this information, in many circumstances permits establishment of the connections present.

Connections

Atrioventricular connections
At atrioventricular level the connections may be categorized as (1) concordant (2) discordant (3) double inlet and (4) absent atrioventricular connection (fig. 2). With

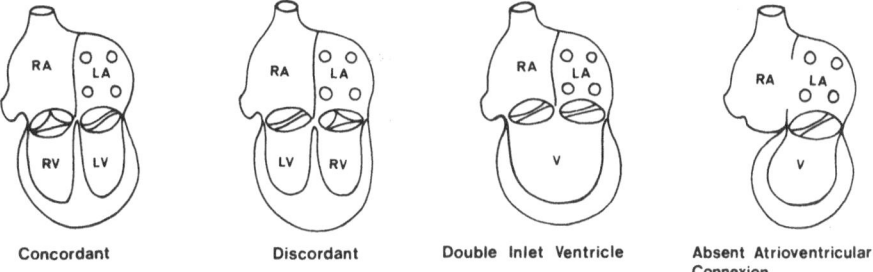

Concordant   Discordant   Double Inlet Ventricle   Absent Atrioventricular Connexion

fig. 2. Diagrams to illustrate atrioventricular connections.

atrioventricular concordance and discordance it is necessary that two atria and two ventricles are present. In atrioventricular concordance the right atrium connects with the right ventricle through a tricuspid valve (fig. 3A). The valve is characterized by a large anterior leaflet, permitted free excursion by its attachment to the anterior papillary muscle, and septal and posterior leaflets more tightly tethered to the ventricular septum and posterior wall (fig. 3C). The left atrium in atrioventricular concordance drains through a mitral valve to the left ventricle (fig. 3B). The valve is characterized by presence of discrete anterior and posterior leaflets, each capable

115

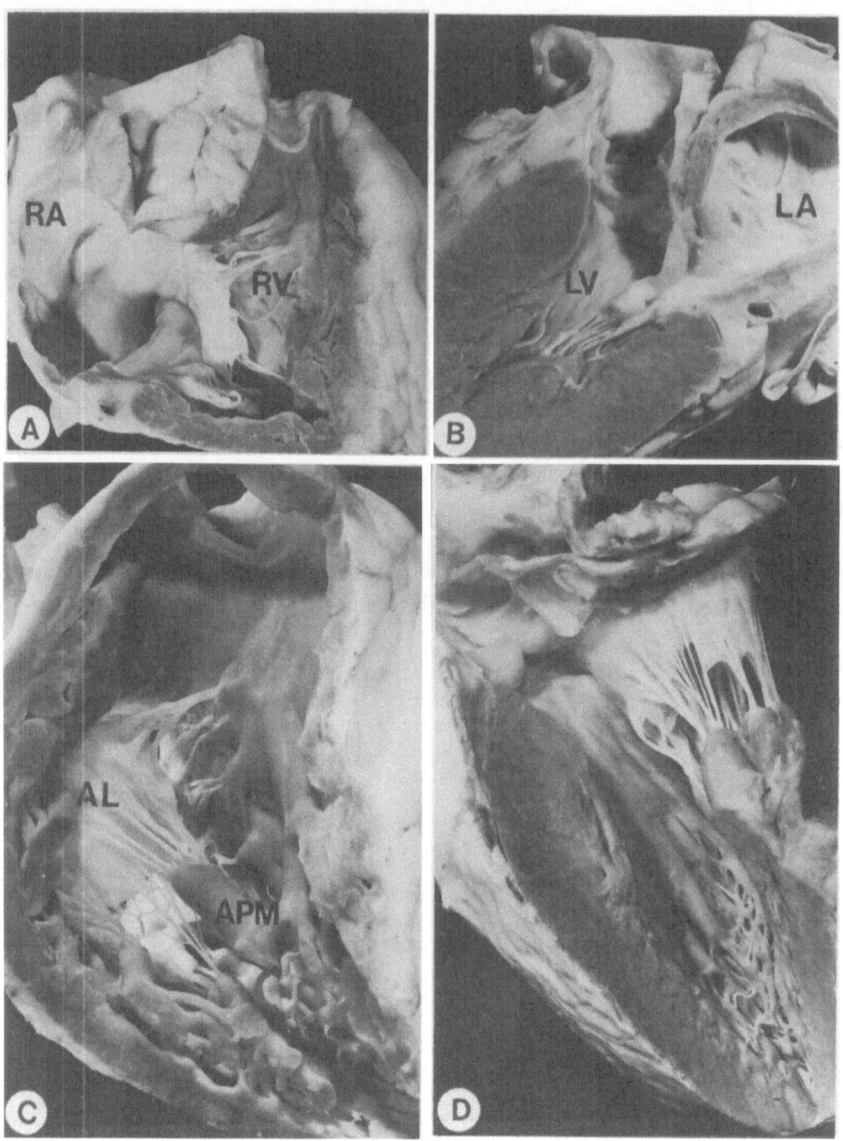

fig. 3. Specimen showing anatomic features of atrioventricular concordance. Fig. 3A shows the opened right side of the heart with the right atrium (RA) connecting to a right ventricle (RV). Fig. 3B shows the opened left side of the heart with the left atrium (LA) connecting to the left ventricle (LV). Fig. 3C shows a detailed view of the right-sided tricuspid valve characterized by a large anterior leaflet (AL), permitted free excursion by its attachment to the anterior papillary muscle (APM), while the septal and posterior leaflets are more tightly tethered to the ventricular septum and posterior wall. Fig. 3D detailed view of the left-sided, mitral valve characterized by the presence of discrete anterior and posterior leaflets, each capable of independent movements, and both tethered to paired papillary muscles.

116

of independent movement, and both tethered to paired papillary muscles (fig. 3D). In most instances, even in congenital heart disease, it is usual to find the tricuspid valve separated from the semilunar valve arising from the right ventricle, whereas the mitral valve is usually contiguous with the semilunar valve arising from the left ventricle (vide infra) In atrioventricular discordance, these features are reversed. Thus the right atrium drains through a valve tethered by paired papillary muscles and usually contiguous with the posterior semilunar valve (fig. 4A), whereas the left atrium drains through a valve tightly tethered to the septum and posterior ventricular wall which is usually separated from the semilunar valve arising from the right ventricle (fig. 4B). It is also usual in atrioventricular discordance for the ventricles to be side-by-side, without the infundibulum of the right ventricle "wrapping" round the left ventricel as in atrioventricular concordance. Thus an unusual relationship of valves or septum should raise the suspicion of atrioventricular discordance.

Double inlet and absent atrioventricular connections are, by virtue of their anatomy, particularly amenable to echocardiographic diagnosis. In double inlet ventricle both atrioventricular valves drain to the same ventricular chamber. It is therefore necessary to categorize also the ventricular morphology present. This can be primitive ventricle, defined as absence of an inflow septum, or double inlet right ven-

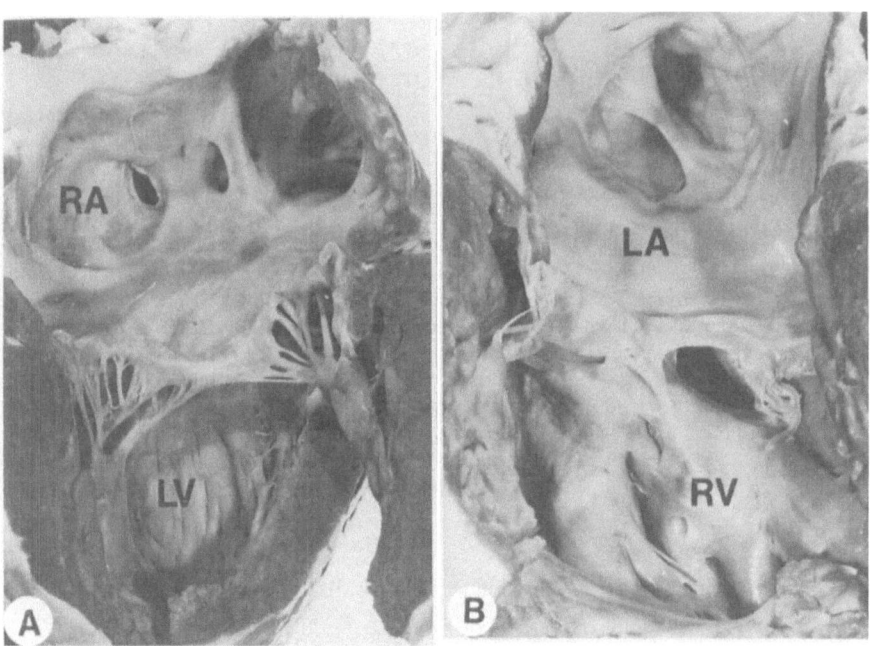

fig. 4. Specimen with atrioventricular discordance. Fig. 4A shows the right atrium (RA) connecting to a left ventricle (LV), through a valve tethered by paired papillary muscles. Fig. 4B shows the left atrium (LA) connected to the right ventricle (RV) through a valve tightly tethered to the septum and posterior ventricular wall.

117

tricle. In both of these anomalies it is usual to find an accessory chamber present, and the site of the septum separating the chamber serves to distinguish them. In primitive ventricle the septum will nearly always be anterior to both atrioventricular valves (fig. 5), whereas in double inlet right ventricle the septum will usually be posterior to the valves (fig. 6). When in double inlet right ventricle the accessory chamber is exceedingly small it may be difficult to distinguish the anomaly from primitive ventricle without accessory chamber. Echocardiography is also exceedingly useful in identifying atrioventricular valves which straddle a septal structure, be it anterior or posterior. Indeed, there is a spectrum of anomalies between straddling

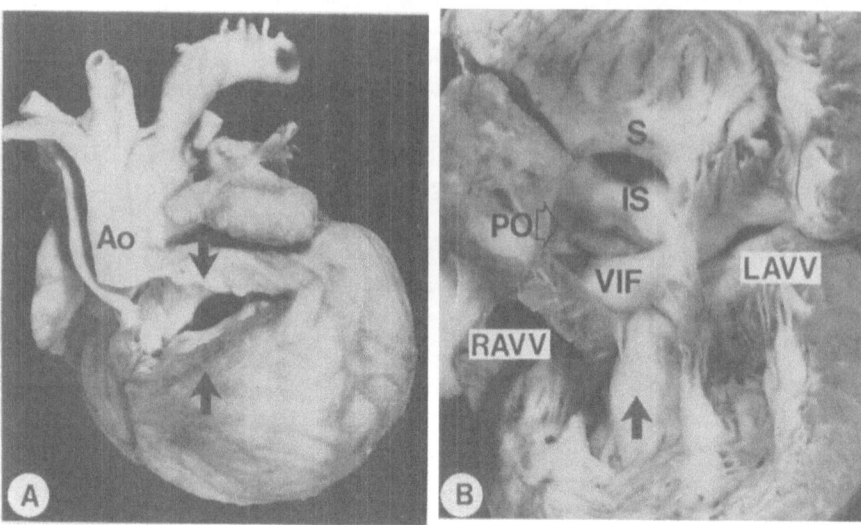

fig. 5. Specimen of univentricular heart, classified as primitive ventricle with outlet chamber. Fig. 5A external view of the heart showing the anteriorly positioned small outlet chamber (between arrows), from which the aorta (Ao) arises. Fig. 5B shows the interior of the heart opened through an incision separating the anterior from the posterior halves of both atrioventricular valves. Between the right atrioventricular valve (RAVV) and the left atrioventricular valve (LAVV) a posterior muscular ridge is identified (arrow). The pulmonary ostium (PO) is separated from the two atrioventricular valves by a muscle bar, the ventriculo-infundibular fold (VIF). The infundibular septum (IS) separates the pulmonic ostium from the defect leading into the small outlet chamber. The septum (S) separating the outlet chamber from the main chamber is positioned anterior to the two atrioventricular valves.

mitral valve with atrioventricular concordance (or discordance) (fig. 6A) and double inlet right ventricle (fig. 6B). Similarly, there is a spectrum between primitive ventricle with outlet chamber and straddling AV valve and atrioventricular concordance (or discordance) and straddling valve. Within our classification, these intermediate specimens are arbitrarily assigned to one or other category, the "cut-off" point being more than half a straddling valve going to a given chamber (fig. 7).

118

As with double inlet connections, absent atrioventricular connections can exist with a variety of ventricular morphologies. Atrioventricular concordance with imperforate valve would present angiographically as absent connection, but echocarciographically it may be possible to identify the imperforate membrane and thus establish the presence of two ventricles.

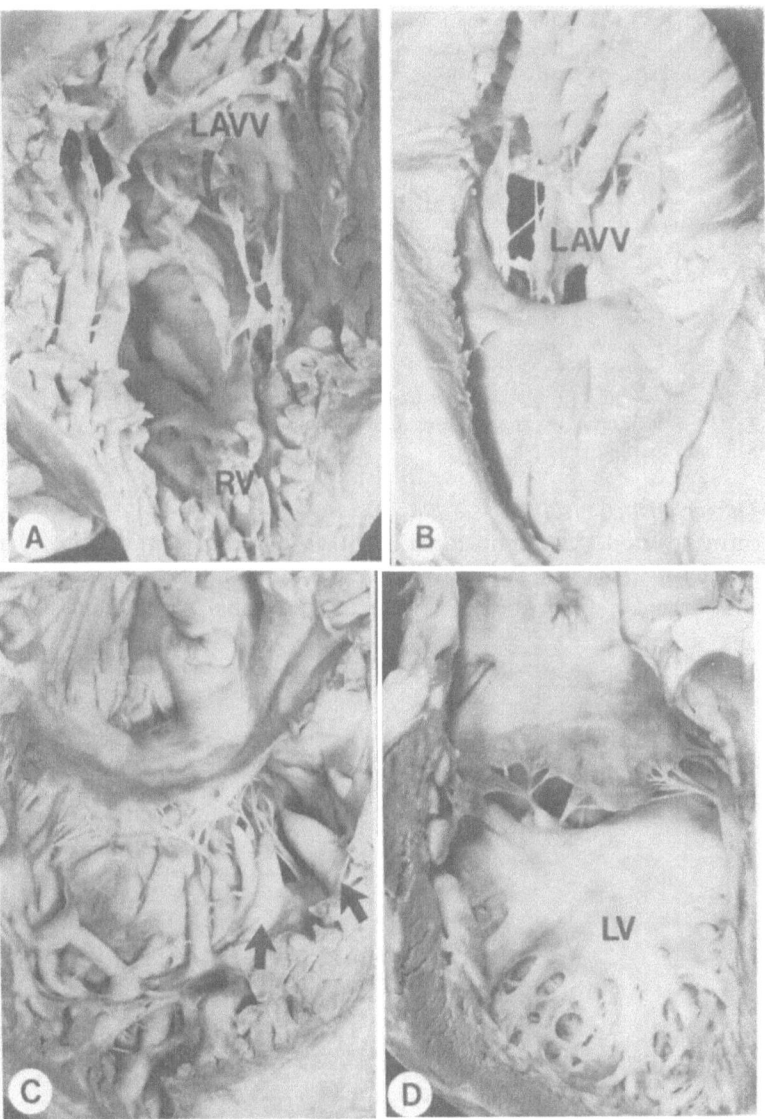

fig. 6. Specimen showing the spectrum between double inlet right ventricle (fig. 6A and 6B) and straddling mitral valve (fig. 6C and 6D). Fig. 6A shows the opened right side of the heart with two perforate atrioventricular valves that drain into the right ventricle (RV). The left atrioven-

119

tricular valve (LAVV) straddles a septum, which is positioned posteriorly to the AV-valves and separates a small left-sided chamber from the main righ-sided chamber. Fig. 6B shows the opened left-sided chamber with the straddling left atrioventricular valve (LAVV). Since the valve opens for more than 50% into the right-sided main chamber, the left-sided chamber is not designated as a ventricle, but instead as a trabeculated pouch (see also fig. 7). Fig. 6C shows the opened right side of the heart in case of a straddling mitral valve. The left atrioventricular valve has the potential to drain into the right ventricle, part of its tension apparatus (arrows) taking origin from the right side of the septum between the two chambers. The opened left side of the heart (fig. 6D) reveals that the major part of the valve opens into this ventricle, which therefore can be designated as a left ventricle (LV).

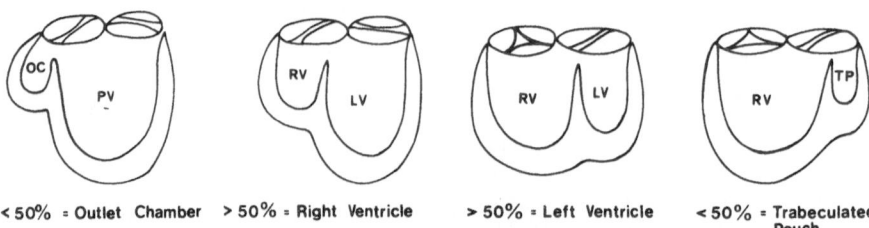

fig. 7. Diagrams to illustrate the chamber classification in case of a straddling atrioventricular valve. A valve is arbitrarily assigned to a chamber when more than 50% of its total circumference opens into that particular chamber.

Ventriculo-arterial connections

The ventriculo-arterial connections can be either (1) concordant (2) discordant (3) double outlet and (4) single outlet (fig. 8). They are much less amenable to echocardiographic diagnosis. Since the relationship of the semilunar valves can vary contin-

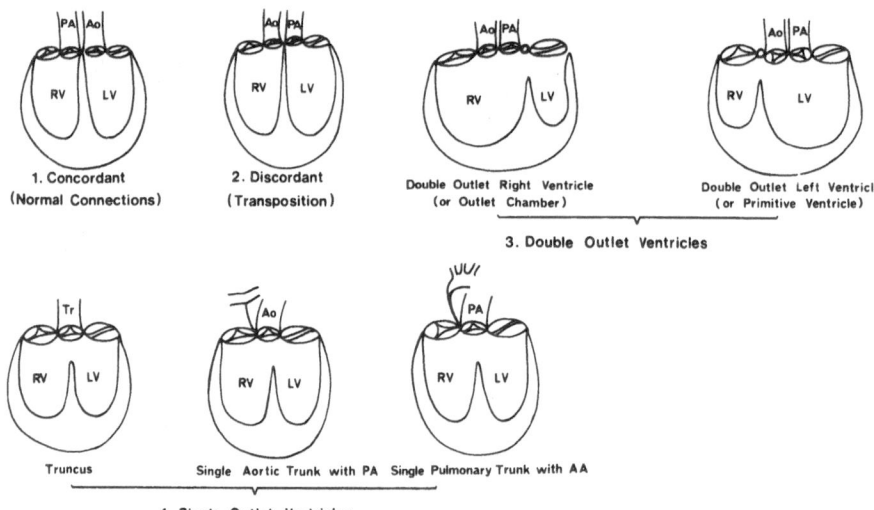

fig. 8. Diagrams illustrating the ventriculo-arterial connections.

120

uously in any connection, it cannot be said that identification of a relationship is diagnostic of any condition. To take an example, demonstration of "normal relationships" with continuity between the posterior great artery and the mitral valve is known to exist in rare cases of complete transposition (ventriculo-arterial discordance). Similarly, in ventriculo-arterial discordance it is known that in only approximately 70% of cases is the anteriorly placed aorta to the right. The presence of discontinuity between a semilunar valve and an atrioventricular valve is also of little value in deciding a ventriculo-arterial connection. This discontinuity, which anatomically is produced by the ventriculo-infundibular fold (that is the inner curvature of the heart, fig. 9), can be present in the left ventricle of hearts with ventricu-

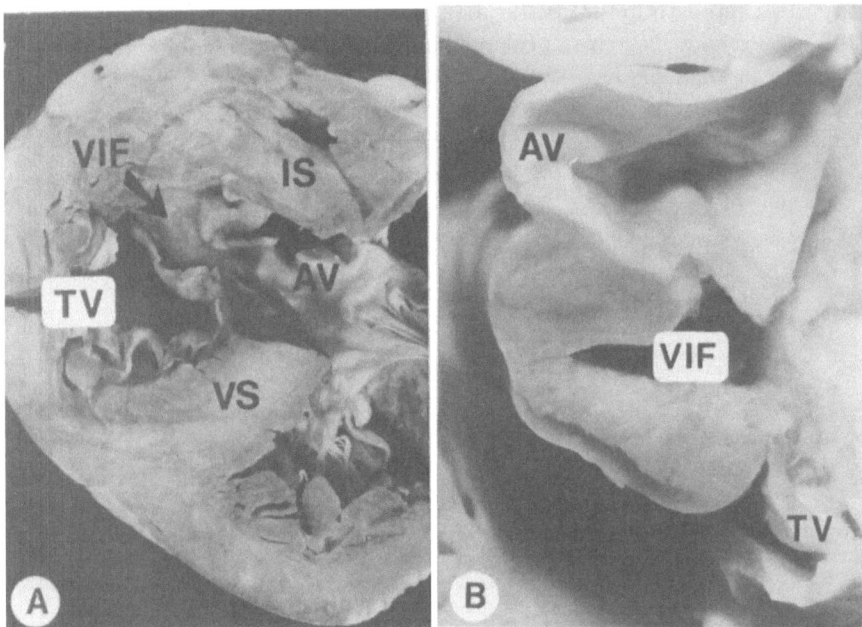

fig. 9. Specimen to demonstrate the ventriculo-infundibular fold (VIF). Fig. 9A shows a specimen of Fallot's tetralogy, looked at from below after cutting away the apical part of the heart. The aortic valve (AV) is separated from the tricuspid valve (TV) by a bar of muscle (VIF). Fig. 9B shows a section through this muscle, which reveals that it actually represents an infolding separating the aortic valve (AV) from the tricuspid valve (TV). This infolding is the ventriculo-infundibular fold (VIF) and represents the inner curvature of the heart. This structure is variable and may account for the presence or absence of semilunar-atrioventricular valve continuity.

lo-arterial discordance (transposition) yet can be absent from the right ventricle of hearts with a double outlet connection. Furthermore, it is known that spectra of anomalies exist between double outlet right ventricle and, on the one hand, Fallot's tetralogy, and on the other hand ventriculo-arterial discordance (transposition). Echocardiography is of value in detecting overriding semilunar valves, and it may be possible to assign the valve to one or other ventricle. As with straddling valves, in our classification an overriding semilunar valve is assigned to the chamber receiving more than 50% of its circumference. Echocardiography should also be of value in distinguishing the single outlet connection, remembering in this instance that it cannot be stated whether the single artery is a persistent trunk, a pulmonary trunk or an aorta. It must also be emphasized that diagnosis of both double inlet and double outlet connections depends upon positive identification of two valves and their position relative to a septum, whereas in diagnosing a single inlet or outlet, the possibility remains that another connection has NOT been identified.

Summary

A segmental approach to the classification of congenital heart disease is of relevance also for the echocardiographer. The method is based upon describing the route of circulation through the heart by recognizing the connections between the various cardiac segments. The important connections are atrioventricular and ventriculo-arterial. Echocardiography may facilitate identification of atrioventricular and semi-lunar valves and ventricular septa, from which, in many circumstances, the type of connection can be established. The anatomic features that may enable this recognition have been discussed.

References

1) Shinebourne EA, Macartney FJ, and Anderson RH: *Sequential chamber localization — logical approach to diagnosis in congenital heart disease.*
British Heart Journal 38: 327, 1976.

2) Van Praagh R: *The segmental approach to diagnosis in congenital heart disease.*
In: Birth Defects: Original Article Series 8: no. 5, p. 4. 1972. Williams and Wilkins, Baltimore.

3) Kirklin JW, Pacifico AD, Bargeron LM, and Soto B: *Cardiac repair in anatomically corrected malposition of the great arteries.*
Circulation 48: 153, 1973.

4) Anderson RH, Shinebourne EA, and Gerlis LM: *Criss-cross atrioventricular relationships producing paradoxical atrioventricular concordance or discordance: their significance to nomenclature of congenital heart disease.*
Circulation 50: 176, 1974.

Echocardiography in
noncyanotic congenital heart disease

by Wim G. van Dorp
Thoraxcentre, Academic Hospital Dijkzigt,
Erasmus University, Rotterdam, Netherlands.

An important differential diagnostic criterion in pediatric cardiology is the presence or absence of cyanosis. Application of this criterion devides the vast spectrum of congenital heart diseases in a cyanotic and an acyanotic group. Cyanosis producing lesions are usually complex: multiple anatomic lesions exist and the "basic floor plan" of the heart is distorted. The term "basic floor plan" (Solinger) may be described as the relative position of, and connections between the atria, the ventricles and the great vessels 1). Acyanotic congenital heart diseases on the other hand are often simple: only one anatomic lesion is present and the basic anatomy of the heart is unaltered. However, exceptions to the above quoted devision in two groups exist, therefore prior to using echocardiography to diagnose any congenital heart lesion, the basic anatomy of the heart must be known, either by echocardiography itself or by any other technique. If the "basic floor plan" of the heart is known, echocardiography provides useful clues to diagnose or differentiate many forms of acyanotic congenital heart disease.

A direct diagnosis in the non-cyanotic disease group is possible in situations where the primary anatomic lesion can be visualized, for instance with atrioventricular- and semilunar valve abnormalities and when abnormal cardiac structures are present.

However, in many other instances (left-to-right shunts etc.) a direct diagnosis is not possible and the lesion may only be suspected on account of demonstration of secondary signs, these are changes in the cardiac configuration or function as a result of the presence of the primary anatomic abnormality.

Direct diagnosis

Mitral valve
Congenital mitral stenosis is rare and seldom exists as an isolated lesion. Lundström 2) reported a reduction of the EF slope of the anterior mitral valve leaflet on the echocardiogram, and a diminished amplitude of this valve leaflet. At least in some patients, the posterior mitral valve leaflet moves anterior in diastole, in the same direction as the anterior mitral valve leaflet 3). Some specific forms of mitral valve incompetence (prolapse, flail mitral valve) may be diagnosed with echo, and are discussed elsewhere in this book.

123

Echocardiology, N. Bom editor, published by Martinus Nijhoff, the Hague 1977.

Tricuspid valve

Ebstein's anomaly of the tricuspid valve is mainly characterized by redundant valve tissue, adherence of the septal and posterior leaflets to the right ventricular wall, resulting in the formation of an atrialized portion of the right ventricle, and a large anterior leaflet. The only absolute diagnostic criterion known at present is late closure of the tricuspid valve: more than 65 msec after closure of the mitral valve, independent from the presence of a right bundle branch block. Suggestive findings are an increased amplitude of the anterior tricuspid valve leaflet and a large right ventricle (fig. 1). Usually echoes of the anterior tricuspid valve leaflet can be recorded over a large area of the left precordium 4).

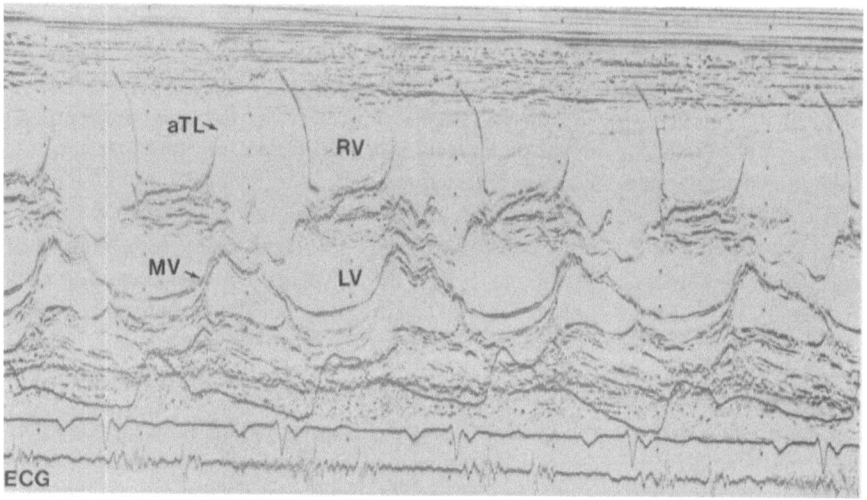

fig. 1. M-mode echocardiogram obtained from a patient with Ebstein's anomaly of the tricuspid valve. The anterior tricuspid valve leaflet (aTL) causes weak echoes and has a large amplitude of motion. The right ventricle (RV) is dilated. Abbrevations: MV = mitral valve, LV = left ventricle.

Common atrioventricular canal

Common atrioventricular canal is the most severe form of the endocardial cushion defect disease spectrum and is characterized by a large defect involving the lower part of the atrial septum, the adjoining proximal ventricular septum and gross abnormalities of the atrioventricular valves. The echocardiographic diagnosis is concentrated on the detection of abnormalities in mitral and tricuspid valve movement 5), 6). When the sound beam is directed toward the mitral valve, a pattern can be recognized in which a common atrioventricular valve leaflet traverses the interventricular septum: parts of this leaflet can be recorded within the left ventricle during systole. From this leaflet echoes appear in the right ventricle during diastole (fig. 2). The limited lateral resolution of the present used echosystems causes pro-

124

jection of the echoes of the valve in the echoes of the interventricular septum. In reality, the valve leaflet crosses the ventricular septal defect, but this defect cannot be demonstrated on the echocardiogram.

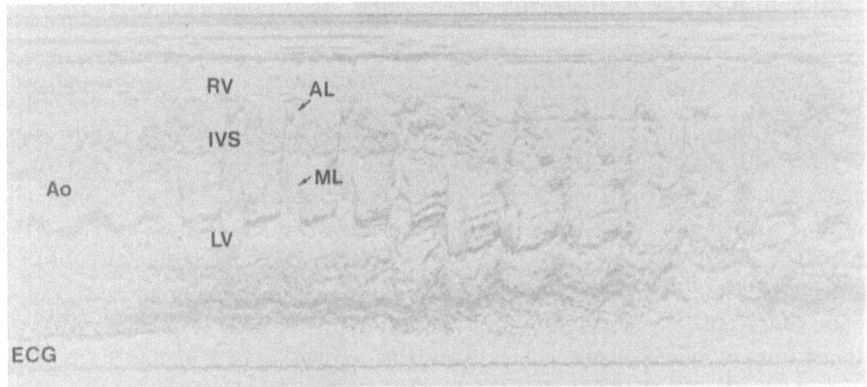

fig. 2. M-mode sectorscan obtained from a patient with a complete atrioventricular canal. At the level of the ventricular septal defect the echoes of the common atrioventricular valve leaflet (AL) "traverse" the interventricular septum (IVS), and are positioned in the right ventricle (RV) during diastole. Echoes of a mitral valve leaflet (ML) are visualized within the left ventricle (LV) during the whole cardiac cycle. Abbrevation: Ao = aorta.

Semilunar valves

In congenital aortic- and pulmonary stenosis the valve is often dome-shaped: the cusps at the base of the dome separate widely, but at the top they adhere. If the ultrasound beam is directed through the properly moving parts of this structure, an almost normal cusp registration may be obtained, despite the presence of severe aortic- or pulmonary stenosis 7).

In some patients with aortic stenosis (especially when the valve is calcified already), multiple diastolic lines and reduced separation of the aortic cusps in systole can be observed. In patients with pulmonary stenosis, a significant increase in amplitude of the pre-systolic motion of the valve may be observed 8).

Eccentricity of the diastolic closure line of the aortic cusps may be caused by the presence of a bicuspid aortic valve, with one large and one small cusp. Often however, this pattern can also be demonstrated in patients with an affected tricuspid aortic valve. Eccentricity therefore merely indicates eccentric positioned commissures of the aortic valve rather than a real bicuspid valve. Empirically it has been demonstrated that an eccentricity index (EI) of more than 1.3 is highly suggestive for a bicuspid aortic valve 9). The EI is calculated as half the width of the aortic lumen, devided by the distance of one cusp to the nearest aortic margin, as measured at the onset of diastole.

125

Supravalvular aortic stenosis

In supravalvular aortic stenosis the echoes of the aorta above the level of the valve may reflect the narrowing of the aortic root. If the transducer is aimed more superior to the stenosis, the aortic lumen widens to its normal diameter 10), 11).

Subvalvular aortic stenosis

In patients with the membranous form of subvalvular aortic stenosis, echoes of this membrane may be recognized within the left ventricular outflow tract 12). In many of these patients, there is also some involvement of the septum in the area of the membrane, resulting on the echocardiogram in a narrowing of the left ventricular outflow tract. The outflow tract diameter is measured at end-systole, at the level of the mitral ring, just below the aortic valve. Secondary signs are: early closure of the aortic valve, fine diastolic fluttering of the mitral valve indicating aortic incompetence and symmetric hypertrophy of the left ventricle 13). In patients with the tunnel form of subvalvular aortic stenosis, the narrowed area is extended (long segment subaortic stenosis) 14). The length of the narrowed part of the outflow tract may directly be recognized in a two-dimensional long axis cross-section through the left ventricle (fig. 3).

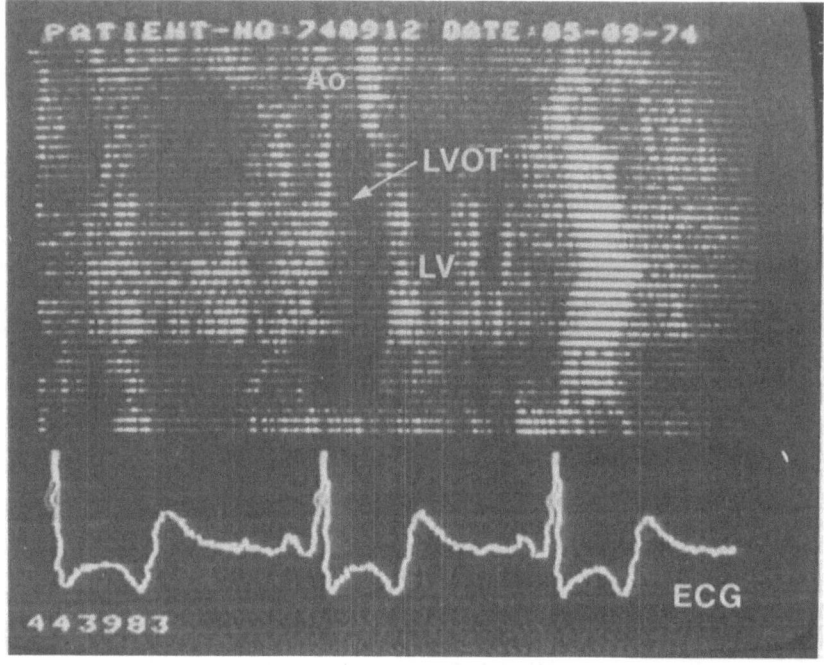

fig. 3. Two-dimensional 40-line image of a cross-section through the long axis of the left ventricle, obtained from a patient with a long segment subvalvular aortic stenosis. Abbrevations: AO = aorta, LV = left ventricle, LVOT = left ventricular outflow tract. The right end of the ECG indicates the phase in the cardiac cycle in which this photograph was taken.

126

Cor triatriatum

Left atrial membranes (cor triatriatum and supravalvular mitral membranes) appear on the echocardiogram as anomalous echoes in the left atrial cavity 15), 16). In two-dimensional images, the attachement of the membrane to the left atrial wall can be visualized. In general, the diagnosis must be made with care, because also in normal subjects echoes of unknown origin may be present in the left atrium.

Occasionally, an interesting observation may be the recognition of abnormal mitral valve motion secondary to a left atrial membrane. We have seen a patient with a normal mitral valve and with a left atrial membrane positioned just above the posterior mitral valve leaflet. This leaflet moved anterior during diastole, imitating a mitral stenosis pattern of the mitral valve (fig. 4). After surgical resection of the membrane, the mitral valve motion returned to normal.

Indirect diagnosis

Atrial septal defect

A left-to-right shunt at the atrial level may cause a volume overload of the right ventricle. Echocardiographically, right ventricular volume overload (RVVO) is characterized by an increased dimension of the right ventricle (fig. 5) and an abnormal, paradoxical pattern of ventricular septal movement.

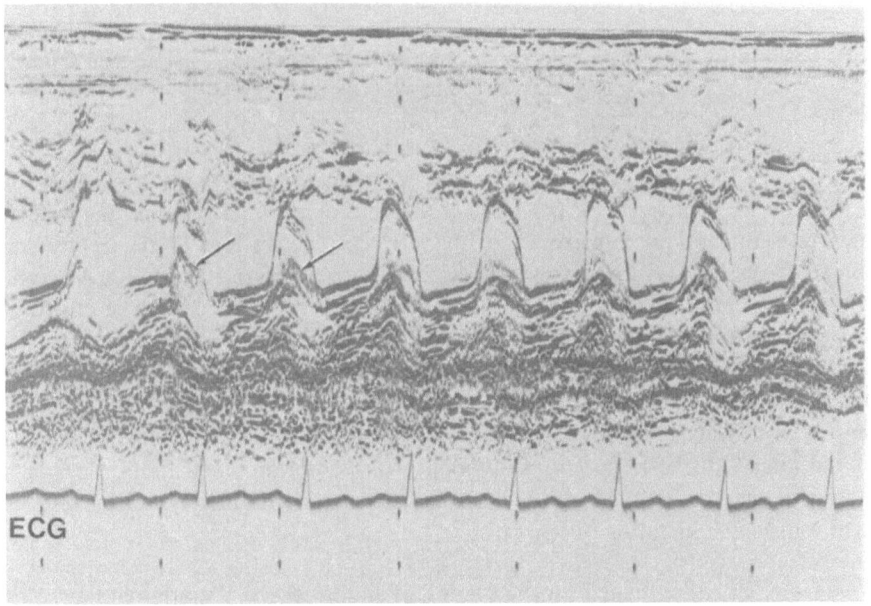

fig. 4. Mitral valve echogram obtained from a newborn with a supravalvular mitral membrane and a normal mitral valve. The posterior mitral valve leaflet (indicated with arrows) shows a fine diastolic flutter and moves anterior during diastole. Post-operatively, the mitral valve movement was completely normal.

127

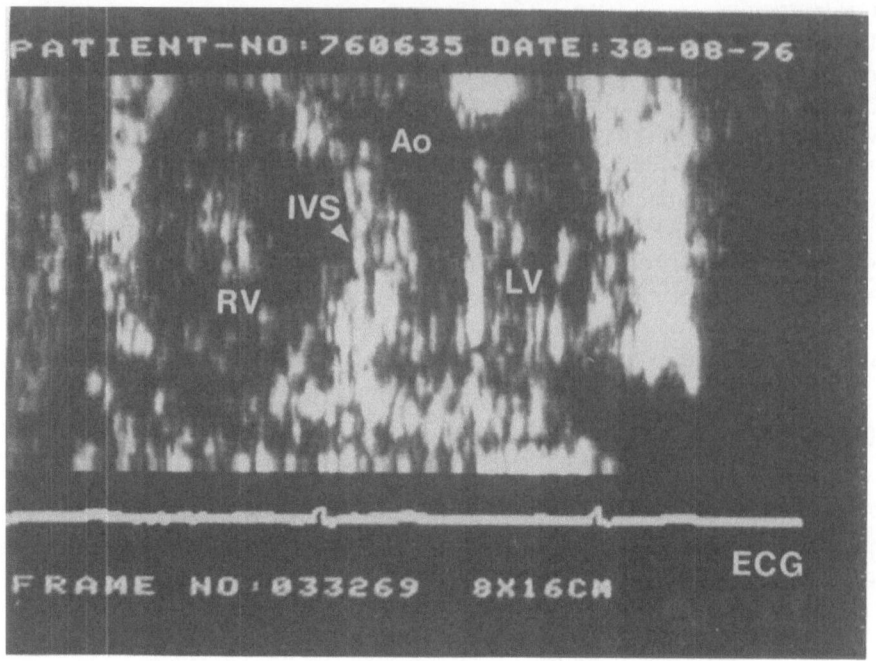

fig. 5. Two-dimensional 320 line image of a cross-section through the long axis of the left ventricle obtained from a patient with an atrial septal defect. Note the enlarged right ventricle (RV): the interventricular septum (IVS) bulges into the left ventricle (LV). Abbrevation: Ao = aorta.

In the normal situation the lower parts of the septum move posterior during systole, and contribute to the contraction of the left ventricle. In RVVO the septum (recorded at the level of the mitral valve leaflets) moves anterior during systole (type A) or has a flattened motion (type B) 17), 18). Recently, the genesis of this paradoxical septal motion became more clear. Pearlman et al. 19) observed that both the direction and magnitude of ventricular septal motion during systole is determined by the intra-cardiac position of the septum at end-diastole. The more the septum is displaced toward the left ventricle, the larger is the paradoxical motion of the interventricular septum. This implies that anterior septal motion is not a diagnostic marker for right ventricular volume overload, but merely reflects relative right ventricular dilatation of any cause.

Weyman et al. 20) evaluated the mechanism of abnormal septal motion in short-axis cross-sectional two-dimensional images of the left ventricle. In patients with dilatation of the right ventricle a change in the left ventricular shape was noted. This change in shape varied from a slight flattening of the left ventricle and the interventricular septum during diastole to a complete reversal of the normal septal curvature (in the normal situation the septum is concave toward the left ventricle). In systole, the septum in patients with RVVO returned to its normal configuration, causing a net motion of the septum toward the right ventricle.

A paradoxical septal motion may thus be present in any condition causing dilatation of the right ventricle. At present, beside in patients with atrial septal defect, this pattern has been described in patients with ostium primum defects (partial endocardial cushion defect) 21), 22), partial and total anomalous pulmonary venous return 23), 24), tricuspid and pulmonary incompetence 25), 26), 27) absence of the pericardium 28), right coronary arterial - right ventricular fistula 29) and even in subjects without apparent heart diseases 30). Unfortunately, the ultrasound examination offers very few criteria to further differentiate these lesions, because the primary anatomic defect usually cannot be visualized.

Helpful observations are in:

Total and partial anomalous pulmonary venous return.
The presence of an echofree space dorsal to the posterior wall of the left atrium, probably representing the common pulmonary venous chamber 24).

Pulmonary incompetence
Fine diastolic fluttering of the tricuspid valve 31).

Ostium primum defect
Narrowing of the left ventricular outflow tract (goose-neck deformity), prolonged approximation of the anterior mitral valve leaflet to the ventricular septum during diastole and a double echo representing the two edges of the cleft mitral leaflet 5), 6).

Ventricular septal defect
In its uncomplicated form this abnormality has almost none distinghuising echocardiographic features. Only one author 32) reports the direct recognition of the defect, using a two-dimensional compound B-scanner. This observation could never be confirmed by other investigators. Only secondary signs may be observed in patients with a large shunt. These are an increase in the left atrial and ventricular dimensions. Lewis et al. 33) demonstrated a linear relationship between the pulmonary to systemic blood flow and the ratio of the echocardiographic left atrial to aortic dimension.

Patent ductus arteriosus
Patent ductus arteriosus also produce an increase in the dimensions of the left side of the heart. Also in this disease entity a correlation was found between the shunted volume and the left atrial size 34). Serial observations in one patient may be worthwile to follow the effect of spontaneous closure or ligation of the patent ductus (fig. 6).

129

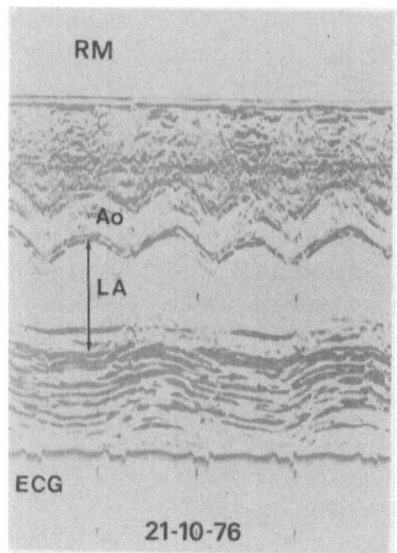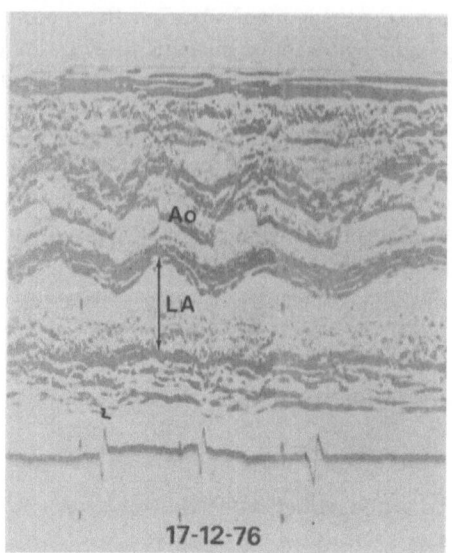

fig. 6. M-mode echogradiograms obtained from a premature neonate. The first echocardiogram (21-10-76) shows an enlarged left atrium due to a patent ductus arteriosus. In the second echocardiogram (17-12-76), the ductus is almost closed, and the left atrial size is markedly reduced. Abbrevations: Ao = aorta, LA = left atrium.

Discussion

Echocardiography is a rather new technique in pediatric cardiology. It offers the possibility to recognize or to differentiate many forms of congenital heart disease. The technique is limited in its diagnostic capabilities, when the primary anatomic lesion, because of its position or small size, cannot be recognized. However, in many instances secundary effects such as volume overload may be observed which are indicative of congenital malformations. Therefore, it may be expected that with a further improvement of the echocardiographic techniques (enhancement of the quality of two-dimensional images, swept focus systems) the range of diagnostic applications can be extended.

References

1) Solinger R, Elbl F, and Minhas K: *Deductive echocardiographic analysis in infants with congenital heart disease.*
   Circulation 50: 1072, 1974.

2) Lundström NR: *Echocardiography in the diagnosis of congenital mitral stenosis and in evaluation of the results in mitral valvotomy.*
   Circulation 46: 44, 1972.

130

3) Murphy KF, Kotler MN, Reichek N, and Perloff JK: *Ultrasound in the diagnosis of congenital heart disease.*
Amer Heart J 89: 638, 1975.

4) Farooki ZQ, Henry JG, and Green EW: *Echocardiographic spectrum of Ebstein's anomaly of the tricuspid valve.*
Circulation 53: 63, 1976.

5) Williams RG, and Rudd M; *Echocardiographic features of endocardial cushion defects.*
Circulation 49: 418, 1974.

6) Sahn DJ, Terry RW, O'Rourke R, Leopold G, and Friedman WF: *Multiple crystal echocardiographic evaluation of endocardial cushion defect.*
Circulation 50: 25, 1974.

7) Goldberg SJ, Allen HD, and Sahn DJ: *Pediatric and adolescent echocardiography.*
Year Book Medical Publishers, Chicago, 1975.

8) Weyman AE, Dillon JC, Feigenbaum H, and Chang S: *Echocardiographic patterns of pulmonic valve motion in pulmonic stenosis.*
Amer J Cardiol 33: 178, 1974.

9) Radford DJ, Bloom KR, Izukawa T, Moes CAF, and Rowe RD: *Echocardiographic assessment of bicuspid aortic valves. Angiographic and pathological correlates.*
Circulation 53: 80, 1976.

10) Williams DE, Sahn DJ, and Friedman WF: *Cross-sectional echocardiographic localization of sites of left ventricular outflow tract obstruction.*
Amer J Cardiol 37: 250, 1976.

11) Nasrallah AT, and Nihill M: *Supravalvular aortic stenosis. Echocardiographic features.*
Brit Heart J 37: 662, 1975.

12) Kronzon I, Schloss M, Danilowicz D, and Singh A: *Fixed membranous subaortic stenosis.*
Chest 67: 473, 1975.

13) Davis RH, Feigenbaum H, Chang S, Konecke LL, and Dillon JC: *Echocardiographic manifestations of discrete subaortic stenosis.*
Amer J Cardiol 33: 227, 1974.

14) Maron BJ, Redwood DR, Roberts WC, Henry WL, Morrow AG, and Epstein SE: *Tunnel subaortic stenosis. Left ventricular outflow tract obstruction produced by fibromuscular tubular narrowing.*
Circulation 54: 404, 1976.

15) Gibson DG, Honey M, and Lennox SC: *Cor triatriatum. Diagnosis by echocardiography.*
Brit Heart J 36: 835, 1974.

16) Nimura Y, Matsumoto M, Beppu S, Matsuo H, Sakakibara H, and Abe H: *Noninvasive preoperative diagnosis of cor triatriatum with ultrasonocardiotomogram and conventional echocardiogram.*
Amer Heart J 88: 240, 1974.

17) Diamond MA, Dillon JC, Haine CL, Chang S, and Feigenbaum H: *Echocardiographic features of atrial septal defect.*
Circulation 43: 129, 1971.

18) Tajik AJ, Gau GT, and Schattenberg TT: *Echocardiogram in atrial septal defect.*
Chest 62: 213, 1972.

19) Pearlman AS, Clark CE, Henry WL, Morganroth J, Itscoitz SB, and Epstein SE: *Determinants of ventricular septal motion. Influence of relative right and left ventricular size.*
Circulation 54: 83, 1976.

20) Weyman AE, Wann S, Feigenbaum H, and Dillon JC: *Mechanism of abnormal septal motion in patients with right ventricular volume overload. A cross-sectional echocardiographic study.*
Circulation 54: 179, 1976.

21) Tajik AJ, Gau GT, Ritter DG, and Schattenberg TT: *Echocardiographic pattern of right ventricular diastolic volume overload in children.*
Circulation 46: 36, 1972.

22) Meyer RA, Schwartz DC, Benzing G, and Kaplan S: *Ventricular septum in right ventricular volume overload.*
Amer J Cardiol 30: 349, 1972.

23) Tajik AJ, Gau GT, and Schattenberg TT: *Echocardiogram in total anomalous pulmonary venous drainage.*
Mayo Clin Proc 47: 247, 1972.

24) Paquet M, and Gutgesell H: *Echocardiographic features of total anomalous pulmonary venous connection.*
Circulation 51: 599, 1975.

25) Seides SF, DeJoseph RL, Brown AE, and Damato AN: *Echocardiographic findings in isolated, surgically created tricuspid insufficiency.*
Amer J Cardiol 35: 679, 1975.

26) Kessler KM, Foianni JE, Davia JE, Anderson WT, Pfuetze K, Pinder T, and Cheitlin MD: *Tricuspid insufficiency due to nonpenetrating trauma.*
Amer J Cardiol 37: 442, 1976.

27) Goodman DJ, Harrison DC, and Popp RL: *Echocardiographic features of primary pulmonary hypertension.*
Amer J Cardiol 33: 438, 1974.

28) Payvandi MN, and Kerber RE: *Echocardiography in congenital and acquired absence of the pericardium. An echocardiographic mimic of right ventricular volume overload.*
Circulation 53: 86, 1976.

29) Verani MS, and Lauer RM: *Echocardiographic findings in right coronary arterial-right ventricular fistula. Report of a neonate with fatal congestive heart failure.*
Amer J Cardiol 35: 444, 1975.

30) Bahler AS, Meller J, Brik H, Herman MV, and Teichholtz LE: *Paradoxical motion of the interventricular septum with right ventricular dilatation in the absence of shunting.*
Amer J Cardiol 38: 654, 1976.

132

31) Feigenbaum H: *Echocardiography.*
Lea & Febiger, Philadelphia, 1972.

32) King DL, Steeg CL, and Ellis K: *Visualization of ventricular septal defects by cardiac ultra-sonography.*
Circulation 48: 1215, 1973.

33) Lewis AB, and Takahashi M: *Echocardiographic assessment of left-to-right shunt volume in children with ventricular septal defect.*
Circulation 54: 78, 1976.

34) Silverman NH, Lewis AB, Heymann MA, and Rudolph AM: *Echocardiographic assessment of ductus arteriosus shunt in premature infants.*
Circulation 50: 821, 1974.

Real-time Assessment of Fetal Dynamics.

by J.W. Wladimiroff,
Department of Obstetrics and Gynaecology,
Academic Hospital Rotterdam-Dijkzigt, Rotterdam.

Two-dimensional imaging systems have opened the possibility of studying the foetus in relation to its dynamics. In our study, the linear array method or Multiscan 1) with dynamically focussing system 2), was used. This system maintains an excellent lateral resolution over the entire depth of scanning.

In diagnostic Ultrasound, focussing over the entire field of viewing provides much more detailed information as to the nature of anatomical structures involved in certain dynamic processes. M-mode facilities create the possibility of recording movements. Finally, data collected on these recordings can be stored on magnetic tape with the view of quantitative evaluation on a computer at a later stage. At present our attention is mainly focussed on:
- fetal movements in general
- fetal heart activity
- fetal breathing movements
- transabdominal fetal blood sampling.

Fetal body movements

In the first half of pregnancy the fetus is surrounded by a relatively large pool of liquor, thus enabling it to change its position within the amniotic cavity at all times. Clinically, fetal movement is a sign of viability; from a physiological standpoint, the frequency and nature of fetal movement is related to the development of its nervous system. It is well-known that anencephalics are more "restless" compared with normally developing foetuses. It is now possible to observe not only movements of fetal head and rump, but also movements of fetal arms, hands, legs and feet as from 8 - 9 weeks of gestation. Currently, we are trying to develop a quantitative method of evaluation of these movements.

Fetal heart activity

In contrast to the adult, in the fetus the primary difficulty lies in the two-dimensional interpretation of various cardiac structures and not in the examination technique. The great variety of fetal positions creates one of the main problems when assessing cardiac structures in relation to their movement. However, the multiscan with focussing system enables us for the first time to combine the excellent anatomical structure recognition on the two-dimensional image with the movements of these structures on the M-mode. Fig. 1 and 2 demonstrate a sagittal section of a fetal heart in two different phases of the cardiac cycle at 31 weeks gestation.

135

Echocardiology, N. Bom editor, published by Martinus Nijhoff, the Hague 1977.

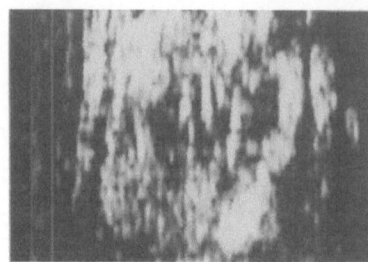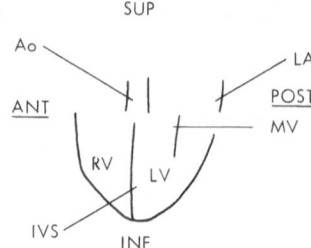

fig. 1. Two-dimensional real-time multiscan image and schematic picture of a sagittal section of the fetal heart at 31 weeks gestation. LA   left atrium; IVS   Interventricular septum; MV Mitral valve; LV   Left ventricle; RV   Right ventricle; Ao   aorta.

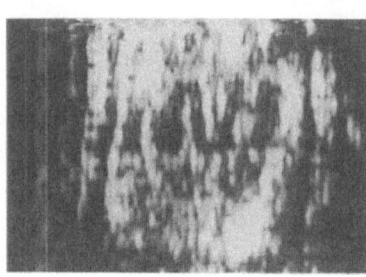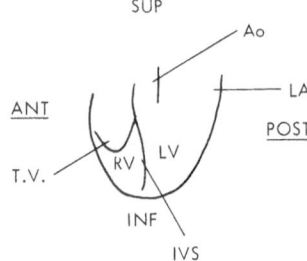

fig. 2. Two-dimensional real-time multiscan image and schematic picture of the same section of the same fetal heart in a different phase of the cardiac cycle. TV   Tricuspid valve.

Fetal breathing movements

Reports on the monitoring of breathing movements in the human fetus have mainly been based on the use of one-dimensional Ultrasound systems. Combining the features of one-dimensional and two-dimensional system produces an accurate means of investigating fetal breathing movements 3). The multi-element transducer is positioned on the patient's abdomen and a real-time cross-sectional image of the fetal chest at the level of the fetal heart is obtained. By using the special time gain compensation, breathing movements can easily be differentiated from movements in adjacent structures, fetal body motion and maternal breathing (fig. 3). The real-time two-dimensional imaging enables the investigator to adjust the position of the transducer to ensure that the line to be selected for M-mode recording is perpendicular to that part of the fetal chest wall showing maximum breathing movements. Fig. 4 shows a normal breathing pattern in a well-oxygenated fetus of 35 weeks gestation, characterized by irregular breathing movements. Fig. 5 demonstrates typical "gasping" often associated with fetal hypoxia.

Transabdominal fetal blood sampling

In recent years increasing attention has been paid to the prenatal diagnosis of genetic defects. The most contributing factor in the recent progress of prenatal genetic

136

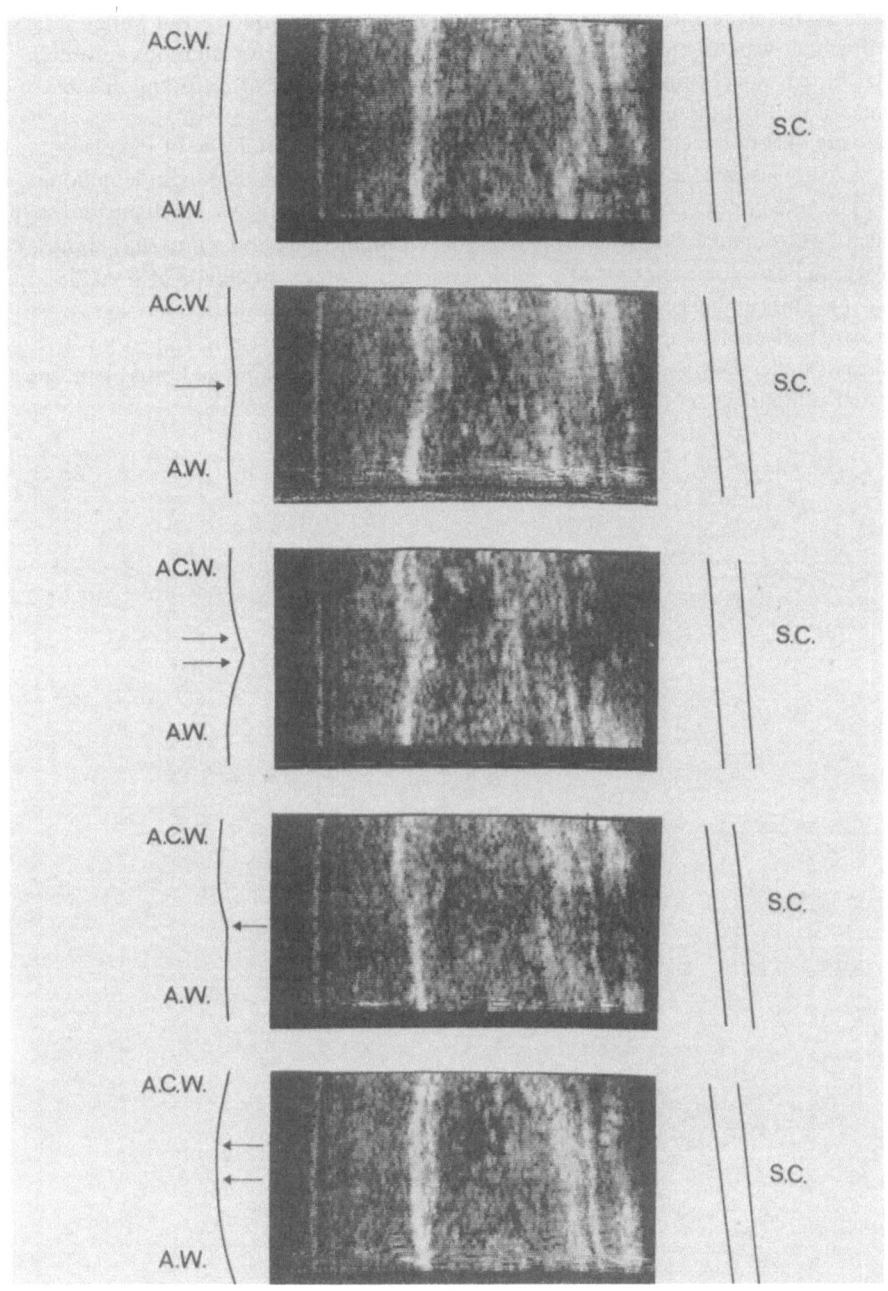

fig. 3. Real-time two-dimensional imaging of a sagittal section of fetus at 35 weeks of gestation showing chest wall movement from expanded to contracted to expanded position again. ACW Anterior chest wall; AW Upper abdominal wall; SC spinal column.

diagnosis has been the availability of liquor. However, the liquor is not purely fetal in origin. It was for these reasons that one began to search for methods to obtain fetal blood. Successful aspiration of fetal blood by means of fetoscopy has been reported by Hobbins and Mahoney 4).

We were able to collect small fetal blood samples from the fetal side of the placenta 5). A 20-gauge needle was used. The tip of the needle can be made visible in liquor and placenta under real-time two-dimensional visualization (fig. 6). Small puffs of so-called "white smoke clouds" arising from the chorionic membrane into the amniotic cavity, indicate the puncture of a fetal vessel and subsequent escape of fetal blood (fig. 7). This can be aspirated. The puncture site closes up within 30 seconds. So far we have collected fetal blood in 3 out of 4 cases. Fetal heart rate stayed positive. All cases underwent abortion for medical or social reasons within 24 hours by means or oral administration of 15 methyl prostaglandine F 2α.

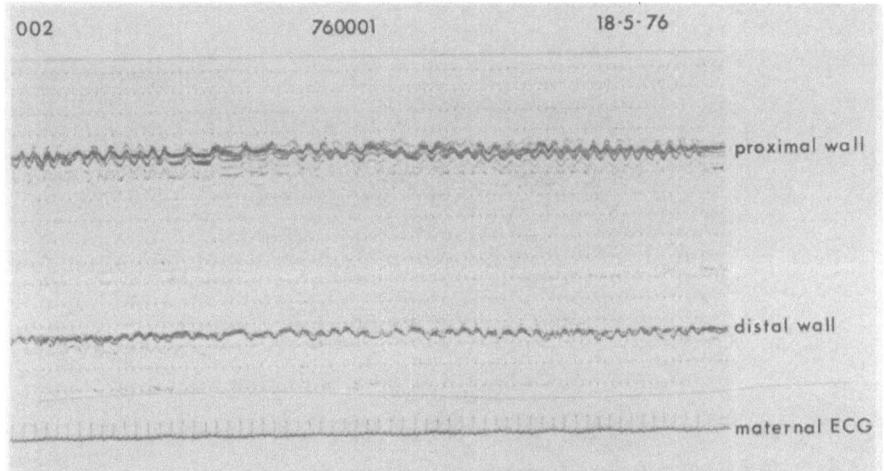

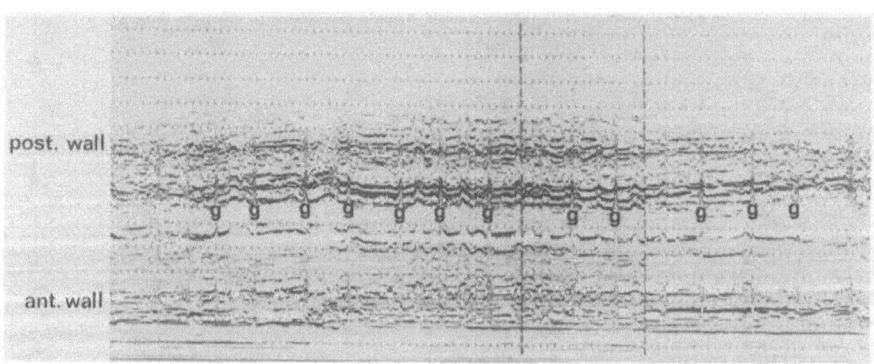

fig. 4 and 5. M-mode recording of normal fetal breathing movements (fig. 4) and gasping (g, fig. 5). Distance between two dots is 0.5 sec. in horizontal and 1 cm in vertical direction.

138

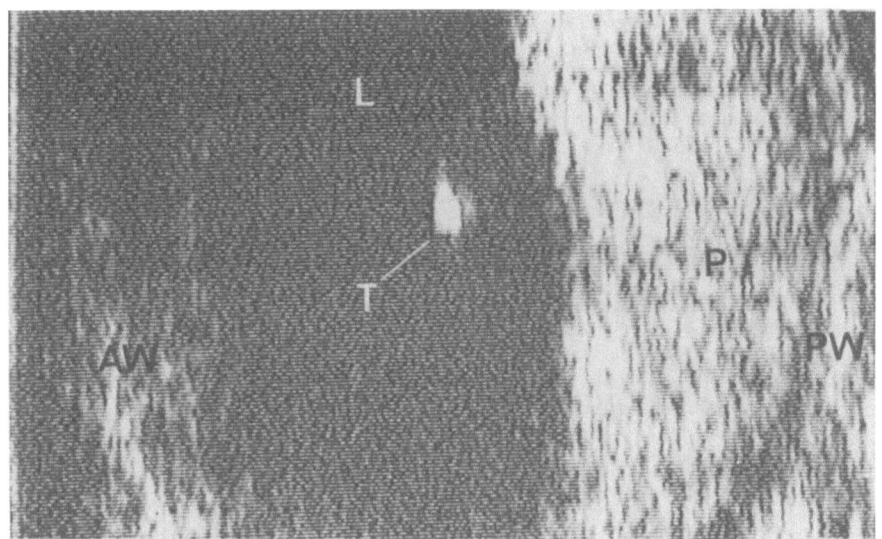

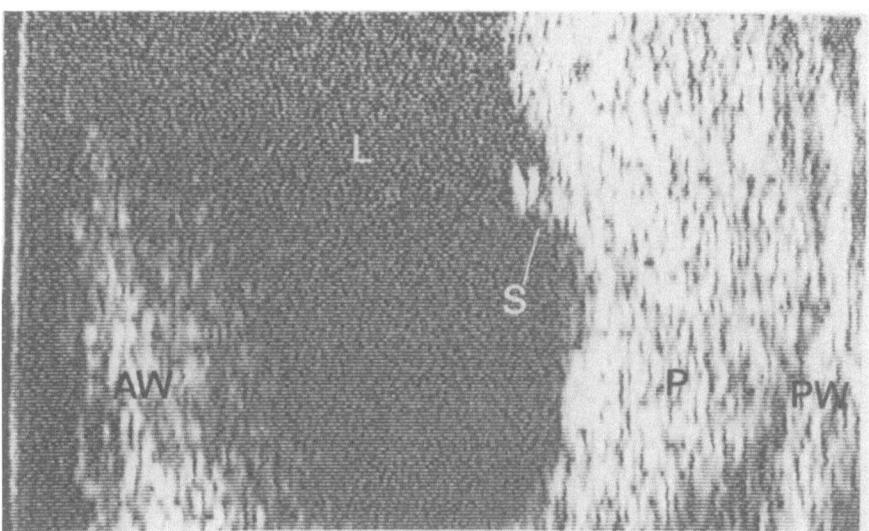

fig. 6 and 7. Tip of amniocentesis needle (fig. 6) and spurt of fetal blood arising from the chorionic membrane (fig. 7). AW   anterior uterine wall; PW   Posterior uterine wall; P   placenta, T   Tip of the needle; S   Spurt of fetal blood.

References

1) Bom N. Lancée CT, van Zwieten G, Kloster FE, and Roelandt J: *Multiscan Echocardio-graphy. I. Technical Description.*
   Circulation Vol. XLVIII, 1066, 1973.

2) Ligtvoet CM, Ridder J, Lancée CT, Hagemeijer F,Vletter WB, and Gussenhoven WJ: *Corresponding chapter in this book!*

3) Wladimiroff JW, Ligtvoet CM, and Spermon JA: *Combined One- and Two-dimensional Ultrasound Systems for Monitoring Fetal Breathing Movements.*
Brit. Med. J. 2: 975, 1976.

4) Hobbins JC, and Mahoney MJ: *Fetoscopy and fetal blood sampling. The present state of the Method.*
Clinical Obstetrics and Gynaecology, 19: 341, 1976.

5) Wladimiroff JW, and Jahoda MCJ: *Real-time scanning and transabdominal fetal blood sampling.*
Lancet 1: 593, 1977.

Echocardiography in a general cardiologic practice
Its practicality and diagnostic usefulness

by R. Vermeulen,
Brussel.

Echocardiography has become an established clinical procedure in large hospitals. On instigation of the Department of Echocardiography at the Thoraxcenter (Rotterdam, the Netherlands), this study was undertaken in an attempt to answer the question whether this technique is practical to perform and helpful diagnostically in general cardiological practice.

The procedure is well suited for use in ambulatory patients; it can be applied without patient preparation, without discomfort or hazard and the results are immediately available. There are some drawbacks too: the equipment is expensive, the examination technique requires special training and is time consuming.

Excluding the financial question, the main problem is the time required for the examination and data analysis. This is mainly dependent upon the skill and experience of the examiner. But, even with considerable experience, the examination itself usually requires 10 minutes and may even require 30 minutes in difficult patients. The quality of the study and the amount of information obtained depends largely on the persistence and the time spent on the examination by the examiner. Poor results are always obtained when one is tired or hurried. Therefore, if echocardiography is to be performed in a general cardiologic practice, a sufficient amount of time must be provided and this will only be possible if a relatively small number of patients are examined.

The following report aims to discuss whether the investment of time and effort is balanced by the clinical benefits to justify the use of echocardiography in a general cardiologic practice based on a clinician's experience during one year.

During 1976, 1420 cardiological examinations, including 745 echocardiograms were performed (table 1). One or more echocardiograms were made in 638 patients, 551 having had one echocardiogram. In 87 patients, serial echocardiograms were performed. Initial evaluation in 568 patients included an echocardiogram in 312 cases. The diagnostic usefulness of the echocardiogram for the patient population examined was evaluated and classified in three categories (table 2). In 25 percent of the patients, it was estimated that the echocardiogram had definite diagnostic value. In a majority of these cases, the clinical diagnosis was confirmed or was defined with more certainty by echo (72 percent). In a smaller number of cases, a new diagnosis was revealed (28 percent).

141

Echocardiology, N. Bom editor, published by Martinus Nijhoff, the Hague 1977.

Table 1.

Cardiological Examinations in 1976		1.420
Echocardiograms		745 (52 percent)
Patients with one or more echocardiograms		638
one echocardiogram	551	
two echocardiograms	68	
three echocardiograms	18	
four echocardiograms	1	
New patients seen in 1976		568
Echocardiograms in new patients		345
New patients with one or more echos		312 (55 percent)

Table 2.

Diagnostic benefit from 745 echocardiograms in 638 patients.

Definite diagnostic value in 158 patients (25 percent)

Suspected diagnosis confirmed	113 patients	(72 percent)
New diagnosis	45 patients	(28 ")

Useful contribution in   356 patients (56 percent)

Diagnosis confirmed	149 patients	(42 ")
Diagnosis excluded	160 patients	(45 ")
New diagnosis of minor importance	47 patients	(13 ")

No help in   124 patients (19 percent)

Echo of insufficient quality	106 patients	(85 ")

In 56 percent of the patients, it was estimated that the echocardiogram made a useful contribution to the final diagnosis. This meant that an already known or strongly suspected diagnosis was accepted because of addditional suggestive and/or supportive data from the echo in 42 percent. In 45 percent, it helped to exclude a suspected specific cardiac disease, whereas in 13 percent the echocardiogram added a new diagnosis of minor or uncertain importance. In 19 percent of the patients, we concluded that the echocardiogram added nothing to our knowledge about the patient, mainly because the echocardiographic recordings were not of sufficient quality to allow firm conclusions (85 percent).

Table 3.

Indications for echo and diagnostic yield

	638 patients		158 patients with diagnostic echo	
	N	percent	N	percent
Myocardial infarction	73	11,4	30	19
Coronary insufficiency[o]	132	20,7	18	11,4
Atypical chest pain	209	32,8	25	15,8
Rhythm disturbance	103	16,1	21	13,3
Hypertension	60	9,4	14	8,9
Heart murmur[oo]	24	3,8	2	1,3
Mitral disease	26	4,1	25	15,8
Aortic valve disease	47	7,4	38	24,1
Heart failure	9	1,4	5	3,2
Congenital disease	7	1,1	4	2,5
Lung disease	14	2,2	3	1,9
Miscellaneous	27	4,2	1	0,6

[o] without myocardial infarction

[oo] other than mitral or aortic, mostly innocent.

The indications for performing an echocardiogram are given in table 3. In the first two columns, the number and percentage of the different diagnoses are given for the total number of patients. In many patients there was more than one diagnosis. As can be expected for a general practice, the majority of patients presented themselves with a problem related to coronary heart disease. Myocardial infarction, coronary insufficiency and atypical chest pain together accounted for 65 percent of these patients. Only 10 percent had valvular heart disease. In the last two columns, the figures are given for the 158 patients in whom the echocardiogram was con-

Table 4.

Diagnostic information obtained in 638 patients by echo.

	638 patients		158 patients with diagnostic echo	
	N	percent	N	percent
LV hypertrophy	48	7,5	23	14,5
LV dilatation	90	14,1	35	22,2
LV hypokinesia	62	9,7	29	18,4
LV aneurysm	13	2,0	10	6,3
ASH	15	2,4	13	8,2
Congestive myopathy	5	0,8	5	3,2
Mitral stenosis	12	1,9	12	7,6
Mitral regurgitation	5	0,8	5	3,2
Mitral prolapse	37	5,8	34	21,5
Decreased E-F slope	60	9,4	32	20,3
Aortic stenosis	18	2,8	16	10,1
Aortic valve thickened	23	3,6	6	3,8
Aortic regurgitation	32	5,0	25	15,8
Bicuspid or dome valve	8	1,3	5	3,2
LA dilatation	57	8,9	32	20,3
RV dilatation	46	7,2	15	9,5
Aortic root dilatation	15	2,4	8	5,1
Pericardial effusion	40	6,3	15	9,5
Prosthetic valve	6	0,9	4	2,5
ASD	2	0,3	1	0,6
Normal echocardiogram	178	27,9	1	0,6
No definite pathology	128	20,1		

sidered to have diagnostic value. The differences in prevalence compared to the total number of patients indicate the difference in usefulness of echocardiography according to the diagnostic problem. The echocardiogram appears to yield maximal profit in the examination of patients with valvular heart disease but its usefulness was also above average in the evaluation of patients with myocardial infarction because of the information obtained on left ventricular size and performance. The diagnostic yield was below average in the evaluation of patients with angina pectoris and atypical chest pain. In 61 percent of these patients, the echocardiogram was found to be normal, or probably normal.

The diagnostic signs demonstrated by echocardiography are given in table 4. In the total series, almost half of the echocardiograms were either normal or did not reveal any definite abnormalities. "No definite abnormalities" includes many patients in whom the recording was not entirely adequate for analysis (72 percent).

In the abnormal echocardiograms, most abnormalities were left ventricular dilatation, hypertrophy, hypokinesis, left atrial dilatation and a decreased E to F slope of the mitral valve. All these findings reflect in some way the condition and performance of the left ventricle. Information on the left ventricular function is important ("road map" for treatment) and this is reflected in the high percentage of patients where this was the major reason for performing an echocardiogram. Also, as 65 percent of the patients examined presented with coronary artery disease and/or chest pain and almost 10 percent with hypertension (these percentages are probably close to the average number of patients seen in private practice), the possibility of evaluating left ventricular function must be considered as one of the major determinants for the usefulness of echocardiography in general cardiologic practice. The number of patients in whom a diagnosis for which echocardiography is a most sensitive indicator and therefore, the first choice method is important as well: pericardial effusion was demonstrated in 6.3 percent (unsuspected in 72 percent), mitral valve prolapse in 5.8 percent, mitral stenosis in 1.9 percent, asymmetrical septal hypertrophy in 2.4 percent and congestive cardiomyopathy in 0.8 percent.

Conclusion

From this experience, it is concluded that echocardiography provides essential and/or useful information in a large number of patients seen in a general cardiologic practice. This improves the diagnostic accuracy which certainly results in better patient care.

In determining the desirability of routine use of echocardiography in general practice, the cost of the examination must also be considered (cost-benefit ratio). This is fairly high and the implementation of echocardiography does appreciably increase the total cost of a cardiological consultation and examination. An increased cost is only justified by an improved quality of patient care but this can only be expected if echocardiography is practiced by careful and well-trained examiners. As with any diagnostic tool, the potential harm from false diagnoses obtained by misuse will be proportional to the potential benefit from good practice. This further raises the problem of training practicing cardiologists in echocardiography and the problem of defining general standards for good quality echocardiography.

Because the performance and analysis of echocardiograms needs an integrated knowledge of cardiac anatomy, physiology and pathophysiology, there is an inherent feed-back which continuously sharpens the diagnostic acumen of the general cardiologist. A last subjective but certainly important reason for considering to perform echocardiography in private practice (and not sending the patient to an echo laboratory), is that it highly serves the cardiologists satisfaction.

Suggested reading

Feigenbaum H: *Educational problems in echocardiography.*
Amer. J Cardiol 34: 741, 1974.

Feigenbaum H: *Hazards of echocardiographic interpretation.*
New Engl J Med. 289: 1311, 1973.

Gramiak R, Fortuin NJ, King DL, Popp RL, and Feigenbaum H: *Report of the intersociety commission for heart disease resources; optimal resources for ultrasonic examination of the heart.*
Circulation 51: A-1, 1975.

Contrast echocardiology.

by Frans Hagemeijer, Patrick W. Serruys and Wim G. van Dorp.
Thoraxcenter, Erasmus University and Dijkzigt Hospital,
Rotterdam, The Netherlands.

Introduction

Echocardiology visualizes heart structures by means of pulsed ultrasound. This direct approach to the cardiac anatomy is most strikingly illustrated by real-time bidimensional cross-sectional imaging methods 1)-7); these pictures immediately bring to mind radiological techniques, more particularly cardiac cineangiography. The only missing item is an injection of ultrasonic contrast material.

Joyner is credited with the introduction of the concept of ultrasonic contrast studies 8), but apparently his work was never published. The first clinical reports 8)-14) deal mainly with intracardiac injections of an acoustic contrast agent for the identification of heart structures. This method also allows qualitative detection of intracardiac shunts during routine catheterization 8), 11), 15)-21); right-to-left shunts can easily be located after an intravenous injection of acoustic contrast into a peripheral vein 20). A review of the literature suggests that contrast techniques can be standardized for applications without catheterization in a laboratory for routine diagnostic echocardiology. This standardization will be described here.

Instrumentation

1. Single crystal M-mode recordings.

This is the standard technique used in most laboratories 22). A single crystal, working alternately as a transmitter and as a receiver, is aimed at a certain part of the heart. Echoes reflected at cardiac interfaces are detected by the transducer and displayed on an oscilloscope. Polaroid photography is no longer acceptable for recording contrast echograms, because it lacks the dynamic capabilities needed for this type of investigation. A M-mode tracing must be recorded throughout the contrast injection, preferably by means of a fiberoptic strip-chart recorder. During the contrast study the probe must be maintained in the desired direction, immobile (no sector scanning) lest movements introduce a second variable where only one is to be studied: the passage of ultrasonic contrast material. Three standardized beam directions can be used for contrast studies 21), 22):

I.   The aortic, traversing the right ventricular outflow tract, the aorta and the left atrium.
II. The mitral, passing through the right ventricle, the interventricular septum and both leaflets of the mitral valve.

147

III. The ventricular beam direction crosses both ventricles and the interventricular septum at the level of the chordae, below the level of the mitral valve itself.

Other beam directions may be selected for special investigations. If different cardiac structures are to be studied with contrast techniques, the injections must be repeated. During each injection the transducer must remain in the same position, and it is recommended that the patient hold his breath in order to minimize extracardiac motion of heart structures.

2. *Multiscan.*

Multiscan 1)-3), 23) was developed in order to obtain bidimensional cross-sectional images of moving cardiac structures. Basically, the system consists of a linear array of at least 20 piezoelectric crystals; fast electronic switching from one element to another allows the ultrasonic examination of moving cross-sections of the heart. An oscilloscope or a television system is used to display the returning echoes line by line in brightness mode. Real-time visualization of a cardiac cross-section is achieved with this technique. Recent development includes a 51 element dynamically focused system 7) and improved display techniques.

For contrast studies, a mere visualization of the heart is inadequate. A videotape is needed to record the multiscan images throughout the injection of contrast. Again, the probe must remain immobile throughout this procedure, aimed at the desired cardiac cross-section, in order to study exclusively the results of the injections of contrast.

The most valuable information can be obtained with two standard transducer positions 13): a) The long axis, visualizing both ventricles, the interventricular septum, both outflow tracts, the aorta and the left atrium, b) A cross-section traversing the pulmonary artery, the aorta and the left atrium.

3. *Sector scanner.*

Sector scanners are essentially single crystal systems 4)-6). We have no personal experience with sector scanners, but they provide excellent contrast images 14). A two-dimensional echocardiogram in real time is obtained by angling rapidly a single transducer through a 30º angle from a fixed spot on the patient's chest 4). Thirty complete frames are generated each second. The recorded echoes are displayed in B_mode on a cathode ray tube. This results in an image resembling a slice of apple pie, with the right ventricle at its apex. Due to the sectorial display method a larger part of the posterior wall of the left ventricle is shown when compared to the anterior wall of the right ventricle. Another, non mechanical method of display is obtained when a small linear array of ultrasound transducers is used to generate tomographic images of the heart in a sector format applying phased array techniques 6), 7). Beam angling during the injection is so rapid that the arguments raised for manually moved single element systems are obviated.

148

For contrast studies, a videotape recording is essential, and the probe aiming may not be changed during the injection, thus the transducer must constantly scan the same cardiac cross-section, e.g. the long axis of the heart or a transverse cross-section of the great vessels.

Contrast

Many substances have been found to generate echocardiological contrast when injected into the heart chambers. The first observations 8)-9) were made after injections of indocyanine green (cardiogreen), but it soon became apparent that virtually any fluid, if injected rapidly, can produce this contrast effect 8)-21), 24), 25). The list includes the following acoustic contrast agents: distilled water, saline, glucose 5 percent in water, blood, indocyanine green, radiological contrast agents, hydrogen peroxide, carbon dioxide and ether.

Obviously the most simple contrast solutions are isotonic saline, glucose 5 percent in water, and the patient's own blood. Ether has been used frequently to measure venous circulation time; it boils vigorously at body temperature and is a very effective contrast agent, even in minute amounts 25). Chemically pure carbon dioxide is a gas easily dissolved in blood; it has been used as a radiological contrast agent 26)-29), more particularly for the detection of pericardial effusion. Carbon dioxide is a safe contrast agent for fluoroscopy 29): even injected in the carotid artery or in the left ventricle in amounts up to 7.5 ml/kg, it produced no deleterious after-effects in the dog 26). Under the same circumstances, air or oxygen killed the animals 27). Carbon dioxide and ether are very strong acoustic contrast agents 25); however, the echoes generated by injections of saline are quite sufficient in clinical practice 8)-21), and the need for gases as echocardiological contrast agents still requires demonstration.

Gas bubbles in blood constitute a strongly reflecting acoustic interface; their detection in circulating blood is easy with ultrasonic techniques 24), 30), 31). However, the presence of bubbles in the injectate is not a prerequisite for the generation of echoes in blood. In vitro experiments and animal studies have shown that slow injections of bubble-free saline produce no echoes; if, however, the same solution is injected rapidly (push injection), abundant echoes are generated 8), 24), 25). This is due to a process called stable cavitation 25), 32), 33), which occurs in the jet stream of rapid injections at catheter tips 33). In the jet stream, the hydrostatic pressure is low (Bernoulli effect), dissolved gases suddenly revert to the gaseous phase, and cavitation microbubbles are formed, consisting mainly of water vapor and other blood gases. These go back into solution as they leave the jet stream and enter the higher pressure of the blood stream. In water, cavitation bubbles may persist during several seconds; in blood, foaming delays the ulterior dissolution of these micro-bubbles which may persist during 15 to 30 seconds. These microbubbles, generated during sudden decompression, constitute an excellent acoustic contrast material; they are carried away by the blood stream, and echocardiological studies may be performed before, during and after the passage of echo-rich blood through a given vascular or cardiac structure 9)-14), 16). The contrast effect is lost during passage through the lungs or systemic capillaries: its appearance across cardiac septa is evidence of intracardiac shunt 8), 15), 17)-21).

Site of injection

Most studies with ultrasound contrast injections have been carried out in the catheterization laboratory: the contrast agents were injected directly into the cardiac cavities. This has allowed echocardiological identification of cardiac structures, visualization of intracardiac shunts, and even of the stem of the left coronary artery.

Actually, echocardiological contrast studies in the catheterization laboratory add very little information to the data obtained with pressure measurements, oxygen saturation determinations, and cardiac cineangiography. Contrast echocardiology will be clinically relevant only if it can be used in the routine diagnostic echocardiography laboratory. A very important contribution came from Valdes-Cruz 20), 21) who showed that cavitation microbubbles generated in an antecubital vein could be detected in the hearts of children, and even of young adults. We were able to confirm this in adults: a push injection of saline (10 ml) through an 18 gauge needle positioned in a basilic vein reproducibly generated echoes in blood flowing through the heart. Injections into the cephalic vein were less effective; injections in the right arm gave better results than injections on the left side. Contrast echocardiological studies can therefore be carried out in a routine laboratory with ambulatory patients, necessitating nothing more intricate than a needle and a push injection of saline.

Standardization

1. Contrast solution: saline (or dextrose 5 percent in water) is effective, non toxic, and is to be preferred over any other solution.
2. Site of injection: the right basilic vein gives the best results; use a standard 18 gauge needle with a three-way stopcock, or a Braunule.
3. Contrast injection: 5 to 10 ml push injection of bubble-free saline.
4. Single crystal studies: M-mode recording on paper by means of a fiberoptic recorder before, during and after the contrast injection, with the axis of the ultrasound beam maintained continuously in the same position. The patient should stop breathing before the injection and breathe again only when the echo-rich blood has left the heart. The contrast injection must be repeated if different ultrasound axes are to be studied. Any scanning movement of the single crystal transducer invalidates the echocardiological contrast study.
5. Bidimensional studies: the images must be recorded on videotape before, during and after the contrast injection for detailed off-line analysis. Cessation of breathing is less important than with a single element transducer. Throughout each contrast injection the multiscan transducer should remain in the same position, e.g. along the long axis of the left ventricle, or cross-sectioning the great vessels. The gain setting should not be modified during a contrast study.

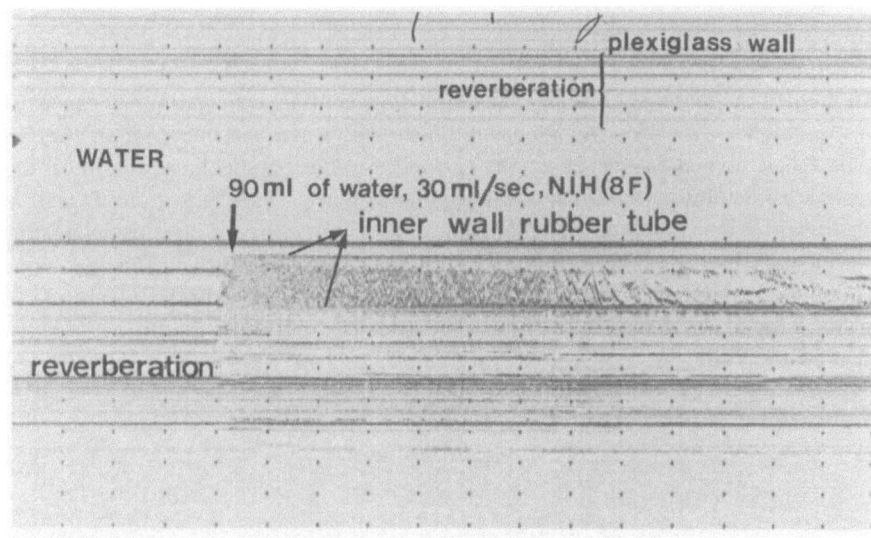

fig. 1. Cavitation microbubbles generated by a rapid injection of water in a water-filled rubber tube delineate the inner walls of this tube.

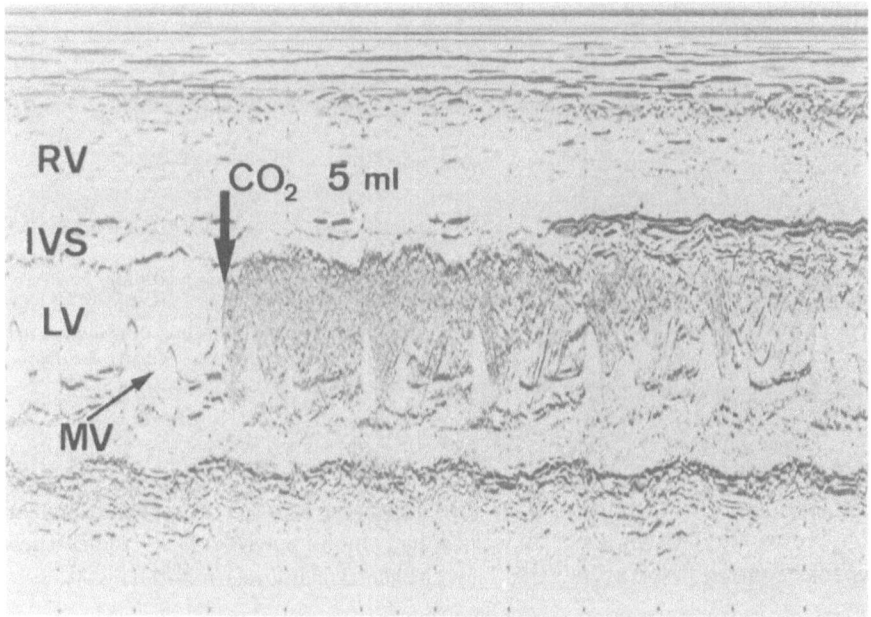

fig. 2. Pig. Single crystal M-mode recording, beam axis directed to the mitral valve (MV). Carbon dioxide (5 ml) injected into the left ventricle (LV) fills this cavity with multiple echoes. Notice that during diastolic opening of the MV, inflowing blood contains no echoes (no mitral regurgitation) RV: right ventricle; IVS: interventricular septum.

Typical illustrations

Structure identification.

An in vitro model (fig. 1) clearly illustrates how contrast echocardiology can assist in structure identification. A rubber tube filled with water was immersed in a water-tank. Single crystal echocardiography showed multiple parallel lines, and it was impossible to determine the inner diameter of this tube. A rapid injection of water in the lumen of the tube produced abundant echoes with clear-cut margins delineating the inner diameter of the tube. Reverberations are also identified. This technique can be used to delineate the left (fig. 2) or right ventricular cavities, e.g. in order to measure the exact thickness of the interventricular septum, or the diameter of the right ventricle (fig. 3).

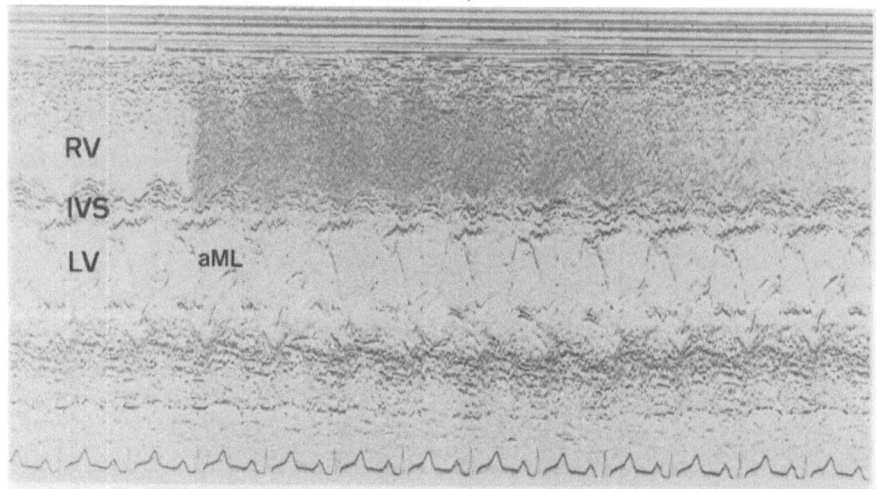

fig. 3. Closure of an atrial septal defect in man. Single crystal M-mode recording, beam axis directed to the mitral valve (aML). The interventricular septum (IVS) is well defined, the anterior wall of the right ventricle (RV) is poorly identifiable. A push injection of glucose 5 percent in water (10 ml) into the right basilic vein generates abundant echoes, clearly delineating the RV cavity. LV: left ventricle.

Detection of intracardiac shunts

Passage of acoustic contrast from the right side of the heart to the systemic circulation proves the existence of an intracardiac shunt. Single crystal studies show whether contrast passes at the atrial or at the ventricular level, or both (fig. 4).

Bidimensional studies (fig. 5) show the passage of a cloud of bright specks through the heart; the images are similar to a cardiac cineangiogram. Right-to-left shunts are easily detected after peripheral vein injections of saline; even in the presence of left-to-right shunting, passage of acoustic contrast from right-to-left may sometimes be observed (fig. 6). Whether gaseous contrast agents (carbon dioxide or ether) are needed under these circumstances still awaits demonstration.

Analysis of flow patterns

The possibility of using microbubbles to study blood flow patterns was first suggested by Gramiak 34). This type of investigation is difficult with single element systems but becomes quite attractive when cross-sectional echocardiological techniques

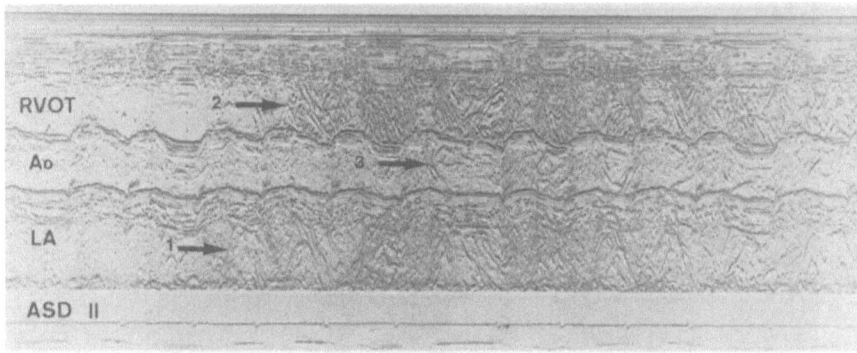

fig. 4. Atrial septal defect with right-to-left shunt. Single crystal M-mode recording, beam axis directed to the aorta (Ao). A push injection of glucose 5 percent in water (5 ml) into the right basilic vein produces snowflake-like echoes in the three cavities crossed by the beam of ultrasound: the right ventricular outflow tract (RVOT), the aorta, and the left atrium (LA). Contrast first appears in the LA (through the septal defect), then in the RVOT and somewhat later (passage through the left ventricle) in the Ao.

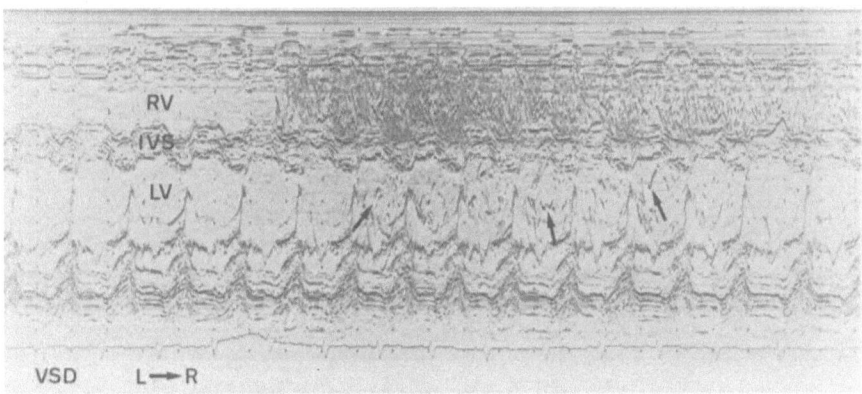

fig. 6. Patient with a ventricular septal defect with left-to-right shunt. Single crystal M-mode recording aimed at the mitral valve. Push injection of glucose 5 percent in water (10 ml) into the right basilic vein. Despite a left-to-right shunt demonstrated during cardiac catheterization, contrast echoes are not confined to the right ventricle (RV) but cross the interventricular septum (IVS) and appear as bright specks (arrows) in the left ventricular outflow tract (LV). On focused multiscan this passage is detected even more easily (illustration not shown).

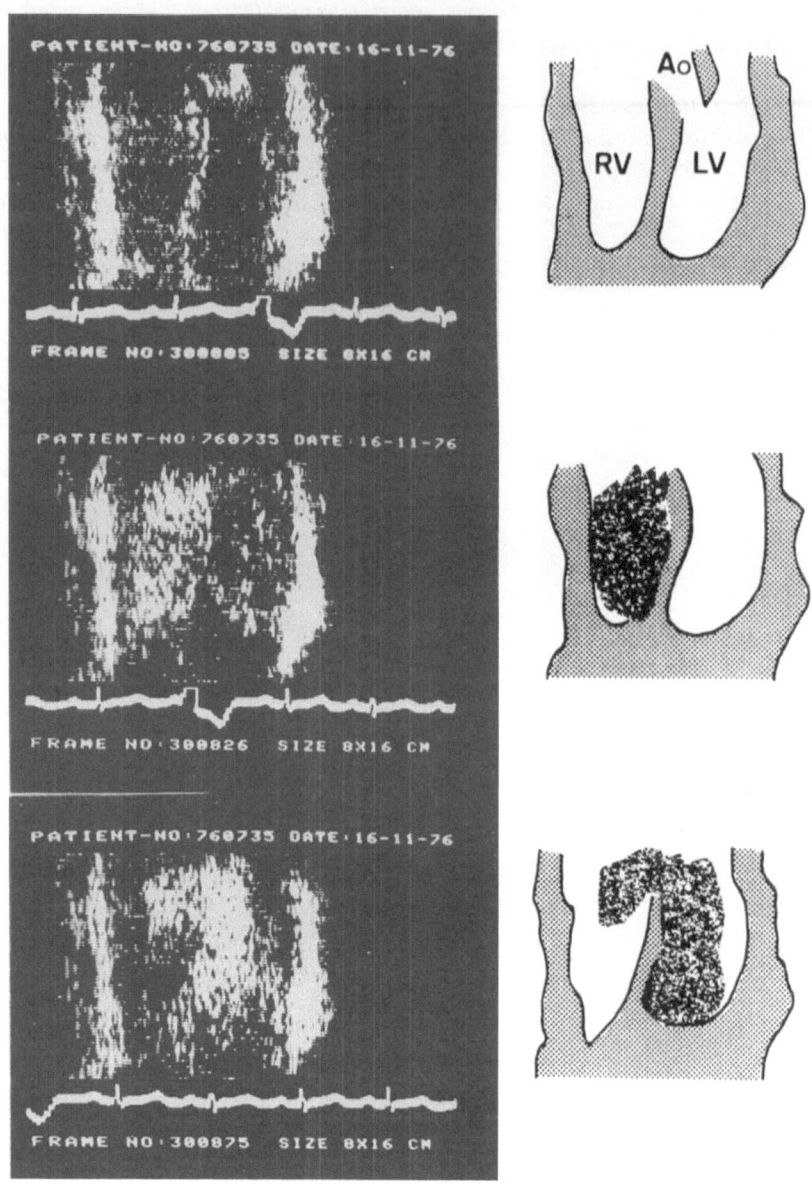

fig. 5. Ventricular septal defect with right-to-left shunt in man. Focused multiscan recording cross-sectioning the long axis of the left ventricle. Before the contrast injection (frame 1), the dilated right ventricle (RV) is clearly visible, separated from the left ventricle (LV) by the interventricular septum. A push injection of glucose 5 percent in water (10 ml) into the right basilic vein generates a cloud of bright specks in the RV (2); at a later stage (3), this echo-filled blood passes into the LV through a ventricular septal defect, and later leaves the ventricles through the aorta (Ao) and pulmonary artery.

154

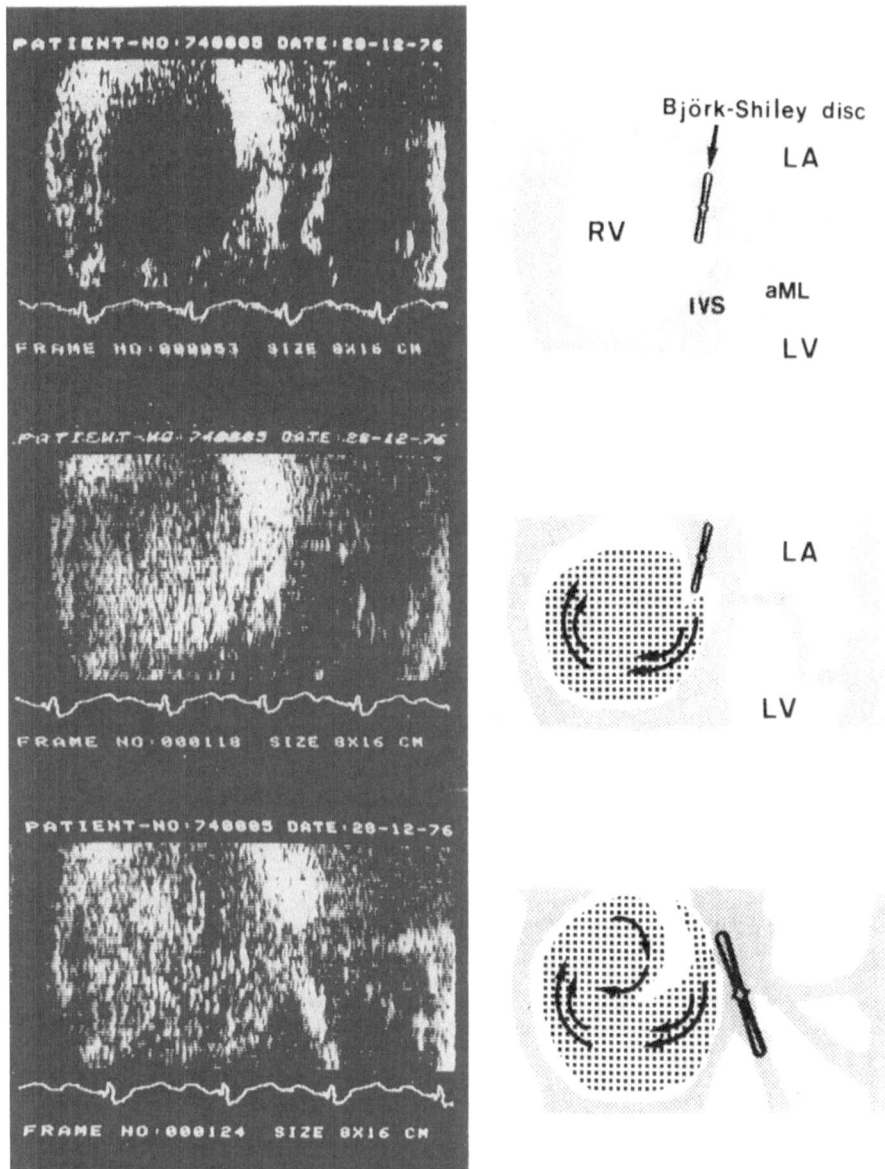

fig. 7. Transverse cross-section through the right ventricle (RV), left atrium (LA), an left ventricle (LV), showing also the interventricular septum (IVS) and the anterior mitral valve leaflet
(aML). Björk-Shiley disc prosthesis in the tricuspid position. A push injection of saline (5 ml)
into the right basilic vein generated a cloud of echoes whirling around the right ventricle during
more than 30 seconds, from where they were progressively whisked away into the pulmonary
artery. The polaroid still frames and the schematic drawing of the whorl pattern on the right
side of the figure bear poor testimony to the striking images seen on videotape.

still awaits demonstration.

Conclusion

Acoustic contrast techniques are now beyond the experimental stages an applied to the heart without catheterization. Studies presently in progress the contribution of peripheral contrast injections to the diagnostic power c clinical echocardiology.

References

1) Bom N, Lancée CT, Honkoop J, and Hugenholtz PG: *Ultrasonic viewer for cros analysis of moving cardiac structures.*
Biomed. Eng. 6: 500, 1971.

2) Bom N, Lancée CT, Van Zwieten G, Kloster FE, and Roelandt J: *Multiscan e graphy. I Technical description.*
Circulation 48: 1066, 1973.

3) Kloster FE, Roelandt J, Ten Cate FJ, Bom N, and Hugenholtz PG: *Multiscan e graphy. II Technique and initial clinical results.*
Circulation 48: 1075, 1973.

4) Griffith JM, and Henry WL: *A sector scanner for real-time two-dimensional e graphy.*
Circulation 49: 1147, 1974.

5) Kisslo J, Von Ramm OT, and Thurstone FL: *Cardiac imaging using a phased (sound system. II Clinical technique and application.*
Circulation 53: 262, 1976.

6) Von Ramm OT, and Thurstone FL: *Cardiac imaging using a phased array ultra tem. I System design.*
Circulation 53: 258, 1976.

7) Ligtvoet CM, Ridder J, Lancée CT, Hagemeijer F, and Vletter WB: *A dynamica, multiscan system.*
(in print).

8) Gramiak R, Shah PM, and Kramer DH: *Ultrasound cardiography: contrast stu tomy and function.*
Radiology 92: 939, 1969.

9) Gramiak R, and Shah PM: *Echocardiography of the aortic root.*
Invest. Radiol. 3: 356, 1968.

156

10) Feigenbaum H, Stone JM, Lee DA, Nasser WK, and Chang S: *Identification of ultrasound echoes from the left ventricle by use of intracardiac injections of indocyanine green.*
Circulation 41: 615, 1970.

11) Goldberg BB: *Suprasternal ultrasonography.*
J. Amer. Med. Assoc. 215: 245, 1971.

12) Gramiak R, Nanda NC, and Shah PM: *Echocardiographic detection of the pulmonary valve.*
Radiology 102: 153, 1972.

13) Sahn DJ, Williams DE, Shackleton S, and Friedman WF: *The validity of structure identification for cross-sectional echocardiography.*
J. Clin. Ultrasound 2: 201, 1974.

14) Weyman AE, Feigenbaum H, Dillon JC, Johnston KW, and Eggleton RC: *Noninvasive visualization of the left main coronary artery by cross-sectional echocardiography.*
Circulation 54: 169, 1976.

15) Kerber RE, Kioschos JM, and Lauer RM: *Use of an ultrasonic contrast method in the diagnosis of valvular regurgitation and intracardiac shunts.*
Am. J. Cardiol. 34: 722, 1974.

16) Seward JB, Tajik AJ, Spangler JG, and Ritter DG: *Echocardiographic contrast studies. Initial experience.*
Mayo Clinic Proc. 50: 164, 1975.

17) Allen HD, Sahn DJ, and Goldberg SJ: *A new echo contrast technique for serial assessment of left-to-right (L-R) patent ductus arteriosus (PDA) shunts in premature infants.*
Circulation 53 suppl II: 47, 1976.

18) Sahn DJ, Allen HD, and Goldberg S: *A serial contrast echo study of cardiac shunts in newborns with heart and lung disease.*
Circulation 53 suppl II: 89, 1976.

19) Seward JB, Tajik AJ, Hagler DJ, and Ritter DG: *Contrast echocardiography in common ventricle.*
Circulation 53 suppl II: 45, 1976.

20) Valdes-Cruz LM, Pieroni DR, Roland JMA, and Varghese PJ: *Echocardiographic detection of intracardiac right-to-left shunts following peripheral vein injection.*
Circulation 54: 558, 1976.

21) Valdes-Cruz LM, Pieroni DR, Roland JMA, and Shematek JP: *Recognition of residual postoperative shunts by contrast echocardiographic techniques.*
Circulation 55: 148, 1977.

22) Feigenbaum H: *Echocardiography.*
Lea and Febiger Publ, Philadelphia, 1976, 512 p.

23) Roelandt J, Kloster FE, Ten Cate FJ, Van Dorp WG, Honkoop J, Bom N, and Hugenholtz PG: *Multidimensional echocardiography. An appraisal of its clinical usefulness.*
Brit. Heart J. 36: 29, 1974.

24) Hipona FA, Sear HS, and Boyle RN: *Precision arteriography with ultrasonic timing.*
Invest. Radiol. 6: 65, 1971.

157

25) Ziskin MC, Bonakdarpour A, Weinstein DP, and Lynch PR: *Contrast agents for diagnostic ultrasound.*
Invest. Radiol. 7: 500, 1972.

26) Oppenheimer MJ, Durant TM, Stauffer HM, Stewart GH, Lynch PR, and Barrera F: *In vivo visualization of intracardiac structures with gaseous carbon dioxide. Cardiovascular-respiratory effects and associated changes in blood chemistry.*
Am. J. Physiol. 186: 325, 1956.

27) Stauffer HM, Durant TM, and Oppenheimer MJ: *Gas embolism. Roentgenologic considerations, including the experimental use of carbon dioxide as an intracardiac contrast material.*
Radiology 66: 686, 1956.

28) Winters W, Wilson M, Chungcharoen D, Stauffer HM, Durant TM, and Oppenheimer MJ: *Use of intravascular carbon dioxide gas to demonstrate interatrial septal defects.*
Am. J. Physiol. 195: 579, 1958.

29) Durant TM: *Negative (gas) contrast angiocardiography.*
Am. Heart J. 61: 1, 1961.

30) Gillis MF, Karagianes MT, and Peterson PL: *Bends: detection of circulating gas emboli with external sensor.*
Science 161: 579, 1968.

31) Rubissow GJ, and Mackay RS: *Decompression study and control using ultrasonics.*
Aerospace Med. 45: 476, 1974.

32) Bove AA, Adams DF, Hugh AE, and Lynch RP: *Cavitation at catheter tips. A possible cause of air embolus.*
Invest. Radiol. 3: 159, 1968.

33) Kremkau FW, Gramiak R, Cartensen EL, Shah PM, and Kramer DH: *Ultrasonic detection of cavitation at catheter tips.*
Am. J. Roentg. 110: 177, 1970.

34) Gramiak R, and Shah PM: *Detection of intracardiac blood flow by pulsed echo-ranging ultrasound.*
Radiology 100: 415, 1971.

Echocardiographic assessment of cardiomyopathies*

by Walter L. Henry and Jeffrey S. Borer,
Cardiology Branch, National Heart, Lung, and Blood Institute
National Institutes of Health, Bethesda, Maryland USA.

Although several noninvasive techniques are useful in evaluating a patient with a suspected cardiomyopathy, none has proven to be as valuable as echocardiography 1). The strength of this technique is its unique ability to noninvasively visualize the left ventricle. In fact, in diseases that diffusely involve the heart (such as the cardiomyopathies), this noninvasive technique rivals invasive procedures as a method for assessing the structure and function of the left ventricle.

Echocardiographic evaluation of the left ventricle

Evaluation of the structure of the left ventricle: Although many early echocardiographic studies stressed abnormalities of mitral valve motion, it soon became apparent that the walls of the left ventricle could be imaged with reflected ultrasound 2)-4). One of the early studies that lead to this realization was by Popp and Feigenbaum, who described a method for visualizing the ventricular septum 3). Once the ventricular septum and posterior free wall were able to be reliably imaged by echocardiography, it was then possible to measure the transverse dimension of the left ventricle in both diastole and systole (fig. 1), and relate these dimensions to the volumes of the left ventricle as determined by angiography 5).

Subsequently, Popp and Harrison derived the relation that the cube of the transverse dimension of the left ventricle was a reasonable estimate of the volume of the left ventricle 6). This simple relation has proved to be a very useful (if only approximate) method for estimating left ventricular volume. Other methods for estimating ventricular volume from echocardiographic measurements have also been published by Fortuin 7) and by Teichholtz 8). However, in order to detect ventricular dilation (as would be necessary in evaluating patients with a suspected cardiomyopathy), the linear transverse dimension of the left ventricle is usually sufficient. In a young adult, the diastolic dimension of the left ventricle (LVTD), ranges from 40 to 54 mm in normal subjects.

During early echocardiographic studies, it also became obvious that the thicknesses of the ventricular septum and posterior free wall of the left ventricle could be measured 9). One of the problems in evaluating free wall thickness was differentiating chordae tendineae from the endocardial surface of the free wall 1). This different-

Echocardiology, N. Bom editor, published by Martinus Nijhoff, the Hague 1977.

iation was accomplished by identifying that the endocardium moves forward toward the chest wall at a faster rate than the more anteriorly located chordae tendineae (fig. 1).

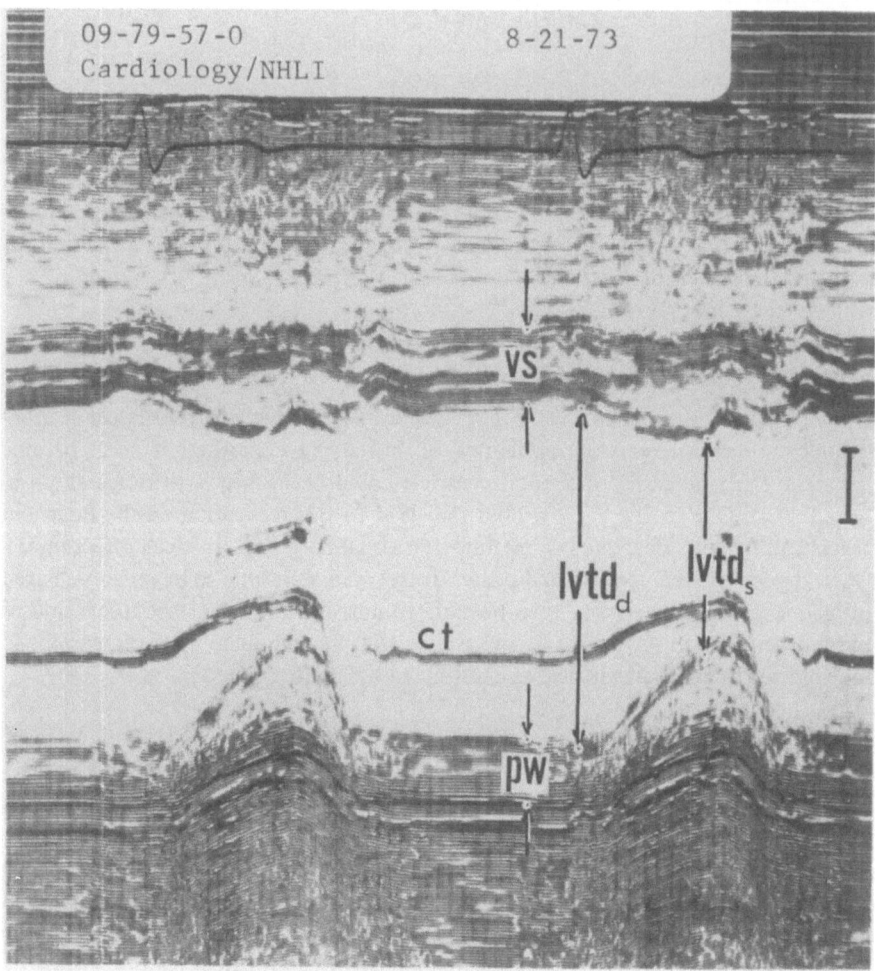

fig. 1. Echocardiogram from a normal subject obtained with the ultrasonic beam being reflected from the left ventricle just caudal to the tip of the mitral valve. The thicknesses of the ventricular septum (VS) and posterior free wall (pw) are measured just prior to atrial systole. The transverse dimension of the left ventricle at end diastole ($lvtd_d$) and end systole ($lvtd_s$) are taken as the maximum and minimum distances between septum and free wall. The echo from the chordae tendinae (ct) is anterior to the endocardium of the posterior wall.

Another problem in determining the thickness of the left ventricular free wall was the identification of the epicardial surface. This problem was solved by rapidly decreasing the gain of the ultrasound receiver until only the strong signal from the epicardial-lung interface was present. This damping technique has been, and still is, an effective method for measuring the thickness of the free wall of the left ventricle. Recently we described a method of electronically switching between high and low amplifer gain settings at a very rapid rate (switched gain) 10). In this method, the switching occurs so rapidly that individual high and low gain regions cannot be seen. However, this rapid switching has the effect of highlighting the epicardium while preserving visualization of the endocardium (fig. 2). In our experience, this modification has simplified measurement of free wall thickness.

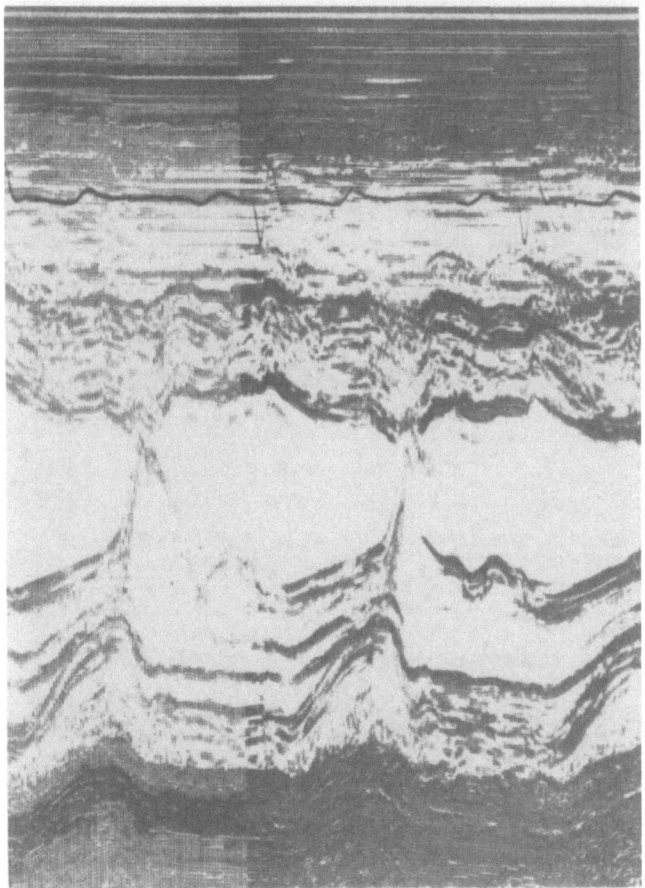

fig. 2. The right side of the figure is an echocardiogram from a patient with an infiltrative cardiomyopathy that was obtained using standard M-mode signal processing. The epicardium is not easily seen in this portion of the echo recording. The left side of the figure was obtained with the switch-gained circuit in operation. Note that the epicardium is clearly seen.

Since the ventricular septum is surrounded on both sides by blood, damping or switched gain techniques are not usually necessary to measure septal thickness. However, it is important to orient the transducer in such a way that the ultrasound beam passes through a portion of the right ventricular cavity before striking the right surface of the ventricular septum. This is accomplished in practice by partially rolling the patient onto his or her left side. In this position, the heart moves laterally from underneath the sternum. This posture change usually allows a larger portion of the right ventricle to be imaged, which in turn improves identification of the right side of the ventricular septum. In a young adult, the thickness of the ventricular septum and posterior free wall of the left ventricle both range from 8 to 11 mm in normal subjects.

Normal values: In order to decide whether a measured dimension or thickness is abnormal, it is necessary to compare it to values obtained from normal subjects. Early normal data were derived largely from young normal subjects and expressed as a range between a lower and an upper limit of normal. However, when data were collected in normal subjects between 2 months and 21 years of age, it was obvious that the data had to be expressed as a function of the size of the subject. The most commonly used method is to relate cardiac dimensions to the body surface area of the subject 11) (fig. 3). A similar relation between cardiac dimensions and body surface area also is found in adults. Thus, normal dimensions for a 5 foot, 100 pound subject will be significantly less than those in a 6 foot 6 inch, 250-pound subject. Therefore, when deciding whether an echocardiographic measurement is normal or abnormal, it is necessary to take the size of the subject into account.

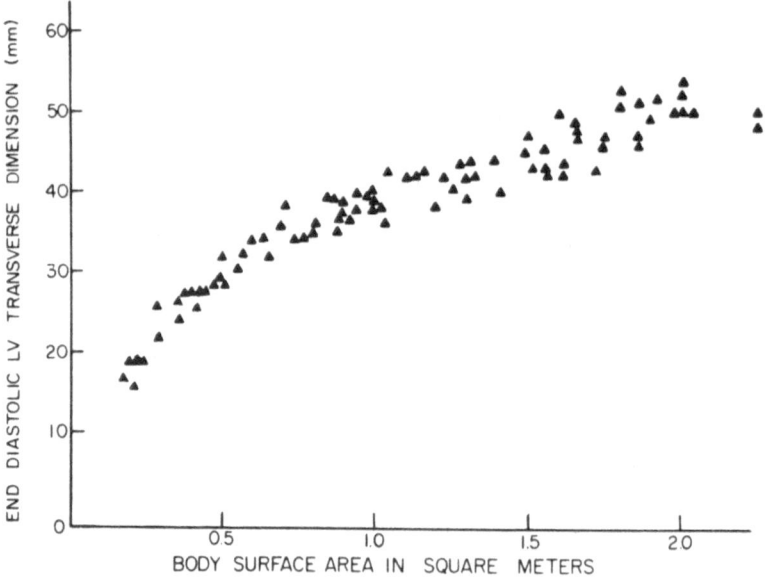

fig. 3. Plot of the transverse dimension of the left ventricle at end diastole (vertical axis) versus body surface area (horizontal axis) for normal subjects ranging from 1 day to 23 years of age.

Several other factors can influence cardiac dimensions. For instance, individuals who engage in competitive athletics have cardiac dimensions that fall outside the normal range. Specifically, individuals who engage in isometric activities (wrestlers, weight lifters), have non-dilated hearts with thick walls, while those who engage in running and swimming have dilated hearts with less wall thickening 12). Aging is another factor that affects cardiac dimensions. Two recent abstracts have indicated that certain echocardiographic measurements are different in younger compared to older normal subjects 13), 14). This is not suprising in view of necropsy evidence that cardiac dimensions change with age.

Thus when evaluating the structure of the left ventricle, it is necessary to take several factors into account. When evaluating a young adult subject of normal size it is probably sufficient to use normal data that are simply expressed as a range between a lower and an upper limit of normal. However, if an adult is unusually large or small, data expressing normal dimension as a function of body surface area should be used. In the future, we can anticipate using normal values that take into account both body surface area and age.

Evaluation of the function of the left ventricle: Several methods have been described for evaluating the systolic function of the left ventricle. Perhaps the most widely used method involves calculating the ejection fraction 1). The equation for the ejection fraction is as follows:

$$\text{Ejection fraction} = \frac{\text{end diastolic volume - end systolic volume}}{\text{end diastolic volume}}$$

Initially these volumes were measured from left ventricular angiograms. However, since left ventricular volumes can be estimated from the echocardiogram, an echocardiographic estimate of ejection fraction can be derived. Any one of the methods for estimating left ventricular volume can be used 6)-8). However, values calculated with each method may differ slightly. Probably the easiest method to use is the cubed assumption 6). Ejection fraction is calculated with the cubed assumption from the following equation:

$$\text{Ejection fraction} = \frac{(\text{LV diastolic dimension})^3 - (\text{LV systolic dimension})^3}{(\text{LV diastolic dimension})^3}$$

The lower limit of normal for ejection fraction calculated from this equation is 65 percent. Because of possible errors in measuring ventricular dimensions, ejection fraction should be below 60 percent before it is considered to be definitely abnormal.

Another method for assessing left ventricular function by echocardiography involves computing the fractional shortening of the left ventricle 15). This computation is similar to that for the ejection fraction. However, the transverse dimensions are used directly in the calculation of fractional shortening, rather than being used to first estimate ventricular volumes. The equation for fractional shortening is as follows:

$$\text{Fractional shortening} = \frac{(\text{LV diastolic dimension}) - (\text{LV systolic dimension})}{(\text{LV diastolic dimension})}$$

This parameter has the advantage of simplicity of computation and does not involve assumptions about the relation of the echocardiographic transverse dimension and the angiographic volume of the ventricle. However, to most physicians this parameter is not as familiar as the ejection fraction. The lower limit of normal for fractional shortening is 28 percent.

The third major echocardiographic method for evaluating ventricular function is the velocity of circumferential fiber shortening (VCF) 16). This parameter is calculated by dividing fractional shortening by the left ventricular ejection time. Although this parameter may have some theoretical advantages over the first two parameters, it has the disadvantage of requiring the measurement of left ventricular ejection time. This additional measurement makes the determination of VCF significantly more difficult. Until studies show a clear advantage of VCF over ejection fraction or fractional shortening, the latter two parameters are recommended because of their simplicity.

Evaluating a patient with a cardiomyopathy

Previous clinical and necropsy studies have indicated that cardiomyopathies can be classified into three groups 17), 18). The echocardiographic features of each of these groups will be described.

Congestive (dilated, hypocontractile) cardiomyopathy:
Individuals with this type of cardiomyopathy are characterized by a markedly dilated heart that contracts poorly 17). Such individuals often have marked congestive heart failure with evidence of low cardiac output. The heart frequently is massively enlarged on chest x-ray. Left ventricular angiography reveals a large and poorly contracting left ventricle. At autopsy, these patients are found to have a left ventricle that is markedly dilated 18).

As expected, the echocardiogram in a patient with this type of cardiomyopathy (fig. 4) reveals a dilated left ventricle (LV diastolic dimension usually greater than 65 mm), and a low ejection fraction (usually less than 50 percent) 19), 20). The separation of the mitral valve leaflets in early diastole is reduced. This latter finding appears even more pronounced because of the dilatation of the left ventricle. This echocardiographic picture of a dilated left ventricle with a reduced ejection fraction cannot be used to infer the etiology of the cardiomyopathy since processes as diverse as diffuse coronary artery disease, chronic and excessive alchohol consump-

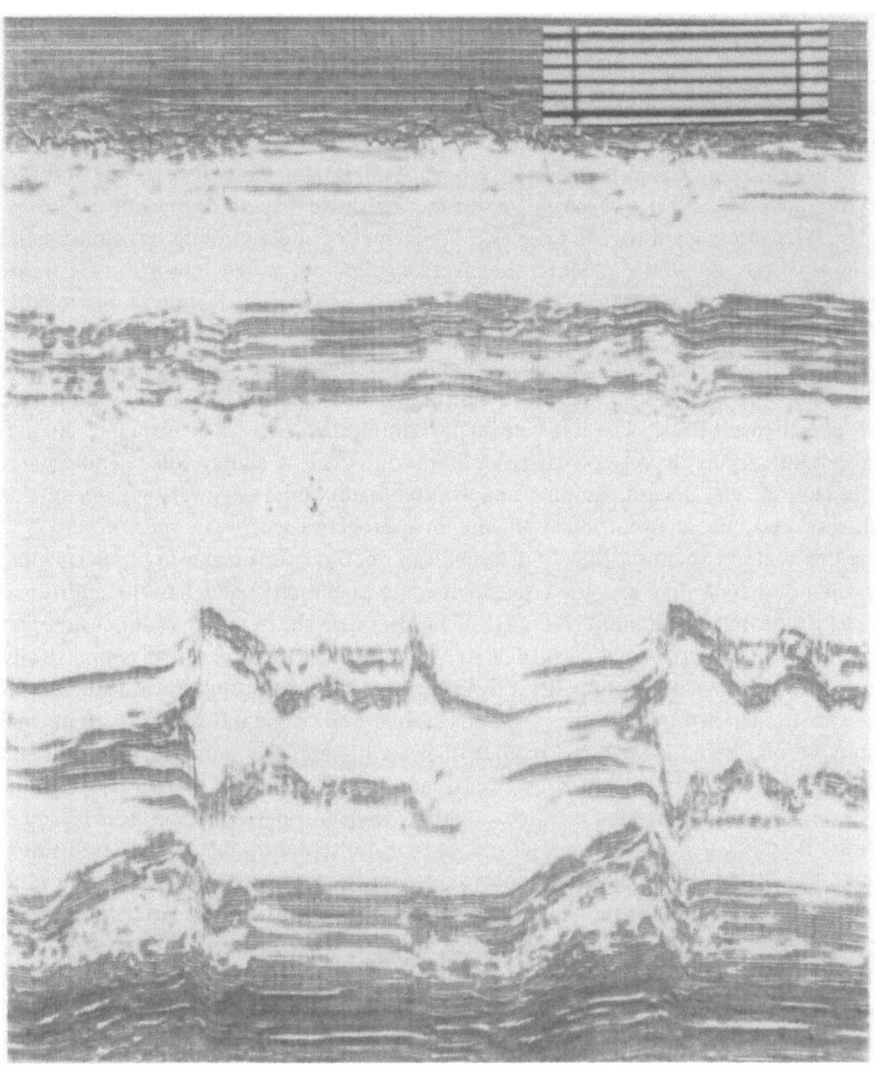

fig. 4. Echocardiogram from a patient with congestive (dilated, hypocontractile) cardiomyo-pathy. The heart is dilated and the ejection fraction is reduced.

tion, and longstanding valvular heart disease can result in this echocardiographic picture. Although the etiology of the cardiomyopathy is unknown in some patients (idiopathic congestive cardiomyopathy), the past medical history of the patient often will suggest the etiology. In addition, information from the echocardiogram may assist in differentiating the dilated cardiomyopathy due to diffuse coronary disease from a dilated cardiomyopathy due to other etiologies 20).

Hypertrophic Cardiomyopathy or Asymmetric Septal Hypertrophy (ASH):

The characteristic feature of this type of cardiomyopathy is marked hypertrophy of the ventricular septum 18), 21). The clinical picture of these patients varies greatly 22), 23). Some individuals are asymptomatic. Others complain of chest pain (both typical and atypical angina pectoris), exertional dyspnea, or presyncope. Orthopnea, paroxysmal nocturnal dyspnea, and fatigue may also be the limiting symptoms. The chest x-ray may be normal, or show varying degrees of cardiomegaly. The electrocardiogram may also be normal or show striking but nonspecific abnormalities. In some patients, the electrocardiogram is characteristic of a transmural myocardial infarction. Cardiac catheterization reveals resting or provokable subaortic gradients in some patients 22). Others have no evidence of left ventricular outflow obstruction 17). The end diastolic pressure of the left ventricle is often elevated, but may be normal. Left ventricular angiography reveals a non-dilated, thick-walled ventricle. The left ventricular silhouette usually is distorted at end diastole and varying degrees of cavity obliteration occur at end systole. In summary, the clinical, electrocardiographic and hemodynamic data may vary greatly in this disease. Only the left ventricular angiogram approaches acceptable specificity.

In this context, echocardiography provides a method for diagnosing hypertrophic cardiomyopathy that has good sensitivity and specificity, and has the additional advantage of being noninvasive 24), 25). Although the transverse dimension and ejection fraction of the left ventricle are both normal, the walls are asymmetrically hypertrophied. This abnormality can be detected by measuring the thicknesses of the ventricular septum and the posterobasal free wall of the left ventricle. In normal subjects and patients with most types of heart disease, the ventricular septum and free wall are equal in thickness (i.e., ventricular septal: free wall thickness < 1.3). In patients with hypertrophic cardiomyopathy, the ventricular septum is at least 1.3 times the thickness of the free wall (i.e. ventricular septal thickness: free wall thickness > 1.3 (fig. 5). Using this echocardiographic marker (i.e., septal-free wall ratio of 1.3 or greater), Clark found ASH in 50 percent of first degree relatives of patients with hypertrophic cardiomyopathy 26). In these first degree relatives, ASH was found equally in both males and females, and appeared to be transmitted as an autosomal dominant trait. Many first degree relatives were asymptomatic and had normal physical examinations and electrocardiograms. Thus, evidence indicates that asymmetric septal hypertrophy is a useful marker of hypertrophic cardiomyopathy that is genetically-transmitted and may be detected by echocardiography in asymptomatic relatives of symptomatic patients 26).

Several conditions may produce disproportionate thickening of the ventricular septum 27). The conditions in which this selective septal thickening occurs most frequently are those associated with severe right ventricular hypertension (primary pulmonary hypertension, valvular pulmonic stenosis) 28). A small number of patients with other types of heart disease may also have septal-free wall ratios that equal or exceed 1.3. In the great majority of these situations the underlying heart disease is recognized from other clinical information. In order to avoid semantic

166

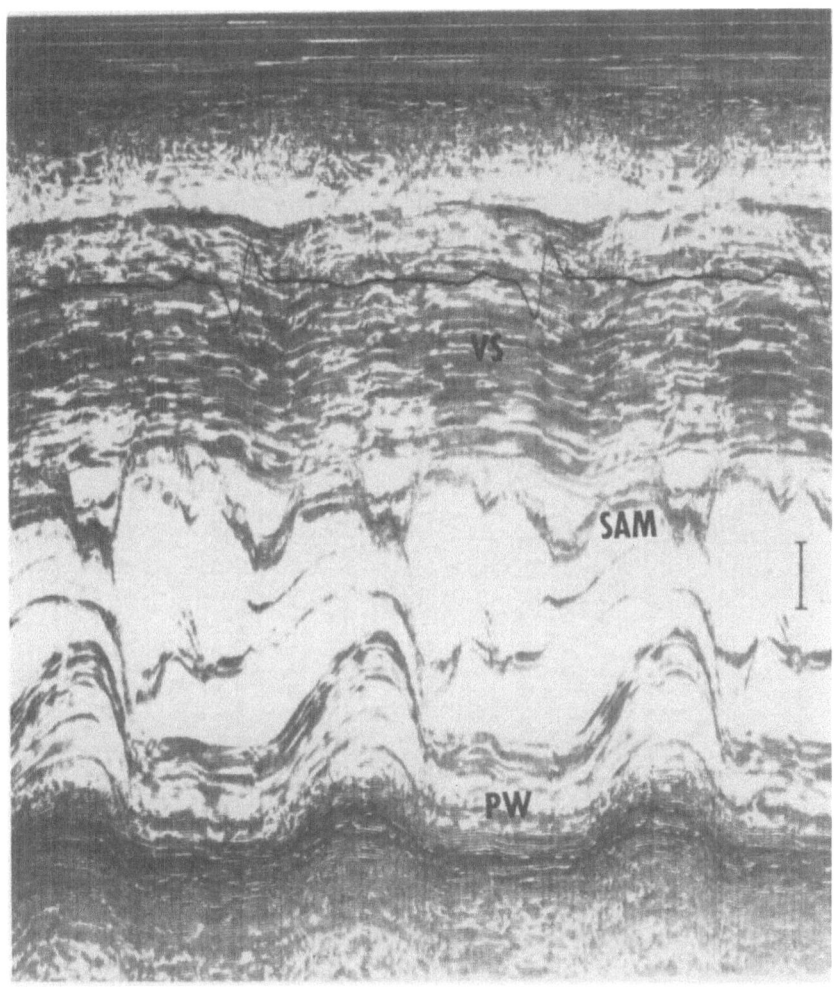

fig. 5. Echocardiogram from a patient with hypertrophic cardiomyopathy demonstrating the marked asymmetric septal hypertrophy (ASH) that is characteristic of this disease. This patient also has systolic anterior motion (SAM) of the anterior leaflet of the mitral valve indicating that left ventricular outflow tract obstruction is present. See legend of fig. 1 for explanation of abbreviations.

confusion, it is suggested that the term *disproportionate septal thickening* 27) be used when referring to patients with septal-free wall ratios greater than or equal to 1.3 who have associated cardiac diseases such as primary pulmonary hypertension. The term *asymmetric septal hypertrophy* (ASH) would be reserved for those individuals with septal-free wall ratios greater than or equal to 1.3 who do not have associated cardiac diseases, particularly when they are members of families in which ASH is genetically-transmitted 26).

167

Another important finding in patients with hypertrophic cardiomyopathy is systolic anterior motion (SAM) of the anterior leaflet of the mitral valve 29), 30) (fig. 5). This abnormal motion pattern almost always occurs in patients who have hemodynamic evidence of left ventricular outflow tract obstruction at rest or with provocative maneuvers (i.e. Valsalva's maneuver, premature ventricular contractions, etc.) 31), 32). Patients without hemodynamic evidence of outflow obstruction usually have no evidence of SAM (fig. 6). In addition to abnormal motion of the mitral leaflets in systole, many patients also have abnormal mitral valve motion in diastole. For example, patients with or without SAM may have a diminished velocity of motion of the anterior mitral leaflet during diastole indicating perhaps that left ventricular compliance is reduced 33).

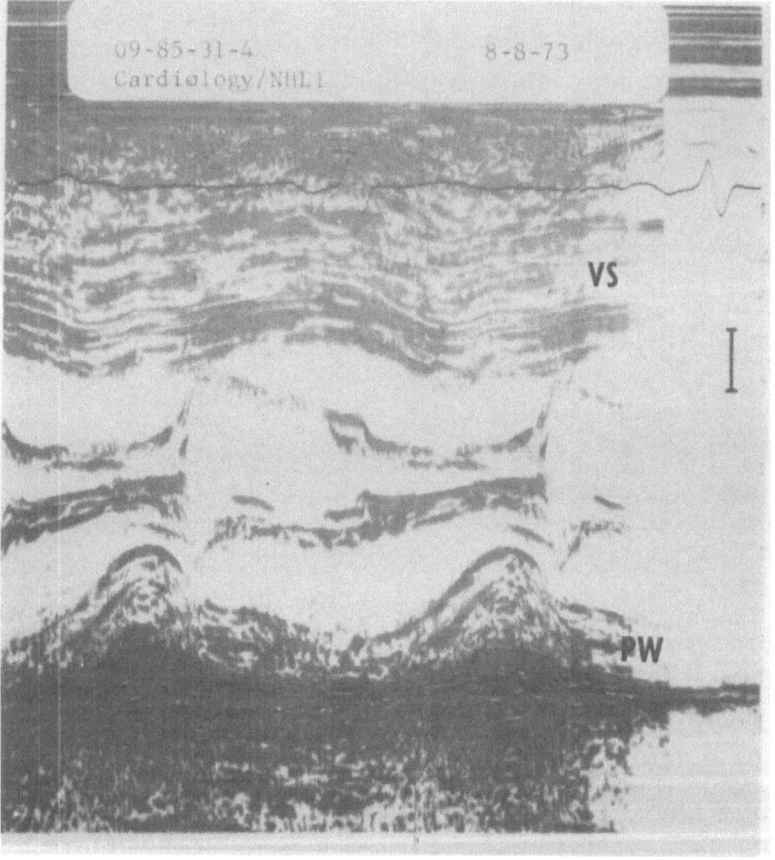

fig. 6. Echocardiogram from a patient with nonobstructive ASH demonstrating the absence of systolic anterior motion (SAM) of the anterior mitral leaflet that typifies the subgroup of patients with hypertrophic cardiomyopathy. Also note that the ventricle is not dilated and ejection fraction appears normal.

In summary, the echocardiogram in patients with hypertrophic cardiomyopathy reveals a ventricular septum that is at least 1.3 times the thickness of the left ventricular free wall (ASH). In these individuals with ASH, the presence or absence of systolic anterior motion of the anterior mitral leaflet is used to determine whether left ventricular outflow obstruction is present. Those with no evidence of SAM usually do not have outflow obstruction and are referred to as *non-obstructive* ASH 34), or *non-obstructive hypertrophic cardiomyopathy*. The majority of patients with ASH fall into this subgroup 26). Those with outflow obstruction almost always have evidence of SAM and are referred to as *obstructive ASH 34)*, or *hypertrophic obstructive cardiomyopathy*. Other names for this less common ASH subgroup are idiopathic hypertrophic subaortic stenosis 22) (IHSS), and muscular subaortic stenosis 35).

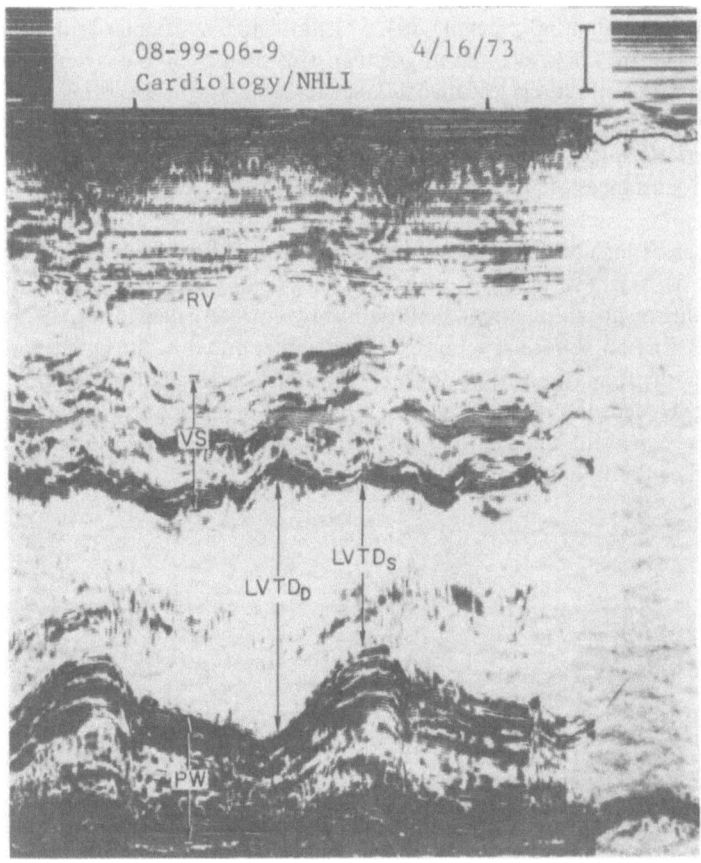

fig. 7. Echocardiogram from a patient with an infiltrative cardiomyopathy. In this type of cardiomyopathy, the walls are concentrically thickened but the ventricle is not dilated and ejection fraction is normal.

Infiltrative or Concentrically-thickened Cardiomyopathy

The hearts in individuals with this type of cardiomyopathy commonly are not dilated and appear to contract normally 18). However, the walls of the left ventricle usually are thick. Although some individuals have congestive heart failure, others may have no cardiac symptoms 17). Both the electrocardiogram and chest x-ray may be normal, or one or both may show evidence of cardiac enlargement. Cardiac catheterization data are not available in large numbers of patients. When obtained, however, the data usually indicate that the end diastolic pressure of the left ventricle is elevated. In the few patients studied, left ventricular angiography has revealed a non-dilated, thick-walled heart that contracts normally. At autopsy, the heart walls are thick. However, the left ventricle may or may not be dilated 18).

In this type of cardiomyopathy, the echocardiogram demonstrates a non-dilated left ventricle (LV diastolic dimension usually less than 55 mm), and a normal ejection

fraction (greater than 60 percent) 36), 37). Both the ventricular septum and posterior free wall are thick, (12 mm or greater). This thickening is concentric and hence the septal-free wall ratio is less than 1.3, see ref. 31). The echocardiographic picture of a non-dilated, thick-walled left ventricle that contracts normally (fig. 7) can be seen in several systemic diseases that result in infiltration of the myocardium with abnormal substances.

These diseases include amyloidosis 36), 37), eosinophilic leukemia 37), and hemochromatosis 37), 38). In this type of cardiomyopathy, etiology is determined not from specific echocardiographic features but by correctly diagnosing the underlying disease. Before an abnormal echocardiogram is attributed to the underlying disease, however, other conditions that produce concentric thickening of the left ventricle must be excluded. In practice, systemic hypertension is the most frequent condition that can produce the echocardiographic features of an infiltrative or concentrically-thickened cardiomyopathy.

Conclusion

In conclusion, echocardiography is useful in evaluating a patient with a suspected cardiomyopathy. By measuring the internal dimensions and wall thicknesses of the left ventricle, and by calculating systolic function, it is possible to classify individuals into one of three categories. Each category has characteristic echocardiographic features and is associated with different etiologies.

References

1) Feigenbaum H: *Echocardiography (2nd Edition)*.
Philadelphia, Lea and Febiger, 1976.

2) Gramiak R, Shah PM, and Kramer DH: *Ultrasound cardiography: contrast studies in anatomy and function.*
Radiology 92: 939, 1969.

3) Popp RL, Wolfe SB, Hirata T, and Feigenbaum H: *Estimation of right and left ventricular size by ultrasound. A study of the echoes from the interventricular septum.*
Amer. J. Cardiol. 24: 523, 1969.

4) Feigenbaum H, Stone JM, Lee DA, Nasser WK, and Chang S: *Identification of ultrasound echoes from the left ventricle using intracardiac injection of Indocyanine green.*
Circulation 41: 615, 1970.

5) Feigenbaum H, Popp RL, Wolfe SB, Troy BL, Pombo JF, Haine CL, and Dodge HT: *Ultrasound measurements of the left ventricle: A correlative study with angiocardiography.*
Arch. Intern. Med. 129: 461, 1972.

6) Popp RL, and Harrison DC: *Ultrasound cardiac echography for determining stroke volume and valvular regurgitation.*
Circulation 41: 493, 1970.

7) Fortuin NJ, Hood WP Jr, Sherman E, and Craige E: *Determinations of left ventricular volumes by ultrasound.*
Circulation 44: 575, 1971.

8) Teichholtz LE, Kreulen T, Herman MV, and Gorlin R: *Problems in echocardiographic volume determinations: echocardiographic-angiographic correlations in the presence or absence of asynergy.*
Amer. J. Card. 37: 7, 1976.

9) Feigenbaum H, Popp RL, Chip JN, and Haine CL: *Left ventricular wall thickness measured by ultrasound.*
Arch. Intern. Med. 121: 391, 1968.

10) Griffith JM, and Henry WL: *Switched gain: A technique for simplifying ultrasonic measurement of cardiac wall thickness.*
I.E.E.E. Transact. on Biomed. Engr. 22: 337, 1975.

11) Goldberg SJ, Allen HD, and Sahn DJ: *Pediatric and adolescent echocardiography.*
Chicago, Year Book Medical Publishers, Inc. 1975.

12) Morganroth J, Maron BJ, Henry WL, and Epstein SE: *Comparative left ventricular dimensions in trained athletes.*
Ann. Internal Med. 82: 521, 1975.

13) Gardin JM, Henry WL, Savage DD, and Epstein SE: *Echocardiographic evaluation of an older population without clinically apparent heart disease.*
Amer. J. Cardiol. 39: 277, 1977 (abstr.).

14) Valdez R, Motta J, Martin R, London E, Haskell W, Popp RL, and Horlick L: *Survey of a normal population with the echocardiogram.*
Amer. J. Cardiol. 39: 277, 1977 (abstr.).

171

15) McDonald IG, Feigenbaum H, and Chang S: *Analysis of left ventricular wall motion by reflected ultrasound: application to assessment of myocardial function.*
Circulation 46: 14, 1972.

16) Cooper RH, O'Rourke RA, Karliner JS, Peterson KL, and Leopold GR: *Comparison of ultrasound and cineangiographic measurements of the mean rate of circumferential shortening in man.*
Circulation 46: 914, 1972.

17) Godwin JF, Gordon H, Hollman A, and Bishop MB: *Clinical aspects of cardiomyopathy.*
Brit. Med. J. 1: 69, 1961.

18) Roberts WC, and Ferrans VJ: *Pathological aspects of certain cardiomyopathies.*
Circ. Res. 34 (Suppl II): II-128, 1974.

19) Abbasi AS, Chahine RA, Macalpin RN, and Kattua AA: *Ultrasound in the diagnosis of primary congestive cardiomyopathy.*
Chest 63: 937, 1973.

20) Corya B, Feigenbaum H, Rasmussen S, and Black MJ: *Echocardiographic features of congestive cardiomyopathy compared with normal subjects and patients with coronary artery disease.*
Circulation 49: 1153, 1974.

21) Henry WL, Clark CE, Roberts WC, Morrow AG, and Epstein SE: *Differences in distribution of myocardial abnormalities in patients with obstructive and nonobstructive asymmetric septal hypertrophy (ASH). Echocardiographic and gross anatomic findings.*
Circulation 50: 447, 1974.

22) Braunwald E, Labrew CT, Rockoff SD, Ross J Jr, and Morrow AG: *Idiopathic hypertrophic subaortic stenosis: I. A description of the disease based upon an analysis of 64 patients.*
Circulation 30 (Suppl IV): IV-3, 1964.

23) Epstein SE, Henry WL, Clark CE, Roberts WC, Maron BJ, Ferrans VJ, Redwood DR, and Morrow AG: *Asymmetric septal hypertrophy.*
Ann. Int. Med. 81: 650, 1974.

24) Abbasi AS, MacAlpin RN, Eber LM, and Pearce ML: *Echocardiographic diagnosis of idiopathic hypertrophic cardiomyopathy without outflow obstruction.*
Circulation 46: 897, 1972.

25) Henry WL, Clark CE, and Epstein SE: *Asymmetric septal hypertrophy (ASH): Echocardiographic identification of the pathognomonic anatomic abnormality of IHSS.*
Circulation 47: 225, 1973.

26) Clark CE, Henry WL, and Epstein SE: *Familial prevalence and genetic transmission of idiopathic hypertrophic subaortic stenosis.*
New Eng. J. Med. 289: 709, 1973.

27) Maron BJ, Clark CE, Henry WL, Fukada T, Edwards J, Mathews E, Redwood DR, and Epstein SE: *Is the disproportionately thickened ventricular septum always genetically transmitted ASH?*
Circulation 55: 489, 1977

172

28) Goodman DJ, Harrison DC, and Popp RL: *Echocardiographic features of primary pulmonary hypertension.*
Amer. J. Cardiol. 33: 438, 1974.

29) Shah PM, Gramiak R, and Kramer DH: *Ultrasound localization of left ventricular outflow obstruction in hypertrophic obstructive cardiomyopathy.*
Circulation 40: 3, 1969.

30) Popp RL, and Harrison DC: *Ultrasound in the diagnosis and evaluation of therapy of idiopathic hypertrophic subaortic stenosis.*
Circulation 40: 905, 1969.

31) Henry WL, Clark CE, Glancy DL, and Epstein SE: *Echocardiographic measurement of the left ventricular outflow gradient in idiopathic hypertrophic subaortic stenosis.*
New Eng. J. Med. 288: 989, 1973.

32) Henry WL, Clark CE, Griffith JM, and Epstein SE: *Mechanism of left ventricular outflow obstruction in patients with obstructive ASH (IHSS).*
Amer. J. Cardiol. 35: 337, 1975.

33) Quinones MA, Gaasch WH, Waisser E, and Alexander JK: *Reduction in the rate of diastolic descent of mitral valve echogram in patients with altered left ventricular diastolic pressure - volume relations.*
Circulation 49: 246, 1974.

34) Henry WL, Clark CE, and Epstein SE: *Asymmetric septal hypertrophy (ASH): The unifying link in the IHSS disease spectrum. Observations regarding its pathogenesis, pathophysiology and course.*
Circulation 47: 827, 1973.

35) Wigle ED, Heimbecker RO, and Gunton RW: *Idiopathic ventricular septal hypertrophy causing muscular subaortic stenosis.*
Circulation 26: 325, 1962.

36) Abbasi AS, Ellis N, and Child J: *Echocardiographic features of infiltrative cardiomyopathy.*
J. Clin. Ultrasound 2: 221, 1974 (Abstract).

37) Borer JS, Henry WL, and Epstein SE: *Echocardiographic observations in patients with systemic infiltrative disease involving the heart.*
Amer. J. Cardiol. 39: 184, 1977.

38) Arnett EN, Nienhuis AW, Henry WL, Ferrans VJ, Redwood DR, and Roberts WC: *Massive myocardial hemosiderosis: A structure-function conference at the National Heart and Lung Institute.*
Amer. Heart. J. 90: 777, 1975.

* Part of this paper will appear in "Practical Cardiology"

Left ventricular wall motion in patients with W.P.W. syndrome studied by echocardiography

by Henk J.M. Dohmen*, Jos Roelandt, Dirk Durrer, Hein J.J. Wellens, University Department of Cardiology and Clinical Physiology, Wilhelmina Gasthuis Amsterdam and University Department of Cardiology, Thoraxcenter, Rotterdam. Interuniversity Cardiological Institute, The Netherlands.

* present address: Department of Cardiology, Groot Ziekengasthuis, 's-Hertogenbosch, The Netherlands.

By echocardiography it is possible to localize both septal and left ventricular posterior wall motion during the cardiac cycle 1)-3). Timing of contraction of any part of the heart is effected by timing of excitation of that particular area. We studied the timing of contraction and the contraction pattern of both septal and posterior wall in patients with W.P.W. syndrome, to gain information about the timing of excitation.

Methods and Material

Using the extra atrial test stimulus method 2) we determined the refractory period of the anomalous pathway and selected 11 patients with a long refractory period of that pathway (table 1).

Table 1

CLINICAL DATA OF PATIENTS STUDIED

W.P.W. syndrome type A and B are defined, according to Rosenbaums' electrocardiographic criteria. *Ajmaline dose*: dose of this drug to be need to block the accessory pathway. Patient 9 showed intermittent pre-excitation.

Pt. nr.	sex	age	WPW type	Ajmaline dose in Mg.
1	♂	20	A	10
2	♂	22	A	12
3	♂	50	A	35
4	♂	35	A	10
5	♀	20	A	
6	♀	44	A	35
7	♂	61	A	21
8	♂	31	A	50
9	♀	22	A	–
10	♀	21	A	37
11	♂	32	B	22

175

No patient had cardiac abnormalities apart from the W.P.W. syndrome. 10 Patients had W.P.W. syndrome type A and 1 patient W.P.W. syndrome type B, according to Rosenbaums' electrocardiographic criteria 5). Out of these 10 patients, 6 were men and 4 were women; their age varied between 20 and 61 years. Echocardiograms were made of all these patients in supine or slight left lateral position, using a commercial available echocardiograph, with a 2,25 MHz transducer, placed along the left sternal border in the third or fourth intercostal space. A conventional M-mode scan (fig. 1) was performed from the aortic root, towards the body of the left ventricle.

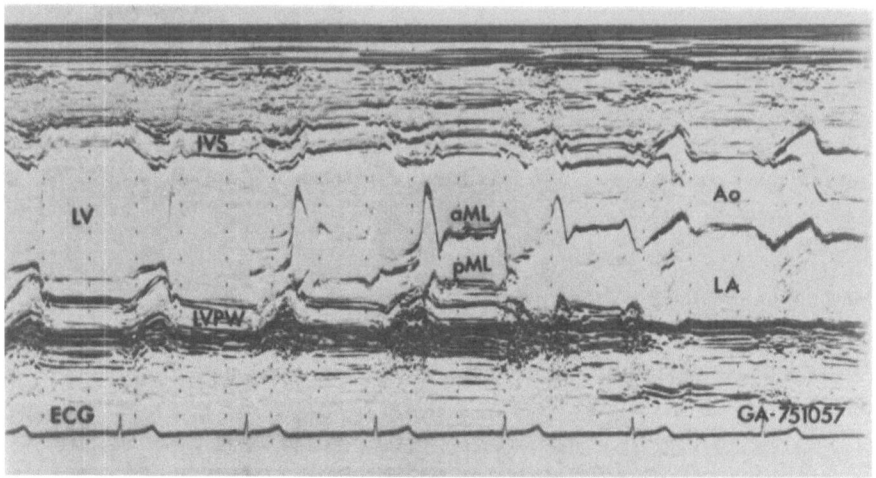

fig. 1. Conventional M-mode scan from aortic root towards body of the left ventricle. Ao = Aorta. La = Left atrium. aML = Anterior mitral leaflet. pML = Posterior mitral leaflet. LVPW = Left ventricular posterior wall. LV = Left ventricle. IVS = Interventricular septum.

The area of the left ventricle where usually ventricular measurements are made 6) was enlarged, and we increased the paperspeed of the stripchart recorder up to 100 mm/sec. Care was taken to keep the same transducer-position. During the investigation the following points were identified on the ventriculo-echocardiogram (fig. 2). Beginning of septal posterior motion was called Bs, and maximal posterior septal excursion Ms. Beginning of posterior wall anterior motion was called Bp and maximal posterior wall anterior excursion Mp.

As reference we selected an electrocardiographic lead with a clear P-wave and QRS complex. We simultaneously recorded continuously lead I, II, III, V_1 and V_5. Ajmaline was then injected intravenously in a dose of 5 mg/min., up to a maximum of 50 mg per patient. As reported before, this drug exclusively blocks conduction over the accessory pathway in patients with a long refractory period of that pathway and does not influence A-V nodal conduction 7). Intervals from beginning of atrial depolarization (P-wave) to Bs, Ms, Bp and Mp were measured during pre-

176

excitation and after normalizing conduction while continuously recording these events (fig. 3, 4 and 5). These intervals were measured in at least 10 consecutive normally conducted beats and averaged (table 2). Statistical analysis was done using the Student-t-test.

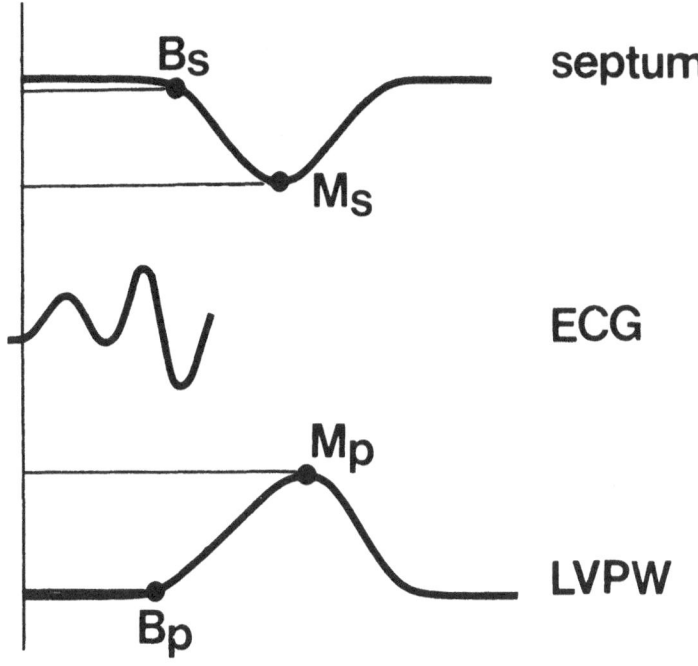

fig. 2. Schematic drawing of septal and LVPW movement related to the ECG. Bs = Beginning of septal posterior motion. Ms = Maximal posterior septal excursion. Bp = Beginning of posterior wall anterior motion. Mp = Maximal posterior wall anterior excursion.

Results

Type A patients:
Interval P-Bs shifted 55, 31 and 30 msec. in patients 1, 3 and 6, respectively, whereas in all other patients there were no significant shifts. P-Ms was often difficult to compare because of the totally different motion pattern on changing conduction. In only 2 patients (pt. 1 and 8) there was a comparable significant shift. Interval P-Bs shifted in 8 patients varying from 26 to 87 msec., whereas in 2 patients this shift was insignificant ($p > 0.05$). All 10 type A patients showed a shift of interval P-Mp, varying from 23 to 119 msec.

Type B patient:
The only patient with W.P.W. syndrome type B, showed on changing from pre- to normal excitation a totally different motion pattern of the septum alone, whereas timing of motion pattern of posterior wall was uneffected.

177

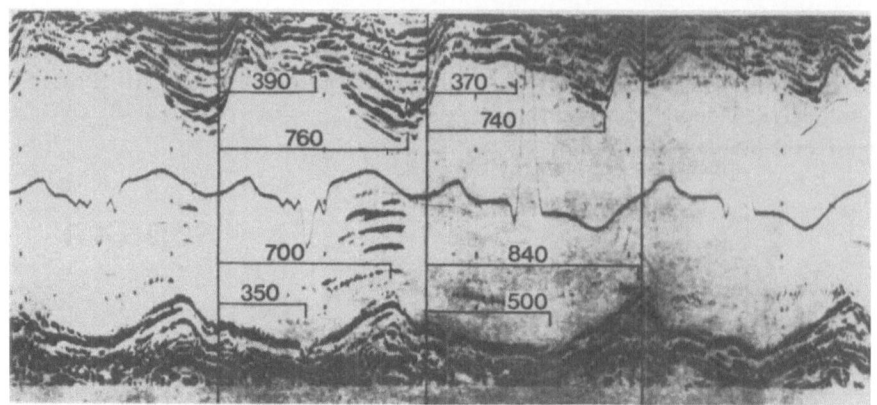

fig. 3. Continuous recording of the change from pre-excitation to normal A-V nodal co
tion. Second beat: pre-excitation. Third beat: normal conduction. No significant shi
intervals P-Bs and P-Ms. P-Bs shifts from 350 to 500 msec. and P-Mp from 700 to 840 mse

table 2

Intervals from P-wave to Bs, Ms, Bp and Mp (see text) were measured in msec
average value during PRE (pre-excitation) and N.C. (normal conduction) are
marized in this table. (asterisk indicates no significant difference between PRE
N.C. with p> 0.05). See text for discussion.

Pt. nr.	P-Bs		P-Ms		P-Bp		P-Mp	
	PRE	N.C.	PRE	N.C.	PRE	N.C.	PRE	N.C.
1	251	306	555	598	327	377*	588	628
2	232	244*	585	591*	260	306	590	654
3	360	391	781	767*	250	337	685	729
4	219	235*	447	446*	201	260	474	580
5	302	279*	611	552*	313	354	528	640
6	215	245	689	662*	237	281	596	668
7	202	202*	483	476*	267	273	551	574
8	186	198*	544	563	224	256	529	558
9	258	264*	632	640*	301	308*	537	602
10	289	207*	589	579*	280	363	537	656
11	233	–	568	–	144	252*	545	545

Discussion

As stated before, septal motion is influenced by several variables (table 3) 8-23

178

INFLUENCES ON SEPTAL MOTION PATTERN

1. Properties of the septal muscle (septal infarction, ASH).
2. Mode of excitation
3. Right or left ventricular volume overload
4. Pulmonary hypertension
5. Post cardiac surgery
6. Abnormal pericardium
7. Site and direction of recording.

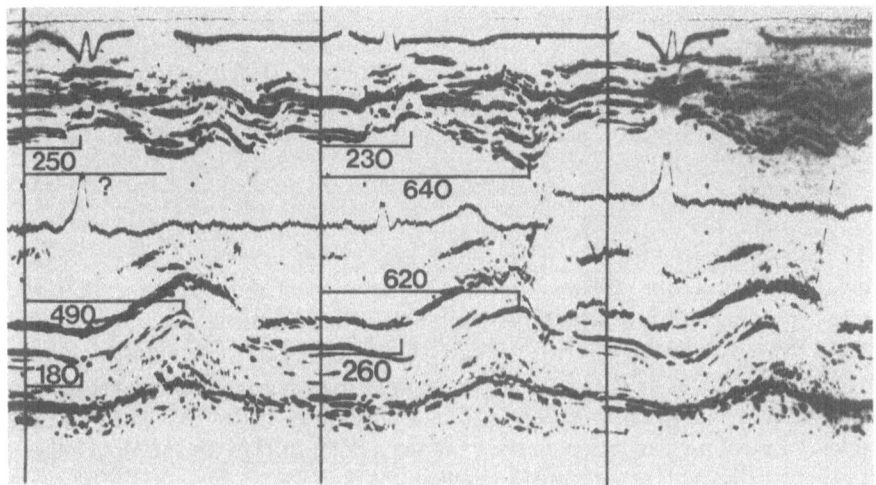

fig. 4. Continuous recording of the change from pre-excitation to normal A-V nodal conduction. First beat: pre-excitation. Second beat: normal conduction. No significant shift of intervals P-Bs whereas interval P-Ms is not comparable. P-Bs shifts from 180-260 msec. and P-Mp from 490 to 620 msec.

Normal septal activation results in normal septal motion whereas in left bundle branch block altered septal activation results in a typical motion pattern 9)-11). During pre-excitation, all our patients had a different septal motion pattern, as compared to normal A-V nodal (e.g. septal) activation. In 3 out of 10 type A patients also a shift of timing of Bs and Ms was seen to a later event varying from 20-55 msec. In these 3 patients, points Bs and Ms were comparable, whereas in the remaining 7 patients these points were not comparable or there was no shift at all, depending on the degree of normal A-V nodal (septal) activation during pre-excitation. When there was significant septal shift one could suppose that septal activation was achieved mainly over an accessory pathway. Patient nr. 1 showed mainly a shift of the septal events and his ECG is suggestive for pre-excitation of the septum (fig. 6).

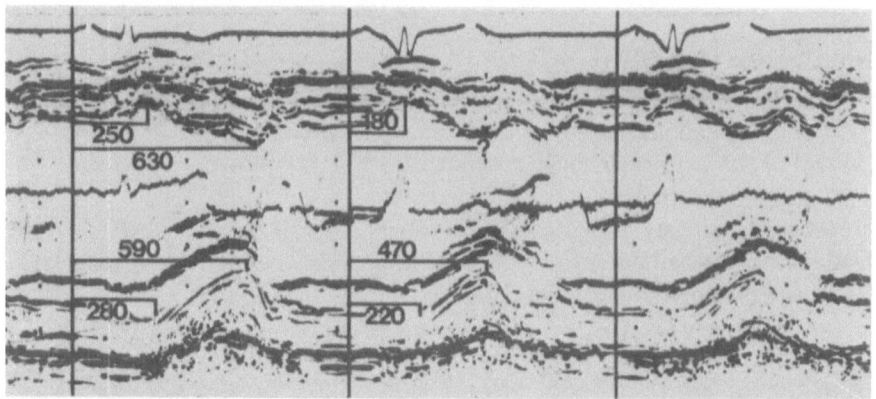

fig. 5. Continuous recording of the change from normal A-V nodal conduction to pre-excitation. First beat: normal conduction. Second beat: pre-excitation. Interval P-Bs shifts from 250 to 180 msec., whereas P-Ms is not comparable. P-Bs shifts from 280 to 220 msec. and P-Mp from 590 to 470 msec.

As far as the posterior wall was concerned a variation of shifts of Bp and Mp was seen, depending on the degree of pre-excitation of that area. It is conceivable that if only a small part of the ventricle is activated over the bypass, these shifts in timing of wall motion will be less conspicious then when a larger area of the ventricle is activated over the accessory pathway. This is illustrated in fig. 7A and B, where a minor degree of pre-excitation on the ECG and a slight shift of Bp and Mp is noticed in patient 2 (fig. 7A), as compared to patient 10 (fig. 7B).

It is our opinion that once posterior wall excitation starts, complete contraction will follow. We never observed "pre-contraction" of that area as demonstrated by DeMaria et al. 22). One can argue against the use of ajmaline to normalize conduction, because of the possible direct effect of this drug on the contraction of the left ventricle. We studied therefore the motion pattern of the LVPW and septum in normal persons (normal AVN conduction) and in W.P.W. patients where we were not able to block conduction over the accessory pathway after injecting 50 mg of this drug. In both groups septum and LVPW motion did not change. Besides that we studied one patient (pt. 9) with intermittent pre-excitation, who shows a beat to beat shift of these events depending on the excitation pattern. A shift of both septal and posterior wall events after maximal pre-excitation is suggestive for location of the anomalous pathway somewhere between the septum and posterior wall of the left ventricle. When only timing of the LVPW motion is affected and septal motion does not change, the anomalous pathway may be located at the posterior wall at a distance from the septum (see fig. 8). The findings of patient 2 and 10 support this theory.

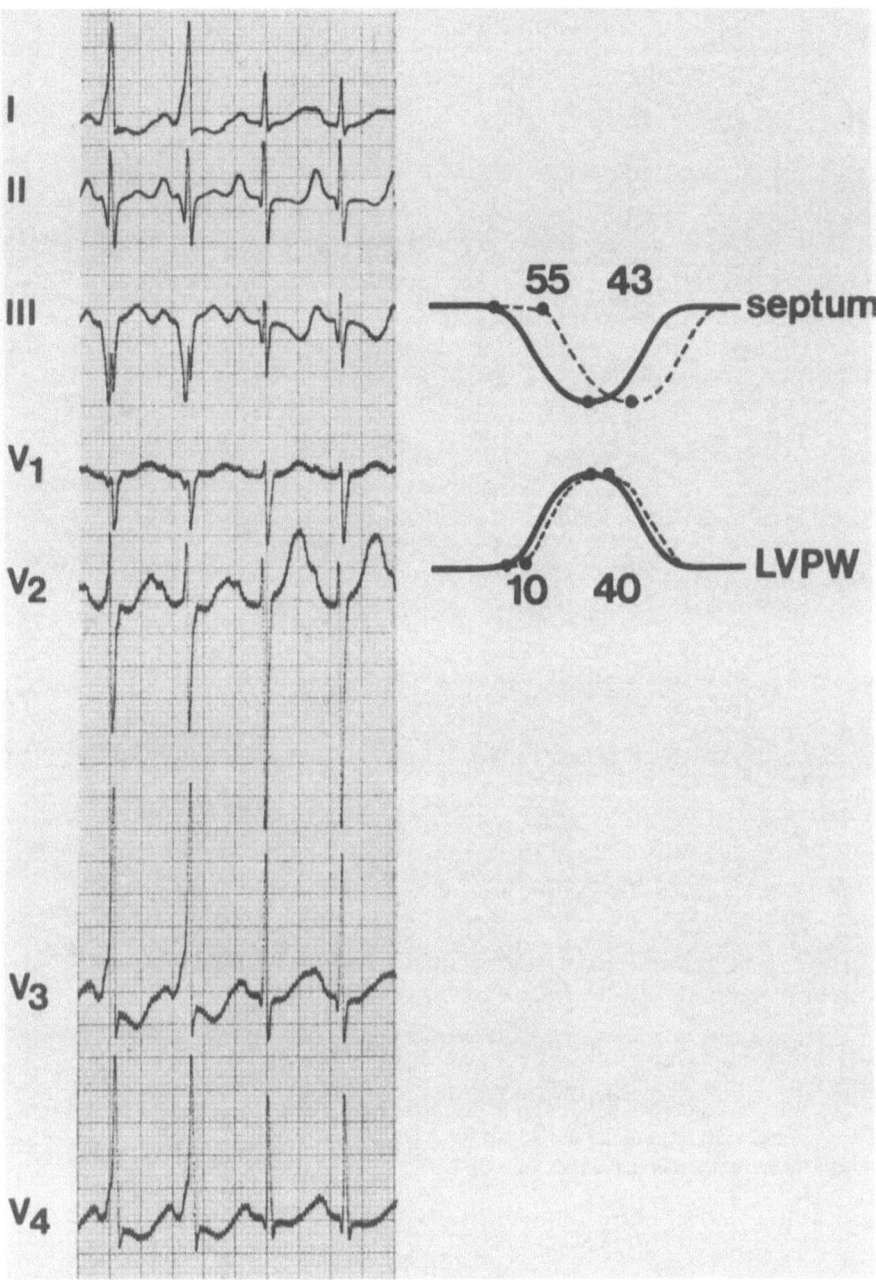

fig. 6. Shift of septal and LVPW motion going from pre-excitation to normal conduction. (pt. 1). ECG is suggestive for pre-excitation of the posterior septal area. Motion shift of the septal and posterior wall is about equal.

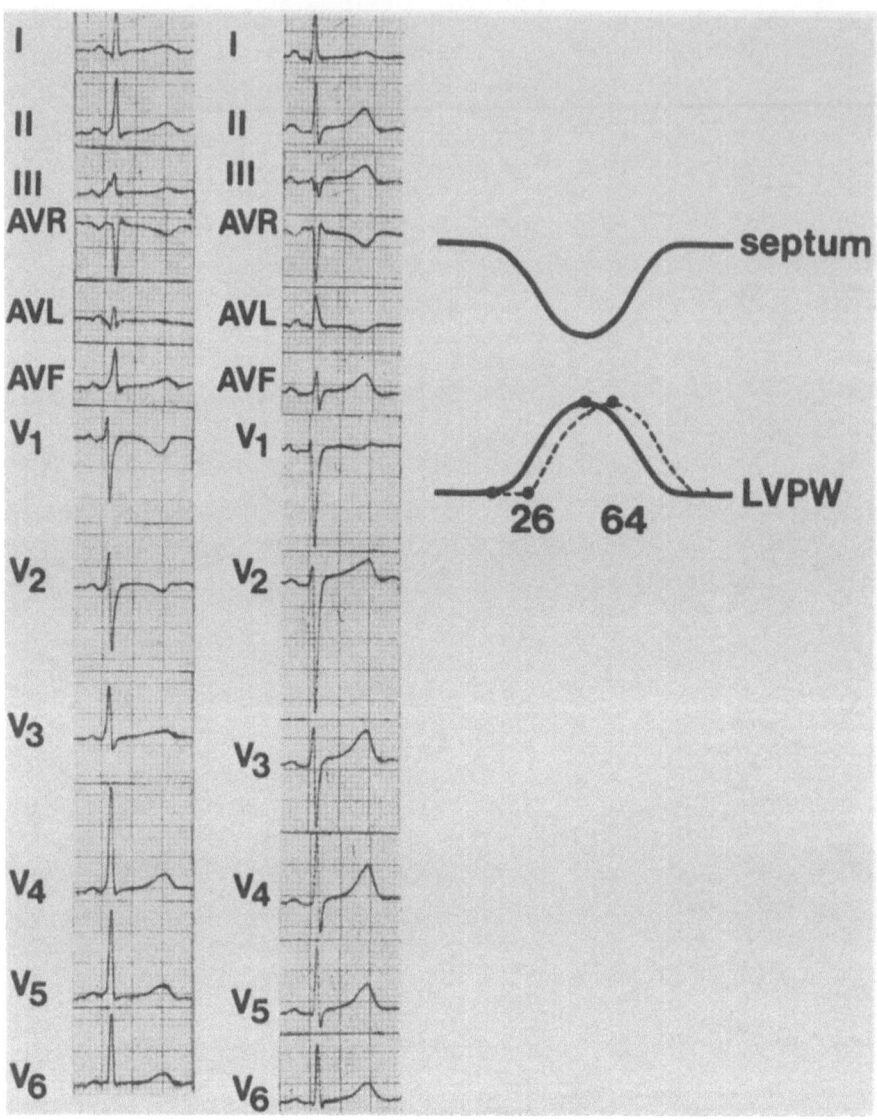

fig. 7A. Minor shift of posterior wall events. ECG is suggestive for a lesser amount of pre-excitation of the posterior wall (patient nr. 2)

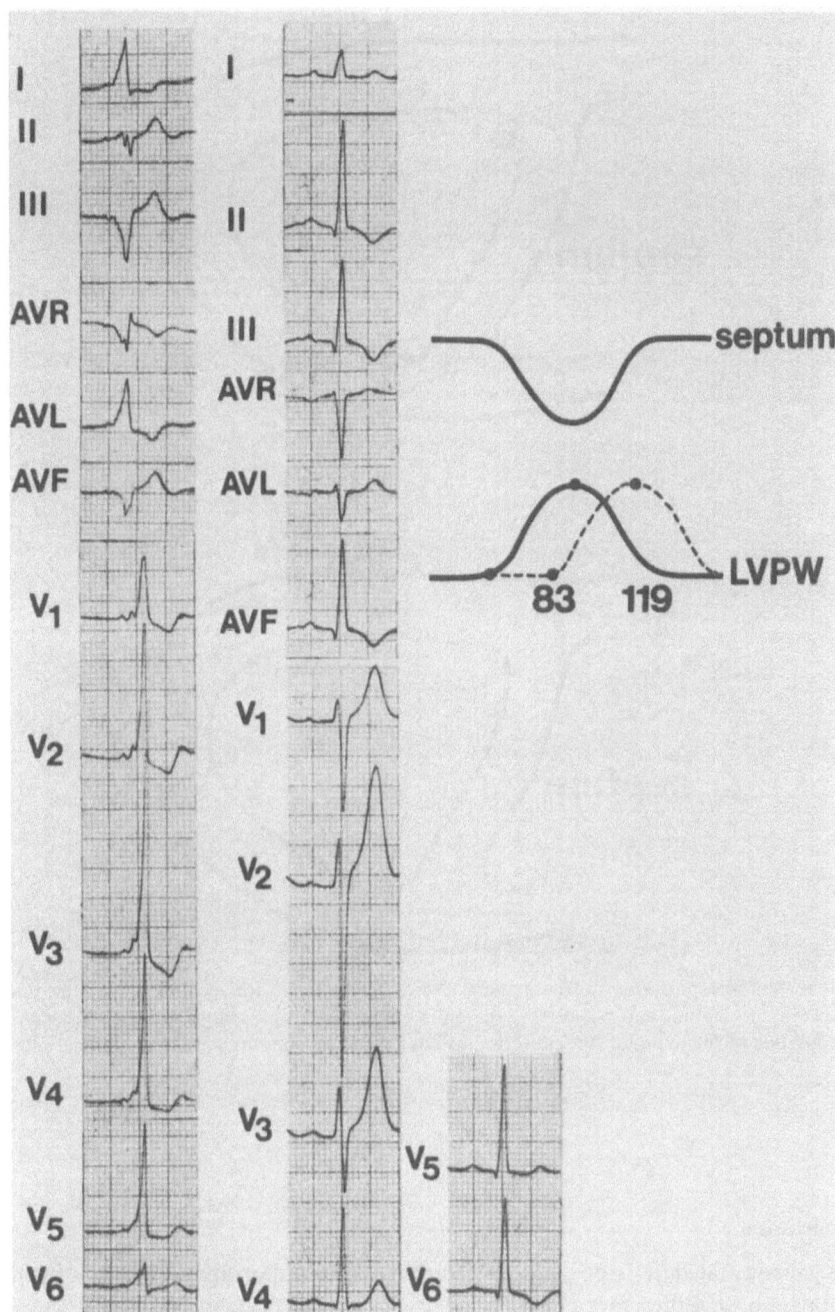

fig. 7B. Maximal shift of posterior wall events. ECG is suggestive for a maximal posterior wall pre-excitation (patient nr. 10).

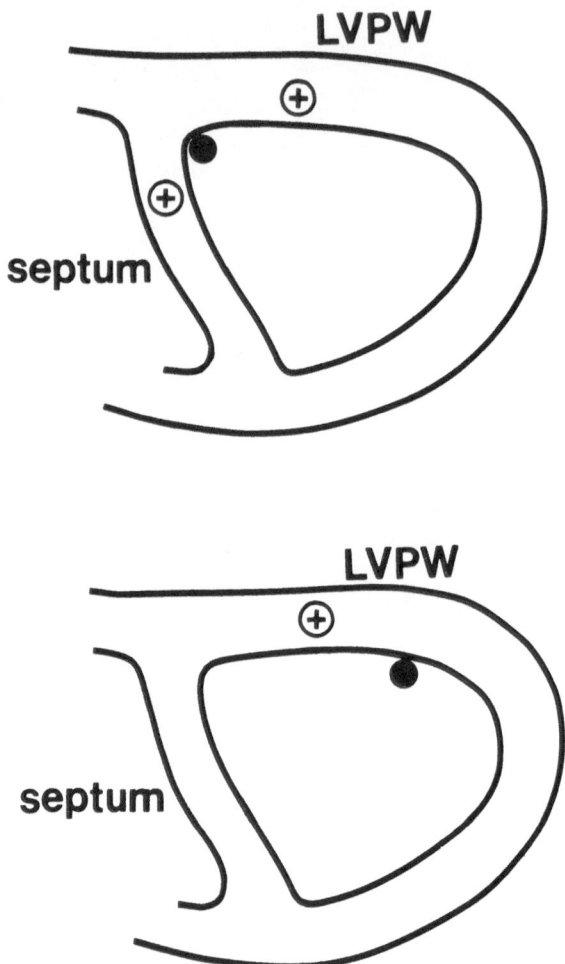

fig. 8. Shift of posterior wall and septal events is suggestive for localization of the bypass between the septum and posterior wall. Shift of posterior wall events alone is suggestive for localisation of the bypass at the posterior wall at a distance from the septum.

Conclusion

As demonstrated it is possible to detect by echocardiography an area of earlier contraction and therefore an area of pre-excitation, by changing the mode of excitation in patients with W.P.W. syndrome. This may give some additional information about the possible localization of the anomalous pathway.

References

1) Feigenbaum H: *Echocardiography.*
   Second edition. Philadelphia, Lea & Febiger, 1976.

2) Feigenbaum H: *Echocardiographic examination of the left ventricle.*
   (Editorial) Circulation 51: 1, 1975.

3) Feigenbaum H: *Clinical applications of echocardiography.*
   Prog. Cardiovasc. Dis. 14: 531, 1972.

4) Wellens HJJ, Schuilenberg RM, and Durrer D: *Electrical stimulation of the heart in pa-tients with Wolff-Parkinson-White syndrome, type A.*
   Circulation 43: 99, 1971.

5) Rosenbaum FF, Hecht HH, and Wilson FN, et al.: *Potential variations of the thorax and the esophagus in anomalous atrio-ventricular excitation (Wolff-Parkinson-White syn-drome).*
   Am. Heart J. 29: 281, 1945.

6) Popp RL, and Harrison DC: *Ultrasonic cardiac echocardiography for determining stroke volume and valvular regurgitation.*
   Circulation 41: 493, 1970.

7) Wellens HJJ, and Durrer D: *Effect of procaine-amide, quinidine, and ajmaline in the Wolff-Parkinson-White syndrome.*
   Circulation 50: 114, 1974.

8) Assad-Morell JL, Tajik AJ, and Giuliani ER: *Echocardiography of the ventricular septum.*
   Prog. Cardiovasc. Dis. 17: 219, 1974.

9) Dillon JC, Chang S, and Feigenbaum H: *Echocardiographic manifestations of left bundle branch block.*
   Circulation 49: 876, 1974.

10) Abbasi AS, Eber LM, Macalpin RN, and Kattus AA: *Paradoxical motion of inter ventricu-lar septum in left bundle branch block.*
    Circulation 49: 423, 1974.

11) McDonald IG: *Echocardiographic demonstration of abnormal motion of the interventri-cular septum in left bundle branch block.*
    Circulation 48: 272, 1973.

12) Winters WL, and Chapman R: *Variations in ventricular septal motion defined by echocar-diography. (abstr.)*
    Circulation 48 and 49 (suppl. IV): 231, 1973.

13) Meyer RA, Schwartz DC, Benzing G, and Kaplan S: *Ventricular septum in right ventricular volume overload.*
    Am. J. Cardiol. 30: 349, 1972.

14) Kerber RE, Dippel WF, and Abboud FM: *Abnormal motion of interventricular septum in right ventricular volume overload.*
    Circulation 48: 86, 1973.

185

15) Tajik AJ, Gau GT, and Schattenberg TT: *Echocardiogram in total anomalous pulmonary venous drainage.*
Mayo Clin. Proc. 47: 247, 1972.

16) Hagan AD, Francis GS, Sah DJ, Karlinger JS, Friedman WF, and O'Rourke RA: *Ultrasound evalution of systolic anterior septal motion in patients with and without right ventricular volume overload.*
Circulation 50: 248, 1974.

17) Jacobs JJ, Feigenbaum H, Corya BC, and Phillips JF: *Detection of left ventricular asynergy by echodardiography.*
Circulation 48: 263, 1973.

18) Chandra MS, Kerber RE, Brown DD, and Funk DC: *Echocardiography in Wolff-Parkinson-White syndrome.*
Circulation 53: 943, 1976.

19) Kanakis Ch, Wyndham CRC, Younce C, Miller R, and Rosen K: *Echocardiographic findings in the Wolff-Parkinson-White syndrome. (abstr.)*
Circulation 51 and 52 (suppl. 11): 11 200, 1975.

20) Francis G, Theroux P, O'Rourke R, Hagan A, and Johnson A: *An echocardiographic study of interventricular septal motion in the Wolff-Parkinson-White syndrome.*
Circulation 54: 174, 1976.

21) Ticzon AR, Damato AN, Caracta AR, Russo G, Foster JR, and Lau SH: *Interventricular septal motion during pre-excitation and normal conduction in Wolff-Parkinson-White syndrome. Echocardiographic and Electrophysiologic correlation.*
Am. J. of Cardio. 37: 840, 1976.

22) Demaria A, Vera Z, Neumann A, and Mason DT: *Alternations in ventricular contraction pattern in the Wolff-Parkinson-White syndrome.*
Circulation 53: 249, 1976.

23) Hishida H, Sotobata I, Koike Y, Okumura M, and Mizuno Y: *Echocardiographic patterns of ventricular contraction in the Wolff-Parkinson-White syndrome.*
Circulation 54: 567, 1976.

186

Chapter 2

DOPPLER INSTRUMENTS

AND

APPLICATIONS

Continuous wave and pulsed Doppler flowmeters - a general introduction

by Robert S. Reneman and Arnold Hoeks,
Departments of Physiology and Biophysics, Biomedical Centre,
University of Limburg, Maastricht, The Netherlands.

Introduction

In the past decades several techniques have been developed to determine cardiac output and blood flow to organs. Most of these techniques are indirect and do not measure blood flow as an instantaneous function of time. This information can be obtained by means of techniques based upon Faraday's law of electromagnetic induction 1)-5), or techniques which make use of ultrasonic waves, e.g. Doppler flowmeters 6)-11). Although very different in principle, their basic objective is similar. Both systems operate by coupling an external field through a vessel wall into the bloodstream and measure, without opening the vessel, a physical parameter which is proportional to blood flow velocity. Doppler flowmeters have some major advantages over electromagnetic flowmeters. Not only because these instruments can be used transcutaneously and in radio-telemetry, but also because some of the difficulties in electromagnetic flowmeters are not met in Doppler systems. On the other hand, quantitative information is still difficult to obtain with Doppler flowmeters. In spite of this disadvantage Doppler instruments have demonstrated their value in the clinical diagnosis of cardiovascular diseases. The aim of the present survey is to summarize the principle, advantages, limitations and applications of Doppler flowmeters.

Principle

In Doppler flowmeters a beam of ultrasonic waves (at the MHz level) is transmitted from a vibrating crystal diagonally through the vessel wall into the bloodstream. Some of the ultrasonic power is reflected by the various structures in the body and received by another or the same crystal. The crystals are mounted in a transducer, either for transcutaneous or for perivascular application or on a catheter for intravascular use. In transcutaneous use, acoustic gel is applied between the crystals and the skin to improve the acoustic coupling (fig. 1).

The ultrasound backscattered from stationary surfaces has the same frequency as the transmitter. In contrast, ultrasound backscattered from particles in the flowing blood, mainly the red cells, is shifted in frequency by an amount proportional to the velocity of the particles. This frequency shift (the Doppler signal = f_d), which is detected by mixing the transmitted and received signals, is in the audio range and equals: $f_d = \dfrac{2 f_t v \cos \alpha}{c}$ in which f_t = transmitter frequency, v = velocity of the par-

Echocardiology, N. Bom editor, published by Martinus Nijhoff, the Hague 1977.

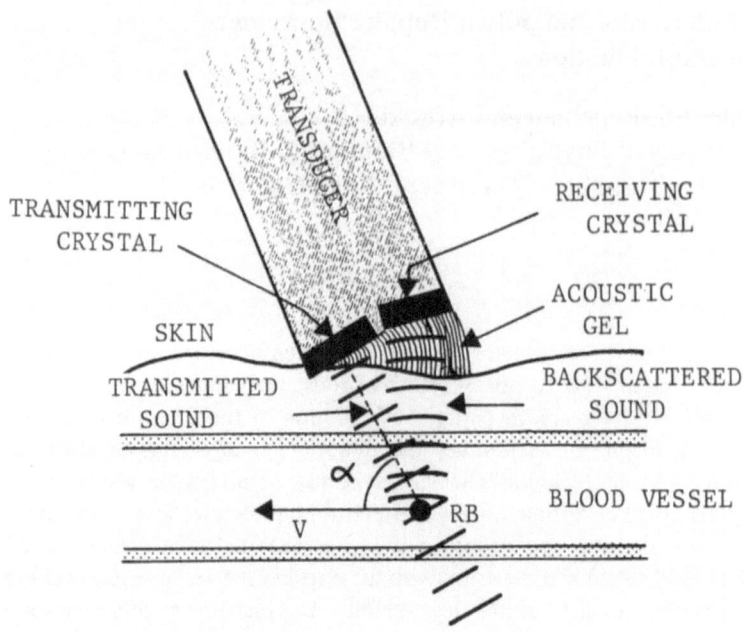

fig. 1. Principle of transcutaneous continuous wave (CW) Doppler flowmetry. The arrow indicates the flow velocity (v) direction. a = the angle between the transmitted sound beam and the direction of flow. RB = red blood cell.

ticles, a = the angle between the transmitted soundbeam and the direction of the velocity of the particles and c = the velocity of sound in the medium (fig. 1).

The Doppler signal does not contain one single frequency, but a spectrum of frequencies (the Doppler spectrum). The variations in frequency distribution depend on such factors as unequal distribution of the red blood cell velocity over the cross-sectional area of the vessel, variations in the red blood cell interspaces, and divergence and nonuniformity of the sound beams, resulting in variations in a (eq 1) when the red blood cells approach the transducer. Changes in the shape of the frequency spectrum caused by beam divergence and amplitude modulation effects are small for the far field region 12). In transcutaneous devices it is usually possible to perform measurements in the far field, which is not the case in cuff probes. Under ideal circumstances, i.e. sharply bounded and uniform sound beams, bathing of the whole cross-section of the vessel in the ultrasonic beam, equal red blood cell and plasma velocity and axisymmetric velocity profiles, the average frequency of the Doppler spectrum is proportional to the average velocity over the cross-sectional area of the blood vessel 13), so that volume flow can be assessed when vessel radius is known.

The amount of power received at the crystals is determined by the amount of reflection from the red blood cell-plasma interface and the quantity of sound ab-

190

sorption by the tissues. The higher the number of red blood cells moving in the ultrasonic beam, the higher the received power. Both the amount of reflection and the quantity of absorption depend on the transmitted frequency. Higher frequencies produce greater reflections since the sound reflection of red blood cells varies with the fourth power of the frequency 14). The absorption of sound by the tissues, however, also increases with frequency. When the effects of reflection and absorption are combined, the backscattering from blood at a given distance is strongest at a particular frequency 12). This theoretical optimal frequency, however, is not very often used because of practical reasons and many devices use a frequency different from the optimum. One should realize, however, that the signal to noise ratio improves when the received power of the velocity information containing frequencies is high.

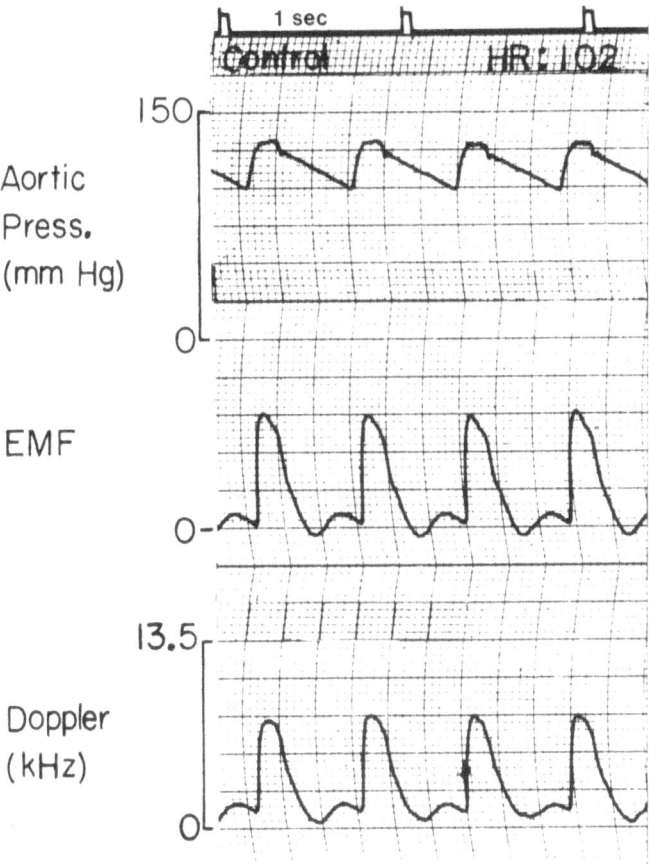

fig. 2. Aortic pressure and instantaneous flow tracings of the descending thoracic aorta as obtained with an electromagnetic (EMF) and a Doppler flowmeter, using a zero-crossing technique. (From Reneman et al., Cardiovasc. Res. 7: 557, 1973).

The received signal does not only contain power backscattered from red blood cells, but also from the vessel wall. Since the vessel wall-blood interface is a much better reflector than the red cell-blood interface, the power reflected from the vessel wall is significantly higher. The high amplitude low frequency signals due to lateral vessel wall motion are often difficult to eliminate, at least without loss of flow velocity induced frequencies.

Analogue signal processing

A simple method to retrieve the Doppler signal (the frequency shift) is mixing of the transmitted and received signals. This demodulation technique has the disadvantage that no information is obtained about the direction of the blood flow (nondirectional system). In directional systems a more complicated demodulation technique is used 15), 16). In this technique the received signal is demodulated with two signals at the transmitter frequency shifted 90° in phase with respect to each other, resulting in two Doppler signals which are 90° out of phase. The sign of the phase shift between both signals indicates the sign of the frequency shift, i.e. the direction of blood flow. To diminish the influence of vessel wall motion signals and noise beyond the Doppler frequency band, the output of the demodulator is passed through a band-pass filter.

Determination of the average Doppler frequency and the conversion of this signal into an electrical signal is usually performed with a zero-crossing meter. The output is an analogue voltage proportional to the number of zero-crossings per unit of time (fig. 2). To avoid the counting of zero crossings not related to blood flow velocity (e.g., random noise), the comparator voltage of the Schmitt-trigger is set at a relatively high level 17). It has been proposed that the output of the zero crossing meter may be assumed proportional to the average velocity over the cross-sectional area of the blood vessel 6), 8). This proportionality is based upon the theory that the shape of the Doppler frequency spectrum is constant regardless of flow speed. In vitro experiments, however, have shown that the shape of the spectrum depends on flow velocity 8), and, for instance, varies during the cardiac cycle. Moreover, Rice 18) and Peronneau and co-investigators 19) showed that the zero-crossing meter does not exactly measure the Doppler frequency corresponding to the average velocity, but a value higher than the Doppler frequency. This systematic error depends on the shape and the width of the received Doppler spectrum; the broader the spectrum the larger the error. The zero-crossing meter appears to be only accurate for a single frequency or a relatively narrow frequency spectrum 19). An additional disadvantage is that the zero-crossing meter output is independent of the amplitude of the audiosignal only at higher input levels. This is especially a problem when the signal to noise ratio is poor 20). Recently an alternative method has been described to determine the mean velocity from the Doppler spectrum 21), 22), 23). This method looks promising because it properly takes into account the spectral distribution of frequencies and avoids the problems encountered in zero-crossing meters.

In directional Doppler flowmeters forward and backward flow in arteries and veins, i.e., flow from and towards the crystals, can be recorded separately. In non-directional systems, all movements of the red blood cells are added and represented as forward flow (fig. 3).

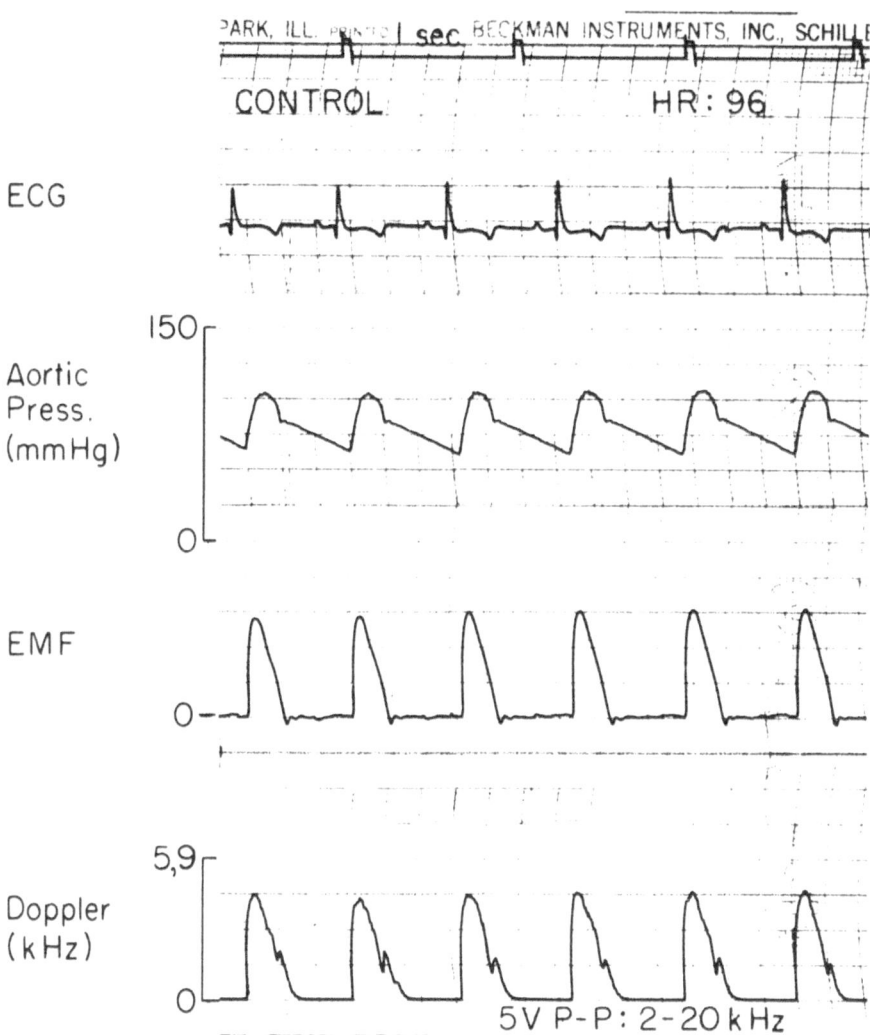

fig. 3. ECG, aortic pressure and instantaneous flow tracings of the ascending aorta as obtained with an electromagnetic (EMF) and a non-directional Doppler flowmeter, using a zero-crossing technique. In the non-directional system back flow in early diastole is represented as forward flow.

On-line spectrum analysis is offered as a possible replacement for the conventional instantaneous analogue velocity signal 24), 25). In this method the Doppler spectrum is recorded as a function of time, while the intensity of the tracing represents the reflected power at a given frequency (fig. 4).

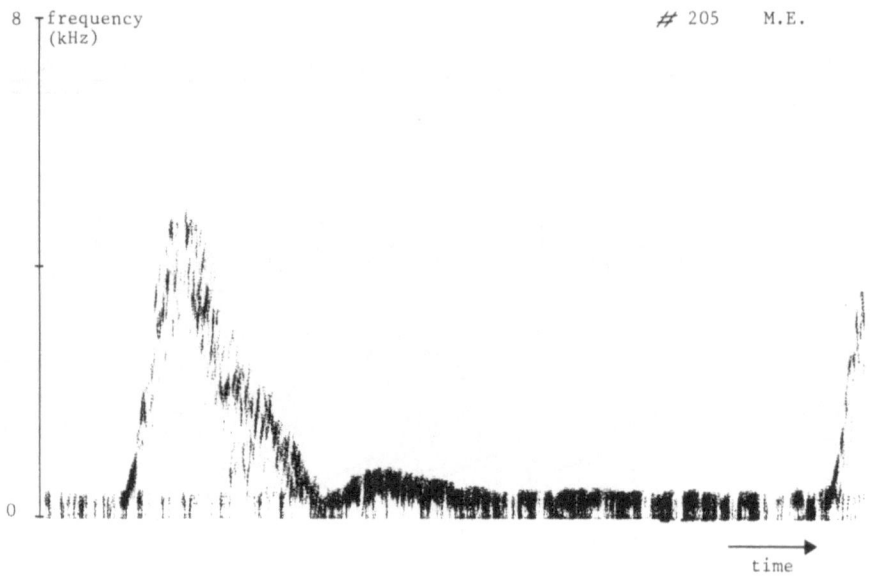

fig. 4. The Doppler spectrum of the brachial artery as a function of time (spectrum analysis). The intensity of the tracing represents the reflected power at a given frequency.

Transmission of ultrasound-continuous wave versus pulsed Doppler systems

In Doppler flowmeters ultrasound can be transmitted continuously (CW Doppler) or intermittently (pulsed Doppler). In CW Doppler flowmeters, e.g. 6), 7), 10), 11), the ultrasonic beam is usually transmitted from one crystal and the backscattered ultrasound received by another one. These systems are easy to build and to operate, but vessel wall motion artefacts are often difficult to eliminate, at least without the loss of flow velocity induced frequencies. The high amplitude low frequency signals due to vessel wall motion influence the shape of the frequency spectrum and, therefore, the accuracy of the determination of the average velocity. Vessel wall motion artefacts can even mask the presence of high velocity information, necessitating the use of a differentiator to weight the amplitudes with respect to frequency before the signal is fed into the zero-crossing meter 20). Moreover, in CW Doppler flowmeters, no information can be obtained about the diameter of the vessel so that volume flow cannot be determined with transcutaneous devices. The principle of CW Doppler systems is shown in fig. 1.

194

In pulsed Doppler flowmeters, e.g. 19), 26), 27), 28), usually one single crystal, operating alternatively as transmitter and receiver, is used. The sound transmission is intermittent (pulsed) so that during the intervals between pulses the crystal receives the backscattered signals from the red blood cells and the vessel wall. An electronic gate allows selection of scatterings either from the vessel wall or from the red blood cells at a given distance from the transducer (fig. 5 and 6).

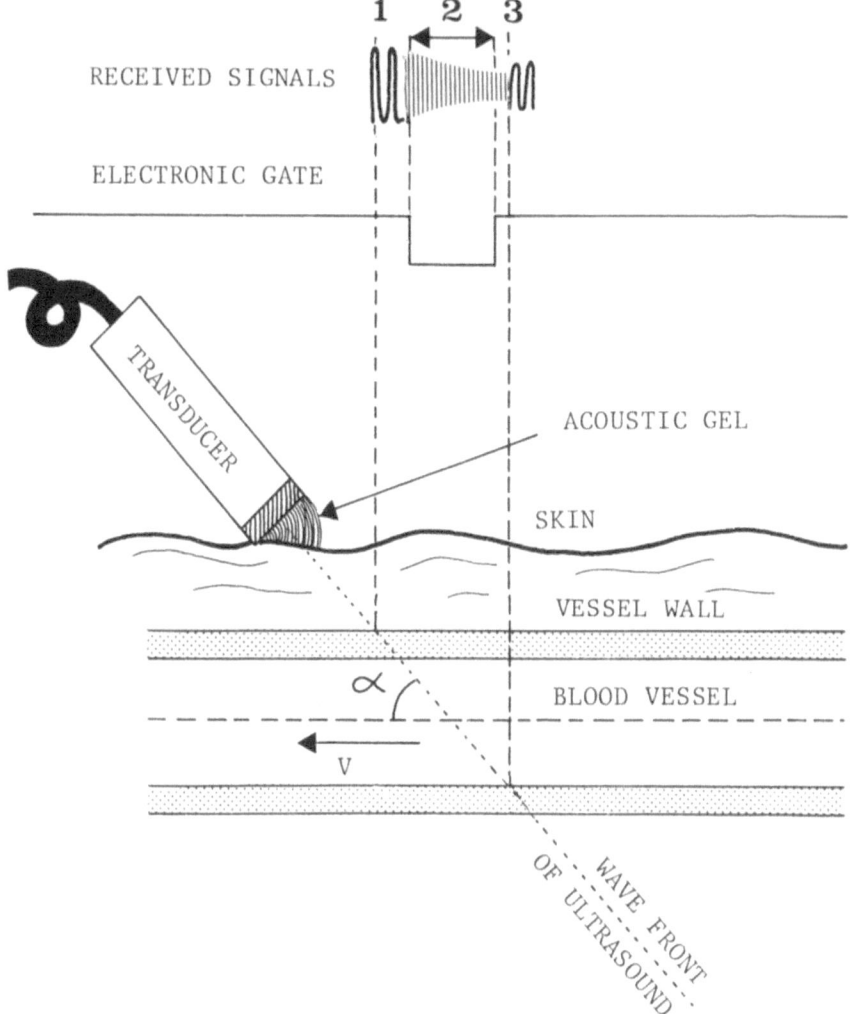

fig. 5. Principle of transcutaneous pulsed Doppler flowmetry. The arrow indicates the flow direction. 1 and 3 = ultrasonic power reflected from the anterior and posterior wall of the vessel, respectively; 2 = ultrasonic power reflected from the red blood cells. The electronic gate is so adjusted that mainly the signal, which contains the blood flow velocity information, is processed.

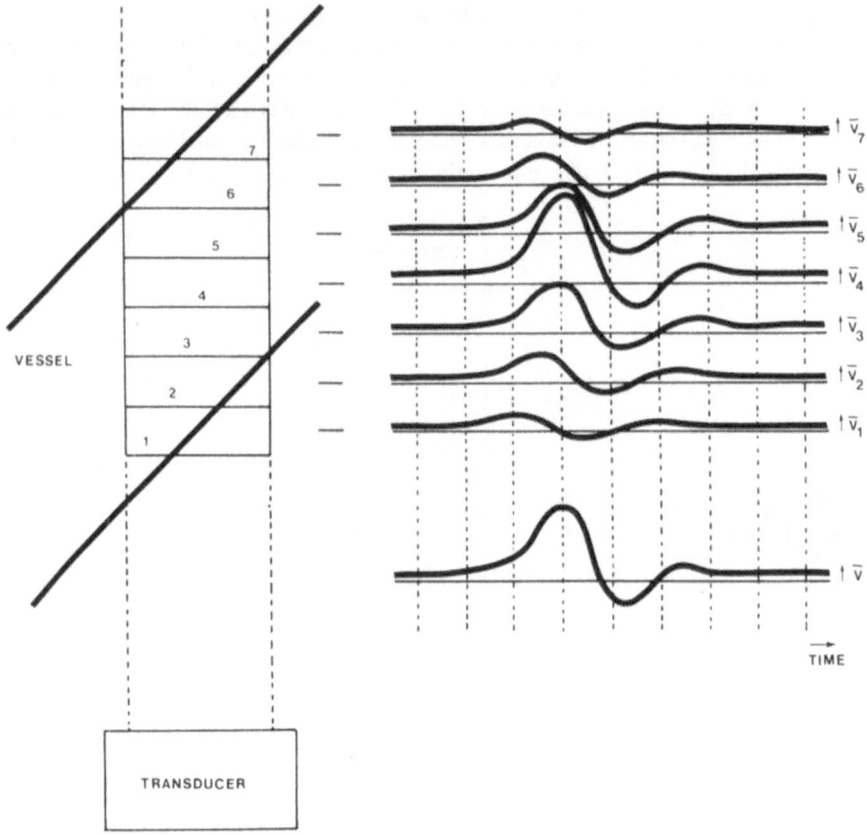

fig. 6. Schematic representation of sampling over the cross-sectional area of the blood vessel with a pulsed Doppler instrument. The instantaneous mean velocity is represented at various sites in the vessel ($\bar{v}_1$ - $\bar{v}_7$). $\bar{v}$ the instantaneous mean velocity in the vessel as determined with a CW Doppler device. The arrow indicates the flow direction.

This makes it possible to assess vessel diameter and velocity profiles 29), 30) and to reduce vessel wall motion artefacts. An additional advantage of pulsed devices is that small volume samples are taken over the cross-sectional area of the blood vessel (fig. 6) so that a narrow frequency spectrum is fed into the zero-crossing meter. Hence this meter can operate in its linear part 19). Recently multichannel pulsed Doppler systems have been developed allowing the simultaneous determination of velocity profiles and vessel wall dimensions per heart beat 31), 32).

Although the advantages of pulsed Doppler systems are obvious, it should be noticed that in these devices problems are encountered which are not met in CW systems. The circuitry of pulsed devices is more complex and the band width of the system is limited. The maximum velocity which can be measured depends on the

196

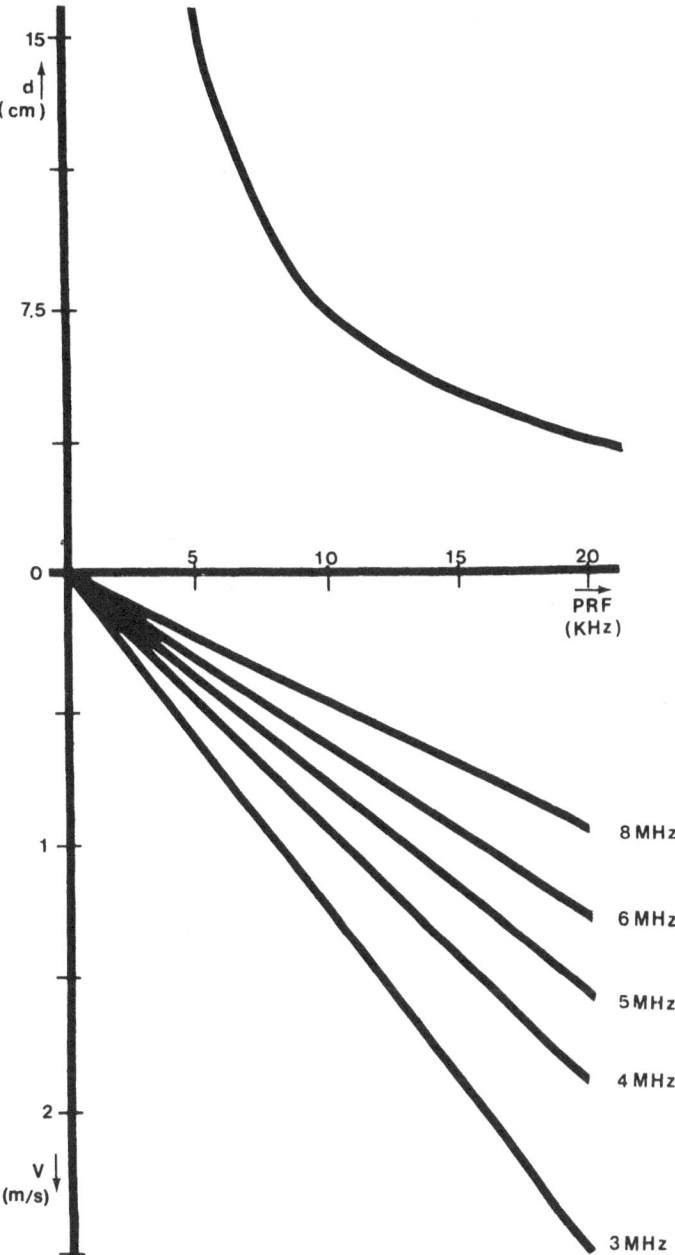

fig. 7. The relation between the maximum measurable velocity (v), the pulse repetition frequency (PRF), the transmitter frequency (3-8 MHz) and the distance between the transducer and the vessel (d). The given relation holds for demodulation by multiplying the transmitted and received signals.

distance between the transducer and the vessel, the repetition frequency of the pulses and the transmitter frequency (fig. 7).

To avoid interference between the received signal and the harmonics of the repetition frequency, this frequency has to be adjusted to the transmitter frequency. In pulsed Doppler devices small sample volumes are taken, resulting in a lower signal to noise ratio than in CW systems. Yet proper positioning of the sample volume is difficult, especially in systems with a fixed gate width. Moreover, the accuracy of the average frequency determination with the zero-crossing meter depends on the effective duration of the measurement. In case of a too short sampling period, the frequency will not be averaged out and a fluttering frequency is fed into the zero-crossing system. Transducer construction is more complicated in pulsed than in CW systems. To obtain a sharp pulse of short duration matching of the characteristic impedance of the crystals to the backing and loading media is more critical than in CW flowmeters.

Advantages and limitations

The major advantage of the ultrasound Doppler technique is its non-invasive application possibilities. In humans blood flow velocity can be measured transcutaneously as an instantaneous function of time in arteries and veins. Pulsed Doppler devices render the possibility of assessing vessel diameter transcutaneously so that volume flow can be determined. With directional Doppler systems forward and backward flow can be recorded simultaneously so that the existence of backward flow can be assessed when the net flow direction is antegrade 16). The delay in Doppler instruments is minimal and mainly determined by the characteristics of the filters in the system. This minimal delay is especially important in phase-relation studies. Close by the heart, as in cuff probes around the ascending aorta or the coronary arteries, the flow signal is hardly disturbed by interference of the electrocardiogram which is the case in electromagnetic flowmeters. A zero flow reference can easily be obtained by disconnecting the input to the analogue signal processing system (e.g. the zero-crossing meter).

In Doppler flowmeters quantitative information is still difficult to obtain, mainly because the angle α (eq 1) between the ultrasonic beam and the direction of velocity of the red cells cannot be determined accurately and precise assessment of the average frequency of the Doppler spectrum is difficult to achieve. In Doppler devices often the whole cross-section of the vessel in not bathed in the ultrasonic beam so that flow velocity is averaged along the diameter rather than the cross-sectional area of the vessel 17), 20). Averaging along the diameter of the femoral artery, for instance, can easily overestimate the velocity by some 33 percent 33).

Applications

Although quantitative information is still difficult to obtain, Doppler flowmeters have shown to be an asset in the diagnosis of cardiovascular diseases. Because of its non-invasiveness, Doppler flowmeters are especially suitable for studies requiring repeated measurements, e.g. epidemiological studies and studies to evaluate the result of surgical or non-surgical treatment.

In peripheral arterial diseases information can be obtained about the site and severeness of the occlusion. This information is derived from the peak velocity readings at various sites along the artery 11), 34), 35), the difference between proximal and distal arterial blood pressure 36), 37), the time delay between proximally and distally recorded velocity pulses 35), and "ultrasonic arteriography" 38), 39). In the lower limbs, analysis of the velocity waveforms renders additional information 40). In cerebral vascular diseases valuable information can also be obtained from the systolic and diastolic amplitudes of the velocity tracings of the common carotid artery 41) and from the flow direction in the ophthalmic artery 39), 41), 42).

When a peripheral artery is completely occluded usually no velocity signal can be recorded at the site of obstruction. In a stenosis (partial occlusion of the vessel) peak velocity is generally increased. Distal to the site of occlusion blood pressure and peak velocity are decreased to a level, depending on the severeness of the obstruction and the amount of collateral circulation.

In ultrasonic arteriography, the Doppler transducer is connected to a mechanical scanning arm. The position of the transducer is electrically sensed by a spot-positioning circuitry which positions the spot on an image storage oscilloscope. The output signal of a directional Doppler flowmeter intensifies the Z-axis of the image storage oscilloscope only for a given direction of flow. By passing repeatedly the transducer over the blood vessel, a two-dimensional picture of the vessel can be made. The image formed is similar to the anatomical display of X-ray arteriography, but represents a functional projection of local blood flow velocities. Ultrasonic arteriography was found to be accurate and especially sensitive in detecting calcified atherosclerotic plaques 39).

Comparison of the effect of respiration, posture and the Valsalva manoeuvre on sublavian venous velocity with that on femoral and popliteal venous velocity gives valuable information about the competence and patency of veins 43), 44), 45).

Because the gas-blood interface is an excellent reflector, Doppler flowmeters are especially suitable to detect aeroembolism, both in decompression sickness of flyers, divers or caisson workers 46), 47) and in open-heart surgery 48).

In clinical cardiology transcutaneous Doppler flowmeters have been used in the diagnosis of right heart diseases 49) and of left-to-right shunts 49), 50) and to determine aortic blood flow velocity 51), 52), 53), a variable which might be useful in the assessment of left ventricular function, especially in the acutely ill patient 54).

Besides valuable information has been obtained with Doppler instruments about cardiac dynamics, for instance, during arrhythmias 55) and about the presence of low intensity cardiac murmurs which were difficult to detect with conventional techniques 51).

Of special importance are the Doppler catheter-tip flowmeters which allow the determination of blood flow velocity in, for example, the mitral ostium 56), the outflow track of the left ventricle or the ascending aorta 57). With these devices it is also possible to assess coronary blood flow velocity in patients 58). Beside the accuracy of zero flow determination and the absence of ECG interference, Doppler catheter-tip flowmeters have the advantage over electromagnetic devices that they can be made smaller and that, using pulsed ultrasound, information can be obtained about vessel diameter 59). In this way volume flow could be determined. Recently a Doppler catheter device for intra-oesophageal use has been described 60). With this device flow velocity signals from the descending thoracic aorta can be recorded.

Summary

In Doppler flowmeters a beam of ultrasonic waves (MHz level) is transmitted continuously (CW) or intermittently (pulsed) from a vibrating crystal diagonally through the vessel wall into the blood stream. Some of the ultrasonic power is reflected and received by another (CW) or the same crystal (pulsed). The crystals are mounted in a transducer either for transcutaneous, or perivascular application, or on a catheter for intravascular use. Ultrasound backscattered from particles in the flowing blood, mainly red cells, is shifted in frequency by an amount proportional to the velocity of the particles. Blood flowing towards and from the probe can be distinguished, using a special processing technique. In the present survey the technical aspects, advantages, limitations, and application possibilities of Doppler instruments are discussed.

Acknowledgements
The authors are indebted to Mrs. B. van der Mars-Pastoors for her help in preparing the manuscript.

References

1) Kolin A: *An electromagnetic flowmeter. Principle of the method and its application to bloodflow measurements.*
Proceedings of the Society for Experimental Biology and Medicine 35: 53, 1936.

2) Wetterer E: *Eine neue Methode zur Registrierung des Blutströmungsgeschwindigkeit am uneröffneten Gefäss.*
Zeitschrift für Biologie 98: 26, 1937.

3) Shercliff JA: *The theory of electromagnetic flow-measurement.*
London, 1962, Cambridge University Press.

4) Spencer MP, and Denison AB Jr: *The square-wave electromagnetic flowmeter: theory of operation and design of magnetic probes for clinical and experimental applications.*
IRE Transactions on Medical Electronics ME-6, 220, 1959.

200

5) Westersten A, Rice E, Brinkman CR, and Assali NS: *A balanced fieldtype electromagnetic flowmeter.*
J. Appl. Physiol. 26: 497, 1969.

6) Franklin DL, Schlegel W, and Rushmer RF: *Blood flow measured by Doppler frequency shift of backscattered ultrasound.*
Science 134: 564, 1961.

7) Satomura S, and Kaneko Z: *Ultrasonic blood reograph.*
Proceedings of the Third International Conference on Medical Electronics, London, 1960, p. 254.

8) Kato K, Motomiya M, Izumi T, Kaneko Z, Shiraishi J, Omizo H, and Nakano S: *Linearity of readings on ultrasonic flow meter.*
6th International Conference on Medical Electronics and Biological Engineering. Tokyo, 1965. Digest of Papers for Scientific Program, p. 284.

9) Franklin DL, Watson NW, Pierson KE, and Van Citters RL: *Technique for radio telemetry of blood-flow from unrestrained animals.*
Am. J. Med. Electr. 5: 24, 1966.

10) Stegall HF, Rushmer RF, and Baker DW: *A transcutaneous ultrasonic blood velocity meter.*
J. Appl. Physiol. 21: 707, 1966.

11) Rushmer RF, Baker DW, Johnson WL, and Strandness DE: *Clinical applications of a transcutaneous ultrasonic flow detector.*
JAMA 199: 326, 1967.

12) Reid JM, and Baker DW: *Physics and electronics of the ultrasonic Doppler method.*
In: Ultrasonographia Medica. Wien, 1971, H. Egermann, p. 109.

13) Arts MGJ: *On the instantaneous measurements of blood flow by ultrasonic means.*
TH-report 71-E-20, Eindhoven University of Technology, Eindhoven, 1971.

14) Wells PNT: *Physical principles of ultrasonic diagnosis.*
London, 1969, Academic Press.

15) McLeod FD: *A directional Doppler flowmeter.*
Digest of Seventh International Conference on Medical and Biological Engineering, Stockholm, 1967, p. 213.

16) Strandness DE, Kennedy JW, Judge TP, and McLeod FD: *Transcutaneous directional flow detection: A preliminary report.*
Am. Heart J. 78: 65, 1969.

17) Reneman RS, Clarke HF, Simmons N, and Spencer MP: *In vivo comparison of electromagnetic and Doppler flowmeters: with special attention to the processing of the analogue Doppler flow signal.*
Cardiovasc. Res. 7: 557, 1973.

18) Rice SO: *Mathematical analysis of random noise.*
Bell System Tech. J. 23: 282, 1944.

19) Peronneau P, Hinglais J, Pellet M, and Léger F: *Vélocimètre sanguin par effet Doppler à émission ultra-sonore pulsée.*
l'Onde Electrique 50: 369, 1970.

20) Reneman RS, and Spencer MP: *Difficulties in processing of an analogue Doppler flow signal; with special reference to zero-crossing meters and quantification.*
In: Cardiovascular applications of ultrasound. Editor R.S. Reneman, Amsterdam, 1974, North-Holland Publ. Co., p. 32.

21) Arts MGJ, and Roevros JMJG: *On the instantaneous measurement of blood-flow by ultrasonic means.*
Med. Biol. Engng. 10: 23, 1972.

22) Roevros JMJG: *Analogue processing of CW Doppler flowmeter signals to determine average frequency shift momentaneously without the use of a wave analyser.*
In: Cardiovascular applications of ultrasound. Editor R.S. Reneman, Amsterdam, 1974, North-Holland Publ. Co., p. 43.

23) Reid JM, Davis DL, Ricketts HJ, and Spencer MP: *A new Doppler flowmeter system and its operation with catheter mounted transducers.*
In: Cardiovascular applications of ultrasound. Editor R.S. Reneman, Amsterdam, 1974, North-Holland Publ. Co., p. 183.

24) Coghlan BA, Taylor MG, and King DH: *On-line display of Doppler-shift spectra by a new time compression analyser.*
In: Cardiovascular applications of ultrasound. Editor R.S. Reneman, Amsterdam, 1974, North-Holland Publ. Co., p. 55.

25) Light LH: *Initial evaluation of transcutaneous aortavelography - a new non-invasive technique for hemodynamic measurements in the major thoracic vessels.*
In: Cardiovascular applications of ultrasound. Editor R.S. Reneman, Amsterdam, 1974, North-Holland Publ. Co., p. 325.

26) Jorgensen JE, Campau DN, and Baker DW: *Physical characteristics and mathematical modelling of the pulsed ultrasonic flowmeter.*
Med. Biol. Engng. 404, July 1973.

27) Baker DW, Johnson SL, and Strandness DE: *Prospects of quantitation of transcutaneous pulsed Doppler techniques in cardiology and peripheral vascular diseases.*
In: Cardiovascular applications of ultrasound. Editor R.S. Reneman, Amsterdam, 1974, North-Holland Publ. Co., p. 108.

28) Peronneau PA, Bournat JP, Bugnon A, Barbet A, and Xhaard M: *Theoretical and practical aspects of pulsed Doppler flowmetry: real-time application to the measure of instantaneous velocity profiles in vitro and in vivo.*
In: Cardiovascular applications of ultrasound. Editor R.S. Reneman, Amsterdam, 1974, North-Holland Publ. Co., p. 66.

29) Peronneau PA, Pellet MM, Xhaard MC, and Hinglais JR: *Pulsed Doppler ultrasonic blood flowmeter. Real-time instantaneous velocity profiles.*
In: Flow, Its measurement and control in science and industry. Vol. 1. Editor R.B. Dowdell, Pittsburgh, 1971, Instrument Society of America, p. 1367.

30) Hagl S, Messmer K, Pfau B, and Meisner H: *Influence of stenosis on the velocity profile analyzed by a pulsed Doppler ultrasonic flowmeter.*
In: Cardiovascular applications of ultrasound. Editor R.S. Reneman, Amsterdam, 1974, North-Holland Publ. Co., p. 216.

31) McLeod FD: *Multichannel pulse Doppler techniques.*
In: Cardiovascular applications of ultrasound. Editor R.S. Reneman, Amsterdam, 1974, North-Holland Publ. Co., p. 85.

32) Brandestini M: *Signalverarbeitung in perkutanen Ultraschall Doppler Blutfuss Messgeräten.*
Dissertation IBT Zürich, 1976.

33) Gessner U: *The performance of the ultrasonic flowmeter in complex velocity profiles.*
IEEE Trans. Biomed. Engng. BME-16: 139, 1969.

34) Strandness DE, McCutcheon EP, and Rushmer RF: *Application of a transcutaneous Doppler flowmeter in evaluation of occlusive arterial disease.*
Surg. Gynecol. Obstet. 122: 1039, 1966.

35) Gosling RG, and King DH: *Continuous wave ultrasound as an alternative and complement to X-rays in vascular examinations.*
In: Cardiovascular applications of ultrasound. Editor R.S. Reneman, Amsterdam, 1974, North-Holland Publ. Co., p. 266.

36) Summer DS, and Strandness DE: *The relationship between calf blood flow and ankle blood pressure in patients with intermittent claudication.*
Surgery 65: 763, 1969.

37) Lewis JD, Papathanaiou C, Yao ST, and Eastcott HHG: *Simultaneous flow and pressure measurements in intermittent claudication.*
Brit. J. Surg. 59: 418, 1972.

38) Mozersky DJ, Hokanson DE, Sumner DS, and Strandness DE: *Ultrasonic visualization of the arterial lumen.*
Surgery 72: 253, 1972.

39) Spencer MP, Reid JM, Davis DL, and Paulson PS: *Cervical carotid imaging with a continuous-wave Doppler flowmeter.*
Stroke 5: 145, 1974.

40) Lewis JD, and Yao ST: *Waveform and pressure measurement with a directional Doppler in the diagnosis and follow-up of peripheral arterial disease.*
In: Cardiovascular applications of ultrasound. Editor R.S. Reneman, Amsterdam, 1974, North-Holland Publ. Co., p. 294.

41) Mol JMF, and Rijcken WJ: *Doppler haematotachographic investigation in cerebral circulation disturbances.*
In: Cardiovascular applications of ultrasound. Editor R.S. Reneman, Amsterdam, 1974, North-Holland Publ. Co., p. 305.

42) Müller HR: *The diagnosis of internal carotid artery occlusion by directional Doppler sonography of the ophthalmic artery.*
Neurology 22: 816, 1972.

43) Sigel B, Popky GL, Wagner DK, Boland JP, McD.Napp E, and Feigl P: *Comparison of clinical and Doppler ultrasound evaluation of confirmed lower extremity venous disease.*
Surgery 64: 332, 1968.

44) Folse R, and Alexander RH: *Directional flow detection for localizing venous valvular incompetency.*
Surgery 67: 114, 1970.

45) Lewis JD, Parsons DCS, Needham TN, Douglas JN, Lawson J, Hobbs JT, and Nicolaides AN: *The use of venous pressure measurements and directional Doppler recordings in distinguishing between superficial and deep valvular incompetence in patients with deep venous insufficiency.*
Brit. J. Surg. 60: 312, 1973.

46) Spencer MP, Campbell SD, Sealey JL, Henry FC, and Lindbergh J: *Experiments on decompression bubbles in the circulation using ultrasound and electromagnetic flowmeters.*
J. Occup. Med. 11: 238, 1969.

47) Spencer MP, Clarke HF, and Simmons N: *Precordial monitoring of pulmonary gas embolism and decompression bubbles.*
J. Aerosp. Med. 43: 762, 1972.

48) Spencer MP, Lawrence GH, Thomas GI, and Sauvage LR: *The use of ultrasonics in the determination of arterial aeroembolism during open heart surgery.*
Ann. Thorac. Surg. 8: 489, 1969.

49) Kalmanson D, Veyrat C, Chiche P, and Witchitz S: *Non-invasive diagnosis of right heart diseases and of left-to-right shunts using directional Doppler ultrasound.*
In: Cardiovascular applications of ultrasound. Editor R.S. Reneman, Amsterdam, 1974, North-Holland Publ. Co., p. 361.

50) Kalmanson D, Veyrat C, Derǎi C, Savier CH, Berkman M, and Chiche P: *Non-invasive technique for diagnosting atrial septal defect and assessing shunt volume using directional Doppler ultrasound. Correlations with phasic flow velocity patterns of the shunt.*
Br. Heart J. 34: 981, 1972.

51) Johnson SL, Baker DW, Lute RA, and Dodge HT: *Doppler echocardiography. The localization of cardiac murmurs.*
Circulation 48: 810, 1972.

52) Light H: *Transcutaneous aortavelography. A new window on the circulation?*
Br. Heart J. 38: 433, 1976.

53) Sequeira RF, Light LH, Cross G, and Raftery EB: *Transcutaneous aortavelography. A quantitative evaluation.*
Br. Heart J. 38: 443, 1976.

54) Buchtal A, Hanson GC, and Peisach AR: *Transcutaneous aortavelography. Potentially useful technique in management of critically ill patients.*
Br. Heart J. 38: 451, 1976.

55) Kalmanson D, Veyrat C, and Chiche P: *Atrial versus ventricular contribution in determining systolic venous return.*
Cardiovasc. Res. 5: 293, 1971.

56) Kalmanson D, Veyrat C, Bernier A, and Witchitz S: *Flow velocity tracings in patients with mitral valve disease. Diagnostic use of the transseptal Doppler catheterization.*
In: The mitral valve. Editor D. Kalmanson, Acton, Massachusetts, 1976, Publishing Sciences Group, Inc. p. 213.

57) Kalmanson D, Toutain G, Nivokoff N, and Derai C: *Retrograde catheterization of left heart cavities in dogs by means of an orientable directional Doppler catheter-tip flow-meter: a preliminary report.*
Cardiovasc. Res. 6: 309, 1972.

58) Benchimol A, Stegall HF, and Gartlan JL: *New method to measure phasic coronary blood velocity in man.*
Am. Heart J. 81: 93, 1971.

59) Martin RW, Pollack GH, and Phillips J: *Stroke volume mearument with an ultrasonic catheter system.*
Proc. first World Federation of Ultrasound in Medicine and Biology, San Francisco, 1976.

60) Duck FA, Hodson CJ, and Tomlin PJ: *An esophageal Doppler probe for aortic flow velocity monitoring.*
Ultrasound in Med. and Biol. 1: 233, 1974.

Pulsed Doppler echocardiography*

by Donald Baker, Gerald Lorch and Simeon Rubenstein,
Center for Bioengineering, University of Washington and
Division of Cardiology, Department of Medicine,
University of Washington, Seattle, U.S.A.

* This work was supported by NHLI Grants   HL-07293 and   HL-05124.

Introduction

Cardiac ultrasound has greatly enhanced our ability to define structural disorders in the heart and great vessels. While certain cardiac diseases lend themselves to firm diagnosis by M-mode echocardiography, many valvular and congenital disorders result in normal or nonspecific echocardiographic findings. In these disorders structural abnormalities clearly exist which cannot be evaluated with present echocardiographic techniques. A range-gated pulsed Doppler device has been developed which can identify blood flow patterns at well-defined intracardiac locations 1), 4). By demonstrating whether intracardiac flow is normal or pathologic, direct inference can be made as to what structural abnormality exists.

Methods

According to the Doppler theory, the frequencies of sound backscattered or reflected from a moving object will be shifted in proportion to its velocity. This effect is known as Doppler shift. Blood scatters ultrasound because it contains particulate matter--namely the blood cells. The pulsed Doppler device uses repetitive bursts, or pulses, of sound in the 3 to 5 megahertz range, much like traditional M-mode echocardiographic systems. While most ultrasonic waves are reflected from the various cardiac structures, a small amount is backscattered by the blood cells within the chambers themselves. These waves can be analyzed using a special Doppler shift detector system. If an ultrasonic beam is directed at smooth, nonturbulent blood flow, the received sound waves will have a fairly uniform Doppler shift. By contrast, sound waves scattered from disturbed, or turbulent, blood flow will show wide fluctuations in Doppler shift.

The pulsed Doppler functions by detecting the Doppler shift from moving blood within the heart or great vessels and provides an output by which blood flow characteristics can be recognized. The primary advantage of the pulsed, as opposed to the continuous wave Doppler, is that blood flow velocities may be evaluated

207

from discrete intracardiac positions. This flow velocity is detected in a teardrop-shaped region called the sample volume, which may be chosen from any depth from 2 to 15 centimeters along the ultrasonic beam through the use of a movable range-gating system. The sample volume measures approximately 2 millimeters in diameter and 4 millimeters in length within the focal zone of the transducer.

The device employs a 3 megahertz piezoelectric transducer with a 1/2-inch diameter crystal focused at 5 centimeters. The transmitter circuit emits 1 microsecond ultrasonic bursts at a pulsed repetition frequency that may be varied between 3,500 and 10,000 bursts per second depending on the depth of penetration desired. The returned signal is divided such that one portion is used to create a traditional A-mode display for orientation, however, the quality of this A-mode Doppler display is not yet comparable to conventional devices due to inherent resolution limitations. The other portion of the returned signal is used for Doppler flow velocity information. The magnitude and direction of the Doppler shift is determined in a special phase detector circuit where the returned frequency is compared to the transmitted frequency. Positioning the transducer in a manner similar to that used in traditional echocardiography and using the A-mode display for orientation, the sample volume is placed at well defined intracardiac locations simply by adjusting the range-gate knob (fig. 1).

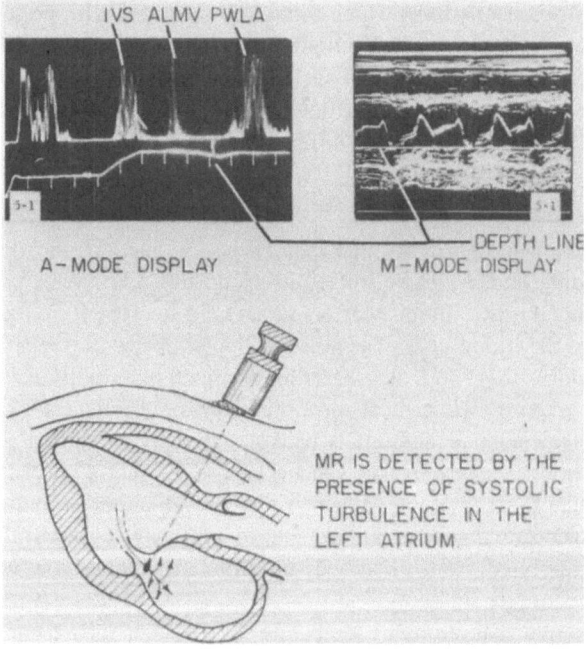

fig. 1. The sample volume is a teardrop-shaped region which may be set anywhere along the ultrasonic beam axis, by adjusting the depth gate. The A-mode and M-mode are used for orientation. The depth line indicates the position of the sample volume.

208

There are two types of outputs available from a pulsed Doppler device. The first provides an audible signal in the range of 400 Hertz to 5 kilo-Hertz which corresponds to the spectrum of Doppler shifts produced by normal or disturbed blood flow. The interpretation is based on evaluating the tonal quality of the signal. Smooth blood flow characteristically has a narrow bandwidth pattern which produces a tonal "music-like" sound whereas disturbed, or turbulent flow has a wide bandwidth pattern which produces a harsh, scatchy sound. This method has been described in detail in previous publications 1)-3). Note: Classical engineering turbulence may not be present in the cardiovascular system, so, use of the word "disturbed" may avoid possible confusion.

The second type of output available is an on-line graphical display of the Doppler shift frequencies which is printed on a fiberoptic-type strip chart recorder. A circuit has been built into the pulsed Doppler detector for performing analysis of flow and creating a display pattern. This circuit creates what is called a time interval histogram (TIH) (see fig. 2), which is a dot pattern by which flow velocity characteristics can be easily identified.

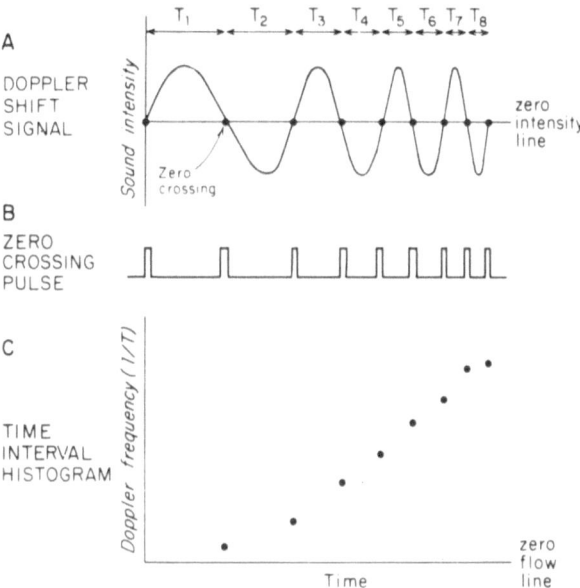

fig. 2. Production of a Time Interval Histogram. A) The Doppler shift frequency signal. Each time the zero intensity is crossed by the Doppler sound wave signal, the time period to the previous zero crossing is measured. This period is the reciprocal of the Doppler shift frequency. T_1, T_2, T_3, etc., successive periods between zero crossings. B) Graph illustrating when the zero crossings occur. C) The time interval histogram. For each zero crossing event of the Doppler shift frequency signal, the time period (T) to the previous zero crossing is measured and a dot is printed. Its distance from the zero flow line is inversely proportional to that time period (T). For longer periods (as in T_1), the dot is printed near the zero flow line. For shorter periods (as in T_8), the dot is printed proportionately farther from the zero flow line. The distance of a dot from the zero flow line is, therefore, directly proportional to the Doppler shift frequency.

The pattern is derived from the zero crossings of the audible signal waveform. A zero crossing is the instant in time when the Doppler shift signal passes through its zero intensity level. It must do this twice for each cycle of the Doppler shift which is detected. Since the Doppler shift contains many frequencies in the range of 100 to 5,000 per second, a complex signal with many randomly spaced zero crossings can occur. The mean frequency of these zero crossing events is the mean Doppler shift or mean velocity. More specifically, the reciprocal of the interval between each zero crossing event is the Doppler shift frequency for that interval. A dot is printed on the strip chart paper for each zero crossing event such that the distance of a particular dot above or below the zero flow velocity baseline is directly proportional to the Doppler shift frequency. For example, if the Doppler shift frequency is relatively low, a dot will be printed near the zero velocity baseline. However, if the Doppler shift frequency is relatively high, a dot will be printed proportionately farther away from the baseline. Any dot printed above the baseline (positive) represents relative blood velocity towards the transducer and conversely, any dot printed below the baseline (negative) represents flow velocity away from the transducer. A dot pattern is thus produced which shows the Doppler shift spectrum, and this pattern is used to identify blood flow characteristics within the sample volume. When laminar flow exists, blood cells within the sample volume may have fairly uniform direction and velocity. Therefore, backscattered sound waves will have a fairly uniform Doppler shift. The time interval histogram produced by this flow has a narrowly clustered dot pattern (narrow band pattern) (fig. 3A). When turbulent, "disturbed", flow exists, the blood cells have varied direction and velocity which produce a time interval histogram with a widely dispersed dot pattern (wide band pattern) (fig. 3B).

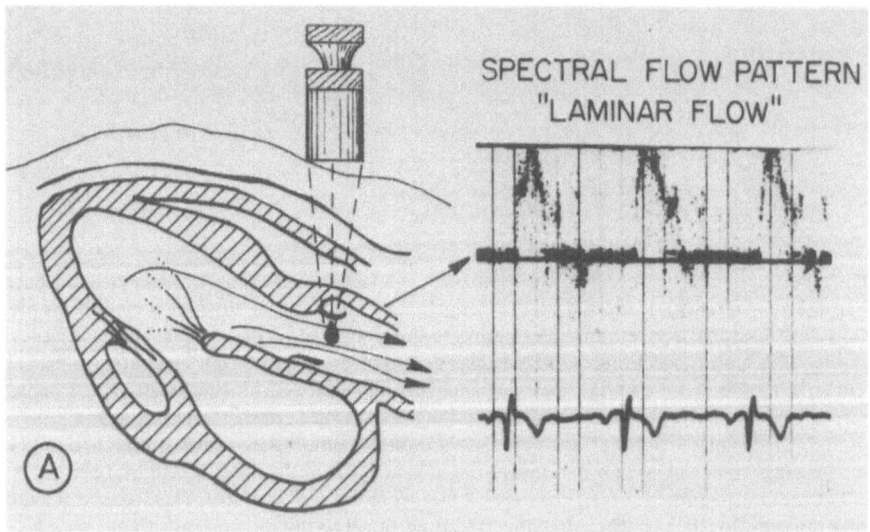

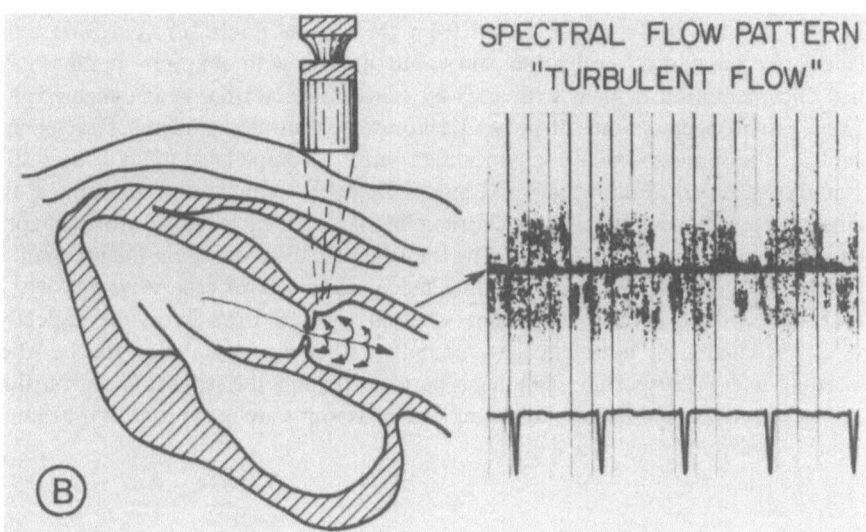

fig. 3. Flow patterns. A) Smooth flow. The dot pattern is narrowly dispersed (narrow band pattern) as a result of uniform Doppler frequency shift. This reflects uniform direction and velocity of blood cells in the sample volume. A cluster of dots above the zero line reflects flow towards the transducer. B) Disturbed flow. Aortic stenosis produces a jet of flow which causes a wide dot pattern centered around a mean value near zero. This reflects marked variation in blood cell velocity and direction, with some blood cells moving towards and others away from the transducer. No net velocity is detected due to the near 90° angle between the sound beam axis and jet.

The time interval histogram analysis also provides a means to follow very rapid changes in flow velocity that may occur during initial ventricular contraction. There are no delays in the response as is characteristic of heavily filtered or smoothed analog flow velocity waveforms. The current device exhibits one principal limitation which hopefully will be remedied with further development. This problem stems from the fact that the zero crossing detection process cannot be made as sensitive or noise immune as the human ear. Because of this, the user may sometimes hear Doppler signals associated with flow disturbances which cannot be written out on the recording. Careful adjustment of the Doppler detector often helps but may not always succeed.

Strip chart records contain simultaneous recordings of 1) the M-mode display of the received Doppler signal (in the form of a traditional M-mode echo display) with a superimposed line indicating the location of the sample volume at any particular time, b) the time interval histogram of the Doppler signal (also called a spectral display), and c) a standard electrocardiogram. It is also possible to record an analog waveform of flow which corresponds to the mean value of the Doppler frequency shift; this can be shown as a separate channel on the recording but has proved of limited value and has been deleted from most later recordings.

Patients for the study were selected from the routine referrals to our ultrasound laboratory for clinical evaluation. Most, but not all, with abnormal findings have had documentation of their pathology by cardiac catheterization and angiography. Each patient seen in our ultrasound laboratory routinely undergoes systematic cardiac ultrasonic examination, beginning with a complete M-mode echocardiographic assessment. Following this a pulsed Doppler examination is performed. Beginning from the suprasternal notch, sampling is obtained from the proximal aorta and the right pulmonary artery 5). The transducer is then placed on the precordium and sampling performed on the inflow and outflow side of each valve and within each valve orifice itself to determine whether forward flow across the respective valve has laminar or turbulent pattern, and whether regurgitant flow exists. When a septal defect is suspected, sampling is performed along the septum on the outflow side of the suspected defect, following which attempts are made to pass the sample volume directly through the defect.

Results

Normal and turbulent flow

Blood flow within a vessel or chamber is usually smooth, or "nonturbulent", and produces a time interval histogram with a narrowly clustered dot pattern (fig. 3A). Turbulent, or disturbed flow, by contrast, produces a time interval histogram with a widely dispersed dot pattern (fig. 3B). With disturbed blood flow velocities, the presence of dots which are widely dispersed both above and below the zero line illustrate the marked variation in blood cell direction and velocity within the sample, with some cells moving towards and others away from the transducer.

Aortic valve flow

With the transducer positioned over the precordium, the systolic flow in or just above the aortic valve is normally laminar or slightly altered (fig. 4). In diastole no flow is appreciated. In aortic stenosis a jet of systolic turbulence is detected within and above the aortic valve and is represented by a broad band Doppler pattern (fig. 5). In diastole a narrow band dot pattern is recorded at or near the zero flow baseline because no flow is present and the Doppler shift is therefore zero.

In aortic insufficiency a regurgitant jet may be detected during diastole within the valve orifice, in the left ventricular outflow tract, and frequently well down within to the left ventricular chamber (fig. 6). When searching for this lesion in the presence of mitral stenosis, diastolic velocity disturbances must be documented within the aortic valve or high left ventricular outflow tract to make a firm diagnosis of coexisting aortic insufficiency. If attempts are made to follow the disturbed flow into each valve orifice, mitral stenosis and aortic insufficiency can be easily differentiated from one another.

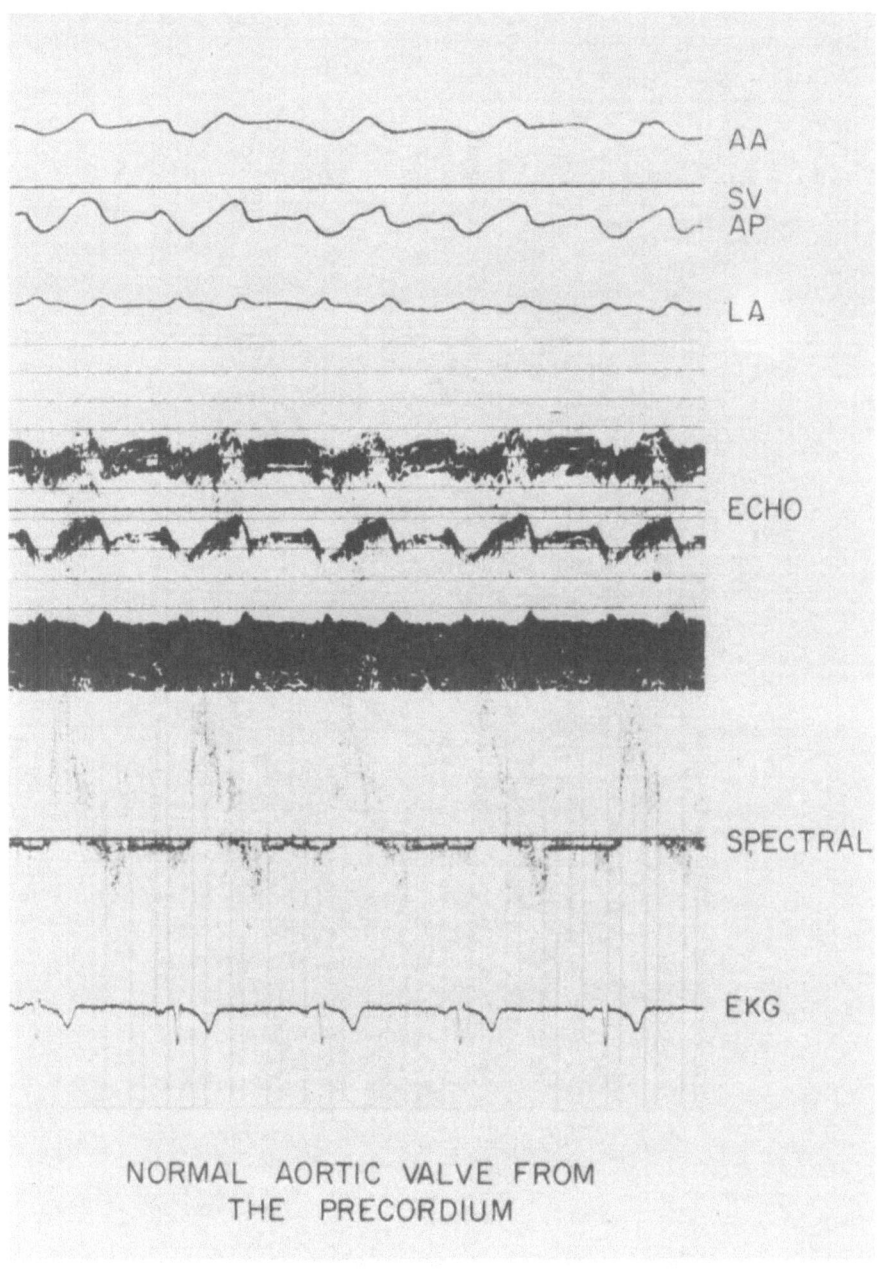

AA

SV
AP

LA

ECHO

SPECTRAL

EKG

NORMAL AORTIC VALVE FROM
THE PRECORDIUM

fig. 4. Aortic valve flow from the precordium. There is a narrow band pattern during systole representing nonturbulent, or smooth, flow. The upper portion of the figure is a schematic drawing of the actual M-mode recording displayed below.

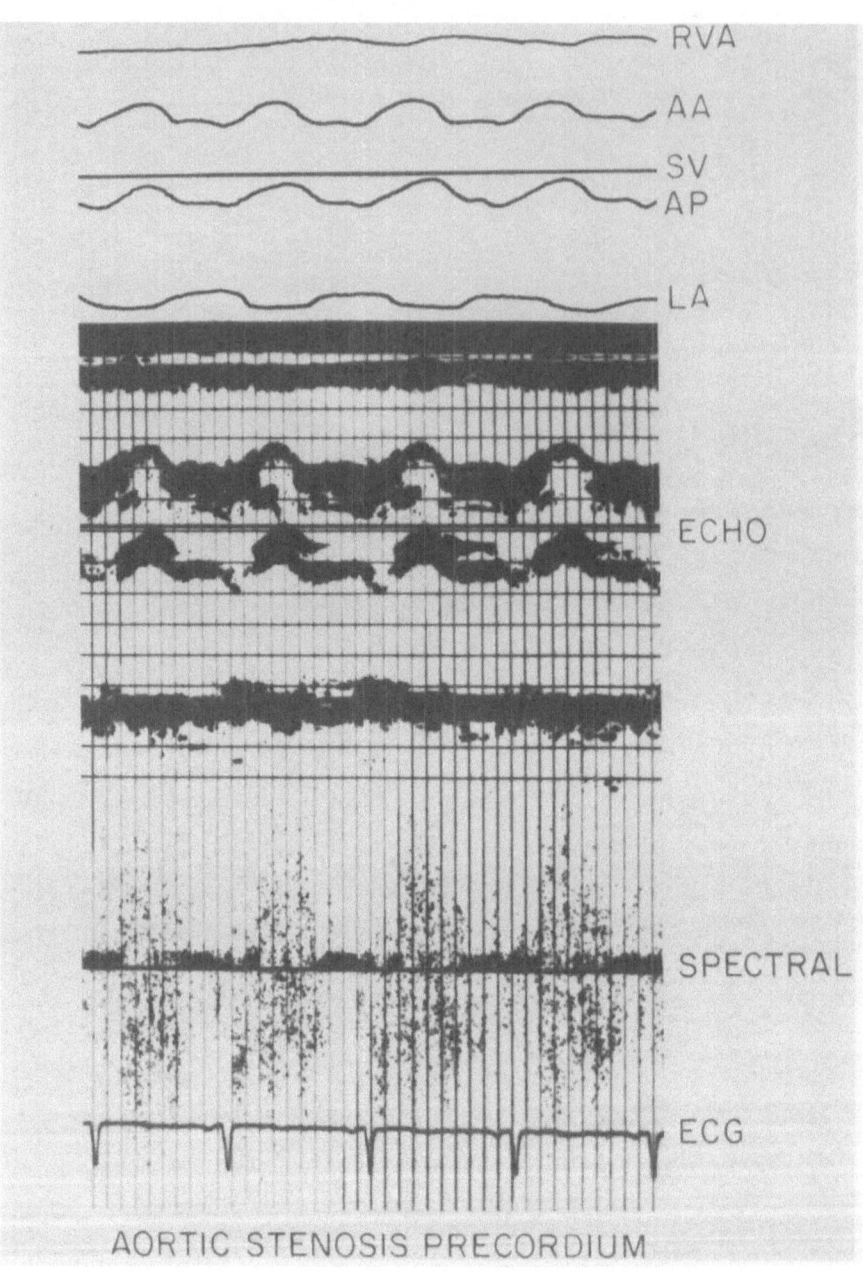

fig. 5. Aortic stenosis produces a wide dot pattern in the spectral "TIH" part of the record. A "harsh" sound would be heard when the sample volume is moved through the jet. Estimates of the degree of stenosis can sometimes be made by using the difference in the sample volume depth as it enters and leaves the jet.

214

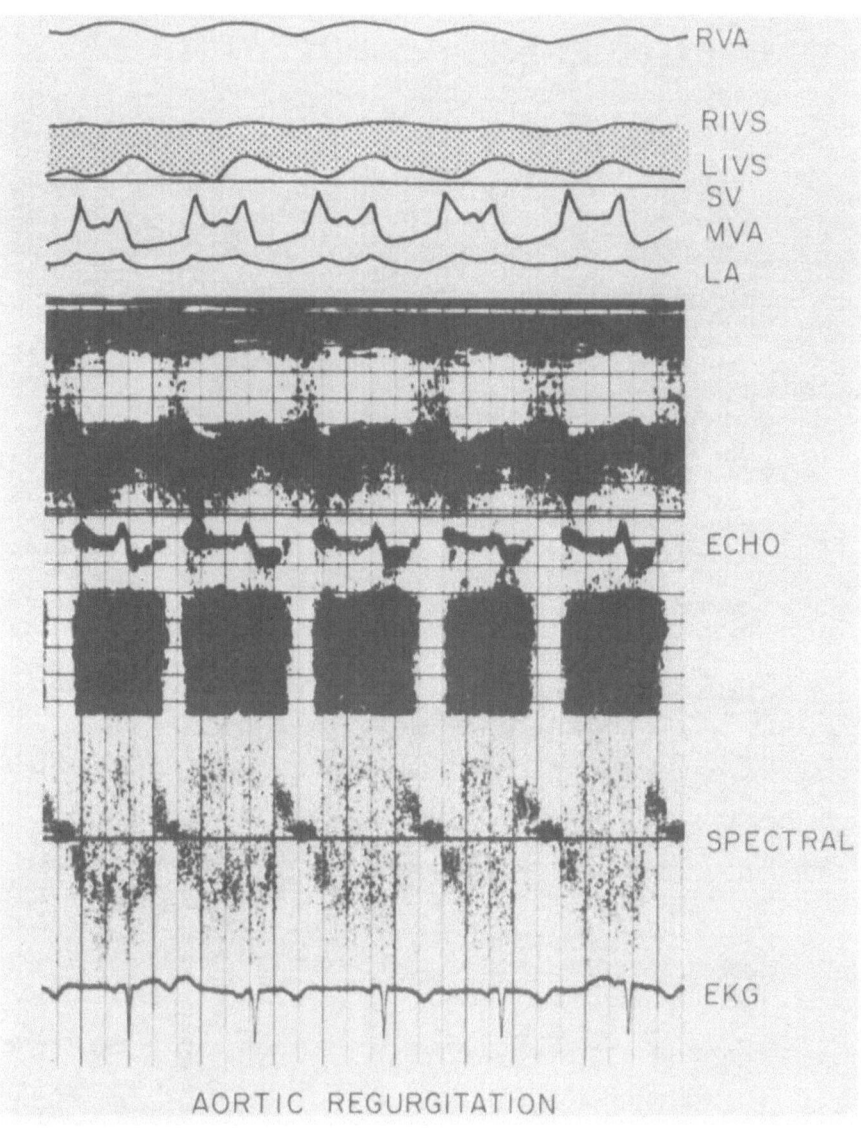

RIVS
LIVS
SV
MVA
LA

ECHO

SPECTRAL

EKG

AORTIC REGURGITATION

fig. 6. Aortic regurgitation disturbances are detected in the LVOT during diastole. The extent of the jet down into the ventricle gives an impression of severity.

Mitral valve flow

If the sample volume is placed in the left ventricular inflow region, nonturbulent, anteriorly directed flow is found to commence with opening of the mitral valve (fig. 7). This flow diminishes, but is sustained until late diastole when a small flow

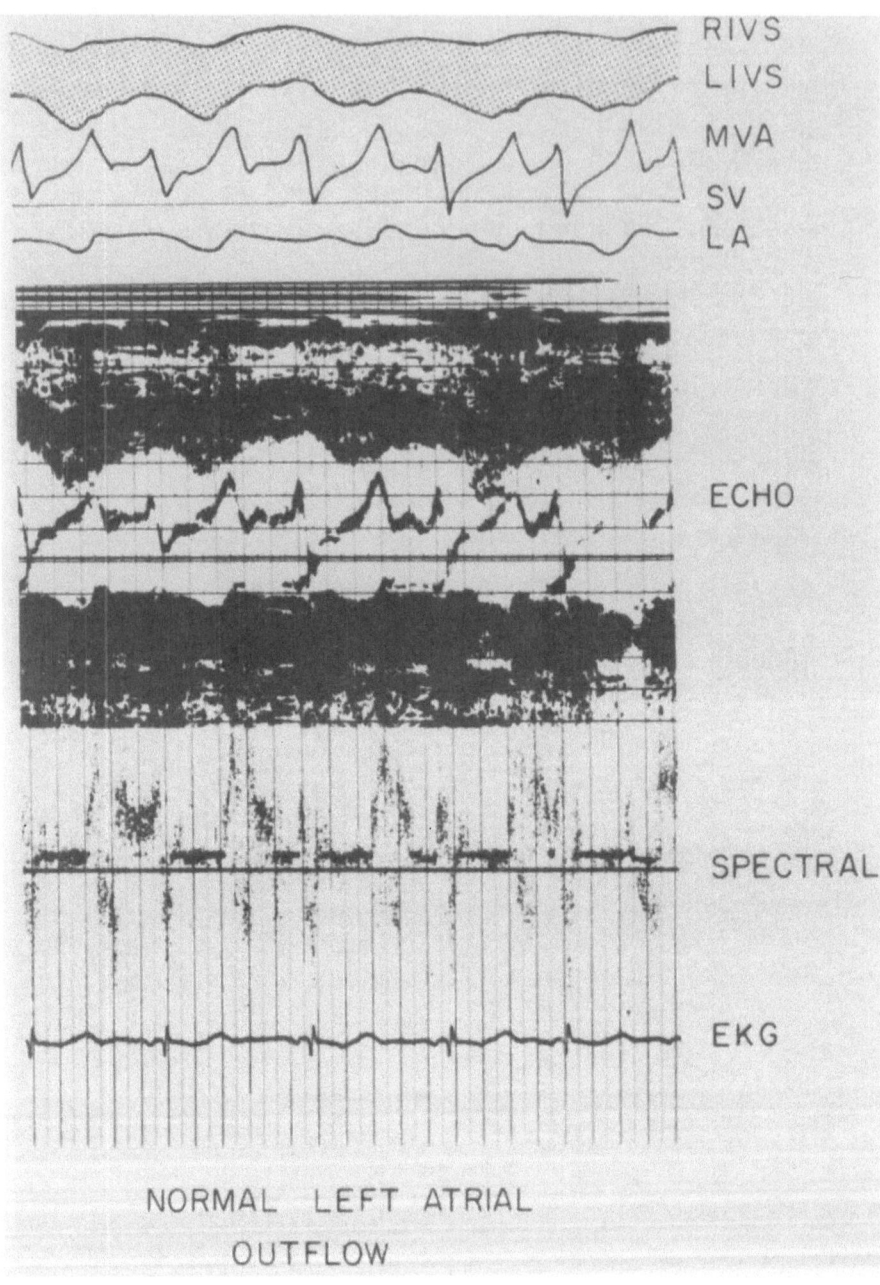

fig. 7. Normal left atrial outflow or ventricular filling with the sample volume placed anterior to the mitral valve. Smooth anteriorly (positively) directed flow velocity denotes the onset of diastole. This flow diminishes, but is sustained, until late systole when a small flow wave occurs coincident with atrial contraction.

wave occurs with atrial contraction. The mitral valve then closes and flow recorded from this position ceases. In mitral stenosis a broad band diastolic pattern is found within the mitral valve orifice, in the left ventricular inflow region, and frequently just posterior to the mitral valve in the left atrial outflow region (fig. 8). Mitral regurgitation is represented by a broad band pattern detected in the left atrial outflow region during systole (fig. 9). This turbulence is frequently confined to the latter half of systole in the presence of mitral valve prolapse.

Pulmonic valve flow
The normal right ventricular outflow tract has a rather characteristic narrow band negatively deflected pattern in systole since flow is directed posteriorly away from the transducer. In pulmonic stenosis a broad band pattern is detected during systole in the proximal pulmonary artery. Pulmonic regurgitation produces a broad band pattern in the right ventricular outflow tract during diastole (fig. 10).

Atrial septal defect
When an atrial septal defect is suspected, the transducer may be directed in such a manner that the sample volume is passed from the left atrial chamber to the right atrial chamber while flow is being assessed (ASD maneuver). If this maneuver is performed several times with the range-gate set at slightly different distances, a sample can usually be obtained from directly within, and on the outflow side of, the atrial septal defect. Intra-atrial shunting generally produces a turbulent pattern with the Doppler detector 6).

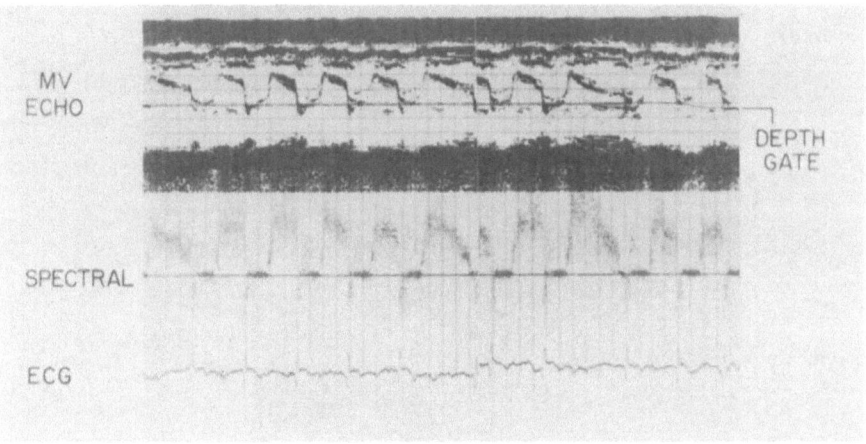

fig. 8. With mitral stenosis, diastolic disturbances are detected within the mitral valve orifice. The spectral pattern is similar in shape to the displacement of anterior leaflet of the mitral valve.

217

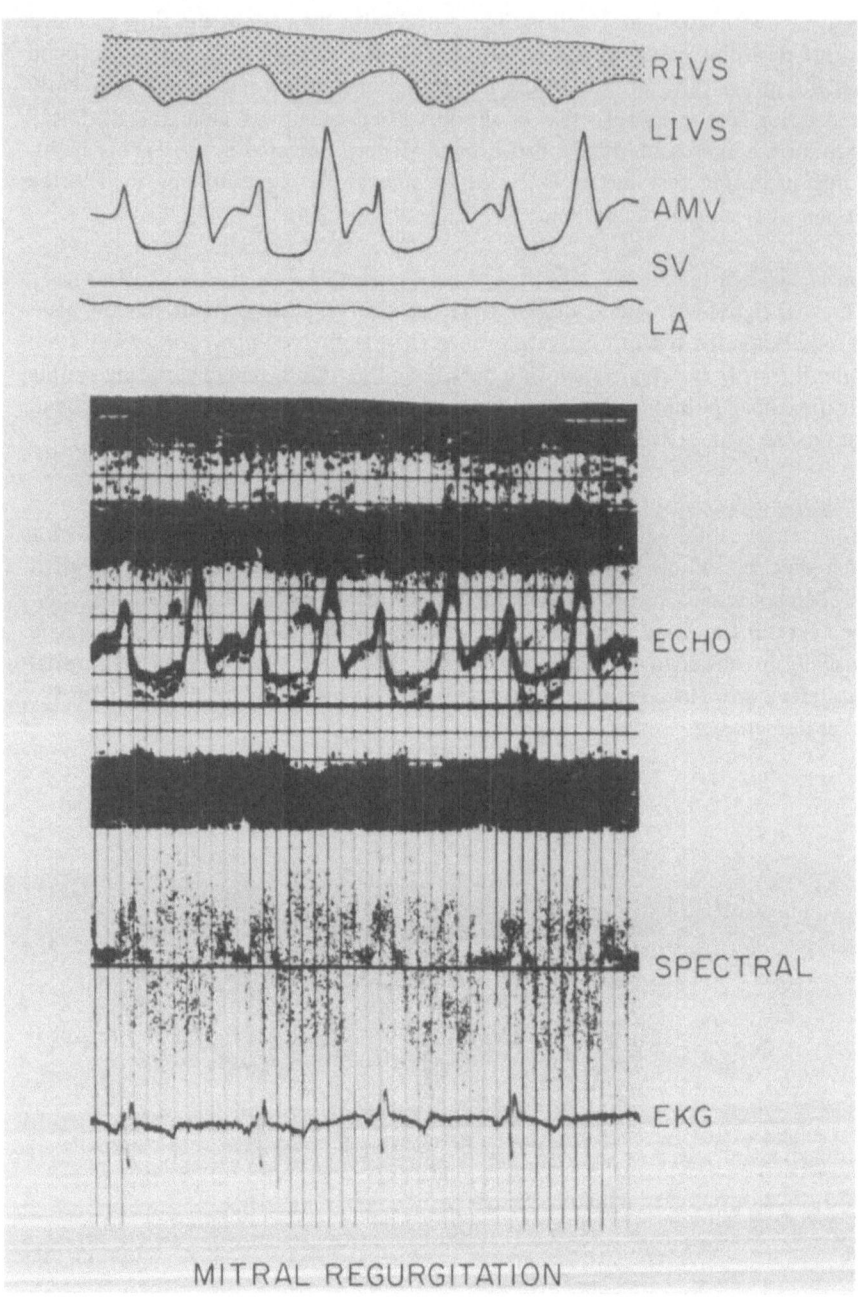

RIVS

LIVS

AMV

SV

LA

ECHO

SPECTRAL

EKG

MITRAL REGURGITATION

fig. 9. Mitral regurgitation produces disturbed flow velocity patterns during ventricular systole. The sample volume is situated in the left atrium just posterior to the mitral valve.

218

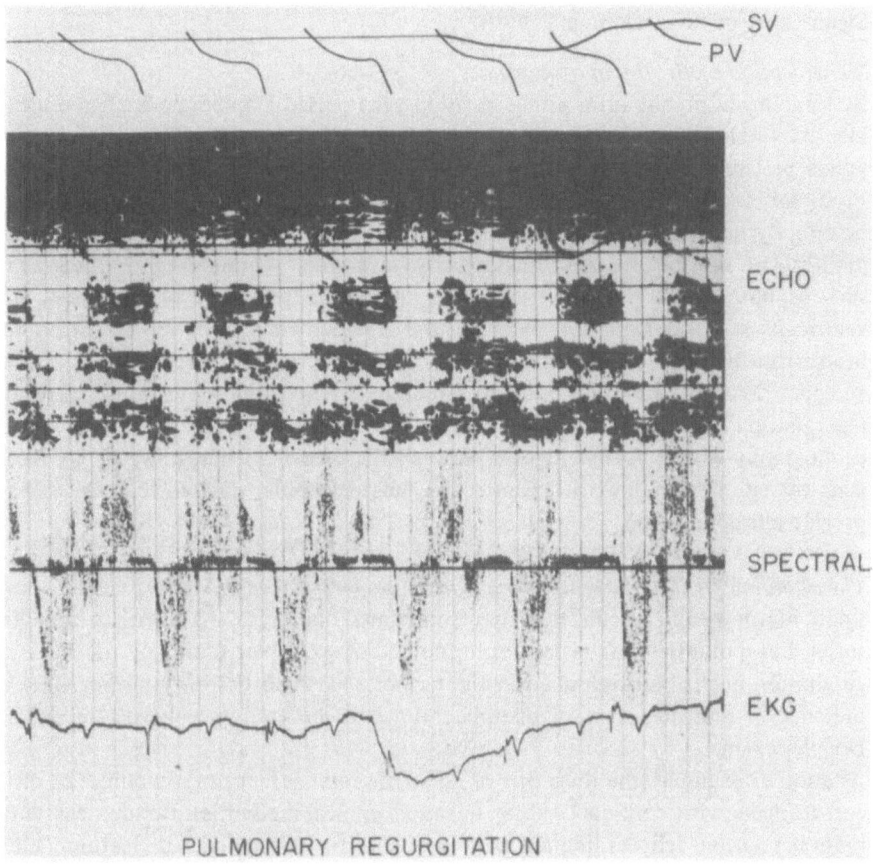

SV
PV

ECHO

SPECTRAL

EKG

PULMONARY REGURGITATION

fig. 10. Right ventricular outflow (RVOT) through the pulmonic valve has a characteristic, negatively deflected pattern detected during systole because flow is posteriorly directed in the RVOT. Pulmonic regurgitation causes a moderately turbulent, positively deflected pattern (a) during diastole.

Ventricular septal defects

Membranous ventricular septal defects are characterized by the presence of a broad band systolic jet in the right ventricular outflow tract. This turbulent jet can frequently be followed through the interventricular septal defect itself. The localization of systolic turbulence to the right ventricular outflow tract and through a portion of the interventricular septum differentiates this lesion from infundibular pulmonic stenosis. In the latter the systolic turbulence is confined to the right ventricular outflow tract.

In the muscular form of ventricular septal defect, a systolic jet exists in the body of the right ventricle. For reasons that are not entirely clear, the jet is frequently difficult to identify and can only occasionally be followed through the septal defect itself.

219

Significance of this technique

Identification of the origin of murmurs

By sampling at precise intracardiac locations, the pulsed Doppler device can reliably identify the location and timing of turbulent blood flow events. The timing corresponds precisely to that heard with stethoscope or recorded on phonocardiogram. From this Doppler information the abnormality causing a particular murmur may be directly inferred. This is especially useful in those lesions which produce either minimal or nonspecific abnormalities by traditional M-mode echocardiography such as mitral regurgitation, tricuspid regurgitation, pulmonic regurgitation, and ventricular septal defects. For example, the development of a new systolic murmur heard from the left lower sternal border to the apex in a patient several days after an acute myocardial infarction could represent a ventricular septal defect or mitral regurgitation from a severe papillary muscle dysfunction. Traditional M-mode echocardiography would not distinguish between these two entities, however, by localizing the site of the flow disturbance, the pulsed Doppler detector can be used to provide a firm diagnosis.

The obtaining of information not recognized on physical examination

Loud murmurs on auscultation may sometimes obliterate the presence of other softer but potentially significant murmurs. For example, mitral or tricuspid regurgitation might be overlooked in the face of a harsh aortic flow murmur, but the presence of multiple areas of disturbed flow can be easily recognized on pulsed Doppler exam.

As another example, the diagnosis of an atrial septal defect can sometimes be difficult to make with confidence using our usual clinical modalities. Paradoxical septal motion seen on echocardiogram is neither specific, nor a constant feature 7), 8), and provides only indirect support for the diagnosis 9). While the flow across an ASD is almost always inaudible by auscultation, it can usually be detected on Doppler examination.

Separation of innocent from pathologic flow murmurs

The significance of systolic flow murmurs in young people is sometimes difficult to assess with the usual noninvasive methods. By Doppler examination innocent murmurs produce minimal or no disturbance, whereas pathologic flow murmurs tend to be quite disturbed. The reason for this is not entirely clear, as presumably some flow disturbances are being produced in the presence of functional murmurs. It may well be, however, that these disturbances are so mild that they are not detected by the pulsed Doppler device. This area of investigation requires further evaluation and validation.

The use of a graphical display depicting the smooth or disturbed state of the intracardiac blood flow adds significantly to the conventional audio output of most Doppler devices. While it is not a total substitute for listening, it makes it possible for those not directly involved with the procedure to identify the flow defect.

More research is required, however, to perfect the optimal flow velocity analysis technique which can contribute as much as the well trained ear.

Acknowledgements

The authors wish to acknowledge the contributions of Vernon Simmons, Robert Olson, and Ronald Daigle from the Ultrasound Program in the Center for Bio-engineering for instrumentation and technical assistance and to Barbara Eyer for typing the manuscript.

References

1) Johnson SL, Baker DW, Lute RA, and Dodge HT: *Doppler echocardiography: the location of cardiac murmurs.*
Circulation 48: 810, 1973.

2) Johnson SL: *Pulsed Doppler Echocardiography.*
Seattle, 1975 Celcom Press.

3) Baker DW, and Johnson SL: *Doppler echocardiography.*
Chap. 19 in Cardiac Ultrasound, R. Gramiak, ed., pages 264-276, C.V. Mosby, St. Louis, 1975.

4) Baker DW: *Pulsed ultrasonic blood flow sensing.*
IEEE Transactions on Sonics and Ultrasonics SU-17 (3): 170-185, 1970.

5) Goldberg BB: *Suprasternal ultrasonography.*
JAM 215: 245, 1971.

6) Kalmanson D, and Veyrat C et al: *Non-invasive technique for diagnosing atrial septal defect and assessing shunt volume using directional Doppler ultrasound.*
British Heart Journal 34: 981, 1972.

7) Hagan AD, and Francis GS et al: *Ultrasound evaluation of systolic anterior septal motion in patients with and without right ventricular volume overload.*
Circulation 50: 248, 1974.

8) Radtke WE, and Tajik AJ et al: *Atrial septal defect: echocardiographic observations.*
Ann. Int. Med. 84: 246, 1976.

9) Solinger RE: *Ultrasound in Congenital heart disease.*
Chap. 13 in Cardiac Ultrasound, R. Gramiak, ed., pages 185-209, C.V. Mosby, St. Louis, 1975.

Applications of pulsed Doppler systems

by P. Péronneau*
Centre d'Etudes des Techniques Chirurgicales,
C.N.R.S., Hôpital Broussais, Paris.
* Maître de Recherches à l'Institut National de la Santé et de la Recherche Médicale.

Introduction

Pulsed Doppler systems appeared some ten years after the first blood velocity measurement involving the Doppler effect induced on ultrasonic-waves by the red cells displacement 1), 2). Previous systems used a continuous emission and quite simple electronics to provide the blood velocity (without or with its sign). Continuous wave apparatus have demonstrated that they are useful tools for non-traumatic cardiovascular investigations and until now, these systems are the more largely used. Nevertheless, the necessity of distance discrimination appeared and was the starting point of the pulsed Doppler systems development. The problem consists in the determination of the position of the moving targets the velocity of which is measured. With continuous wave systems, this discrimination is only provided by the ultrasonic beam of the probe.

Principle

The principle of pulsed Doppler systems is a combination of echographic and Doppler methods: series of coherent pulses are emitted by the transducer in the direction of observation defined by the ultrasonic beam. Between the emitted pulses, the transducer operates as receiver and an electronic gate allows the selection of signals reflected by the red cells at a settled distance from the transducer. The position d of the red cells is known from the relation $d = 0.5 \, ct$ (c velocity of sound, t, reception time) and their velocity v is extracted by detection circuits according to the well known Doppler relationship. A given duration of the electronic gate corresponds to a thickness of the measurement volume (or sample volume) along the beam axis; particularly, a small gate duration will provide local velocity measurement. Here two points have to be underlined:
1. By using a gate duration equal to the repetition period spatial characteristics similar to those of continuous wave systems are obtained and can be used for a preliminary study of the vessel.
2. Multiple gate detection has to be used if multiple points of velocity measurements are needed (it can be demonstrated 3) that a fast moving single gate is not adequate for pulsatile flows studies). Recent digital technology affords one to build systems with a large number of simultaneous points of detection along the ultrasonic beam 4).

As for any instrumentation system, it is obvious that some theoretical and technical problems arise in the definition of performances and design of the apparatus, and

223

Echocardiology, N. Bom editor, published by Martinus Nijhoff, the Hague 1977.

they have to be taken into account according to the purpose of the application. As a matter of fact, some points are common for continuous wave and pulsed systems: sensitivity, incidence of the beam angulation on the vessel for the velocity calibration, conversion of Doppler frequencies into velocity signal. Nevertheless two important problems are specific of the pulsed Doppler systems: the ambiguities induced by the periodic process of exploration and the sample volume definition. Ambiguities occur both in time/distance and frequency/velocity domain 5). The maximum unambiguous range d_{max} and maximum unambiguous velocity in the direction of the ultrasonic beam are related by: $d_{max} \cdot v_{max} = c^2/8$ Fe, Fe being the emission frequency. Actually the practical limits are depending on the vessel-beam angulation, the width of the Doppler spectrum and the choice of the emission frequency. The latter is related to sensitivity factor and a compromise has to be chosen: low frequencies are used for deep examinations (2-4 MHz) and higher values (8 MHz) for peripheral measurements. (For example, for 4 MHz emission frequency and 45° angulation, one has d_{max} (cm) x v_{max} (cm/s) =1000). The currently used pulsed emission described here is not the single time-coded emission type which yields the distance discrimination. Other systems have been studied as well such as frequency or phase modulation and pulsed random process 6). They can overcome the ambiguities but often with some loss of sensitivity. Progress will probably be made along this way.

The definition of the sample volume and its interference on the measurement accuracy is described by several authors 3), 5), 7), 8). The dimensions of the sample volume depend on the shape of the beam and, in the direction of observation, on the emission and gate durations. The resolution is given by the smallest actual durations; in other words it is determined by the overall bandwidth including the probe; typical resolution is 0.5 to 1.5 mm in the direction of the beam. In the case of velocity profile determination, a distortion is induced by the finite size of the sample volume and procedures of correction involving deconvolution have been suggested by several authors 3), 9). It should be noticed that if fine resolution is not desired, the greater the sample volume, the better the sensitivity.

Cardiovascular examinations

Numerous applications of pulsed Doppler systems are now developped. They can be classified in five groups: velocimetry and flow-rate determination in peripheral vessels, velocimetry of moving structures, vessel imaging and experimentation studies.

Blood flowmetry in peripheral vessels

It is obvious that most investigations performed with a continuous wave system can also carried out with a pulsed system. It is not the point of major interest and specific possibilities are afforded by the distance discrimination ability: separation of vessels close to each other within the ultrasonic beam, determination of velocity profiles, measurement of the flow rate. From the technical point of view within a range of about 4 cm few problems arise: the sensitivity is good, the ambiguities do

224

not occur, except possibly at the level of very strong stenoses and the resolution is good enough for drawing profiles.

A velocity profile with a resolution better than 1 mm can be obtained either by a multiple point velocimeter 11) or by moving the observation gate along the beam axis and off-line reconstruction of the profile if instantaneous full evolution of the velocity distribution is needed 12). The simplest way is the automatic scanning of the probe field by the gate with the storage on a C.R.T. screen of the peak to peak velocity recorded according to the position of the gate 13); an example of such a tracing is given on fig. 1. The tracing of velocity profiles can be a useful tool for the vascular obliterans examination.

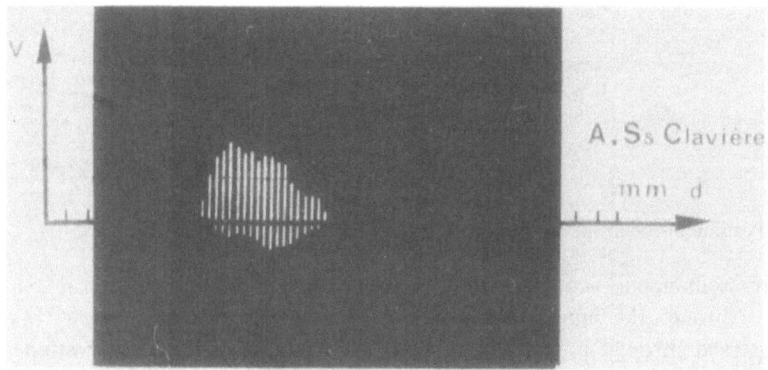

fig. 1. Peak to peak velocity profile recorded in the left sub-clavian artery by an automatic scanning of the observation field with a step of 0.35 mm.

Correction of the angulation error has been described elsewhere 5), 7), 13) and can quite often be applied in order to achieve absolute measurement of velocities and diameters. Bench tests and angiographic checkings have demonstrated regression coefficients better than 0.95 for flow-rate and diameter measurements (the accuracy on its determination can reach 0.7 mm) 13), 14). It seems that a new field of application is now offered.

Blood velocimetry in heart and deep vessels
Numerous investigations of deep vessels and outflow tract of valves have now been performed with pulsed Doppler systems 7), 15), 18). For this field of application, the distance discrimination and the included echographic system are very important positive factors to eliminate contaminating information from other vessels and get anatomic data. On the other hand, technical problems are severe.

Sensitivity and ambiguitie problems arise. This calls for a careful choice of repetition and emission frequencies. To increase the sensitivity focalisation of the beam and large longitudinal size of the sample volume are used and subsequently the resolution becomes poor (several mm). For the same reason, spectral analysis is sometimes employed to analyse the Doppler signal, as its signal to noise ratio ranges between 0 and 20 dB. A great difficulty to obtain proper blood velocity signals is the interference of the Doppler signal caused by movement of vascular or cardiac walls. Strong filtering of low Doppler frequencies has to be performed with adjustable cut-off. In practise, care must be taken for the proper adjustment of the sample volume and for the threshold which is introduced on the measured velocity.

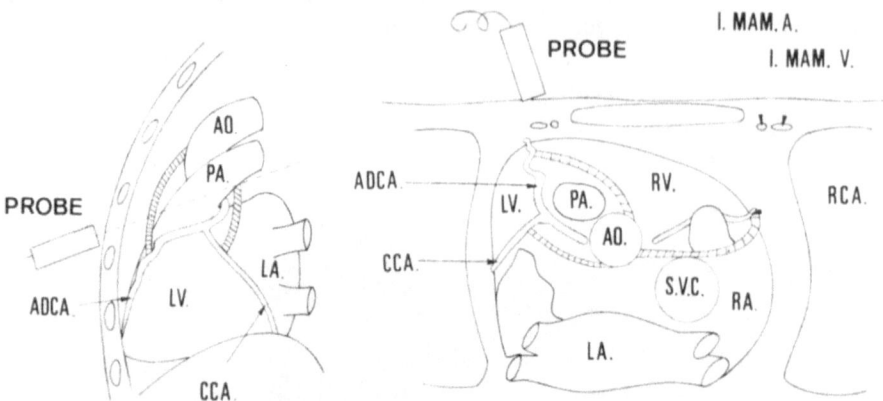

fig. 2. Position of the probe used to investigate the aorto-coronary grafts.

Few transcutaneous acoustic windows are available. The aortic arch is generally reached through the suprasternal notch, other main vessels and outflows of valves are observed through precordial windows. As example of deep observation, fig. 2 shows the pathway (within lateral and transversal cross-section), we use for the study of the permeability of aorto-coronary bypass 17). Such grafts can have several locations inside the thorax, but the diastolic characteristics of the flow and the spatial detection of major flows help to locate the by-pass. The pulmonary outflow is easily recorded (fig. 3); the aortic flow is observed just behind and to the right.

The mammary vessels are fixed along the internal thoracic wall and close to the heart during expiration. The artery is differentiated by its systolic flow, but the vein is the major cause of errors for anterior grafts detection. Its flow is diastolic and the velocity wave looks like a coronary one. The spatial discrimination and respiratory test (the vein doesn't move in respect of the thoracic wall during inspiration) lead up to a good assurance to detect the anterior graft. Generally speaking according to the position of grafts, some interference can occur with different vessels for instance with pulmonary artery or coronary arteries. Great care has to be taken for this examination with various positions of the patient. As summary of preliminary results for 51 patients investigated, a correlation of 74 percent was found with angiographic results with 5 negative falses, 5 positive falses. We have to mention that no calibration in terms of velocity was done.

The difficulty of quantification of measurement is a general problem for deep flows examinations 7), 16). This is particularly due to the lack of multiple acoustic windows to reach a given site. Some possibilities are apparently present at the level of the aortic arch: one is the determination of the normal incidence to the aorta and

226

known rotation of the probe, the other could be the Doppler imaging of the arch. Nevertheless, the measurement of absolute values of flow-rate (through quantified velocity profiles or cross-section averaged velocity measurement which assumes uniform illumination of the area) remains until now somewhat uncertain.

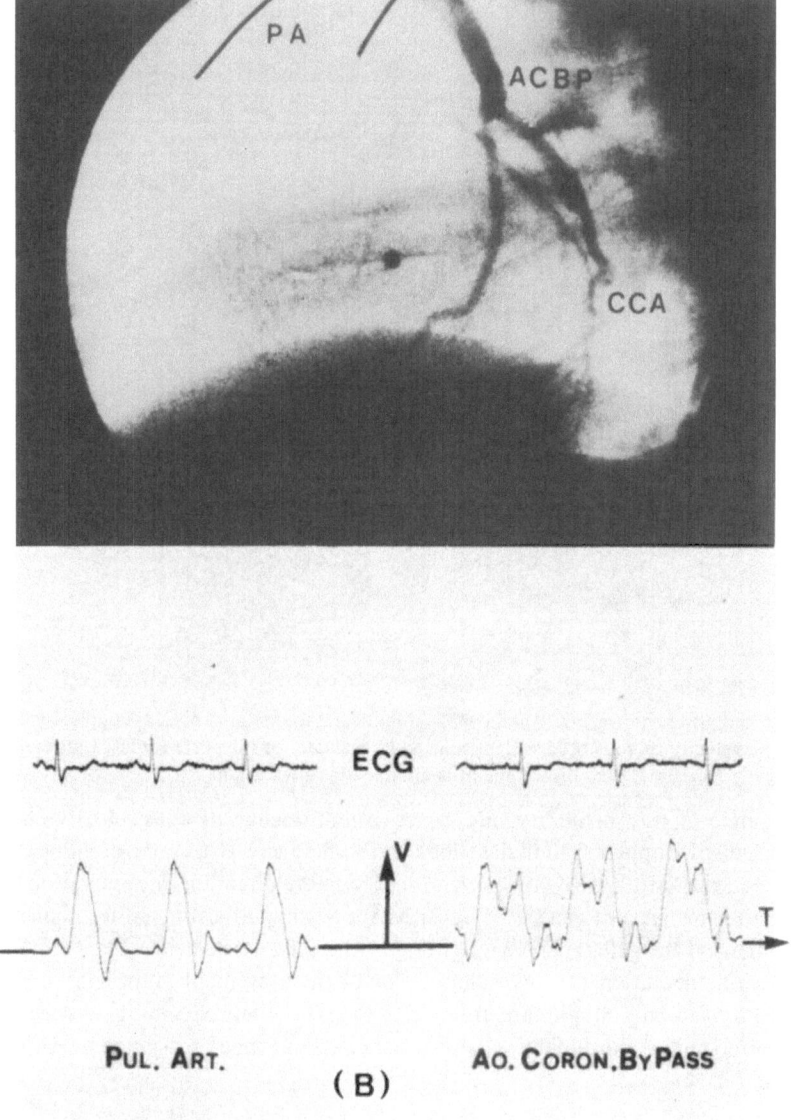

fig. 3. Investigation of an aorto-coronary graft.
    (A) angiographic view
    (B) velocity tracings recorded in the pulmonary artery and the graft.

Velocimetry of moving structures

The blood is not the single moving structure of interest in the body and since a long time recordings of the movement of cardiac structures (valves and walls) and of their pathological alterations have been a widely used tool for the diagnosis of cardiopathies. These investigations are made with A, or B-mode echographic systems and few direct measurements of structures displacement velocity are performed by Doppler effect.

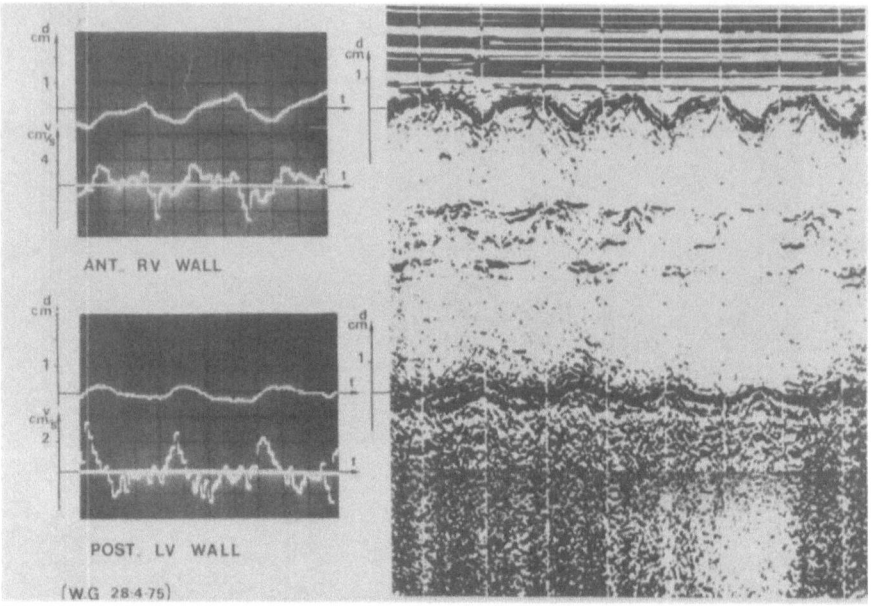

fig. 4. Comparison of tracings obtained in M-mode (at right) and pulsed Doppler system (at left): the velocity of the anterior right ventricular wall and of the posterior left ventricular wall are directly measured, their displacement is obtained by integration.

As example of this possibility, fig. 4 gives direct tracings of walls velocity obtained with a pulsed Doppler system described somewhere else 18). Anterior and posterior walls are selected by two gates, operating along the direction of observation. Technical problems are not caused by sensitivity or ambiguities but rather concern the adjustment of the gates and the weighting of the echoes selected.

Differential measurement allows elimination of the movement of the heart in respect of the thoracic wall. Studies are in progress to test the reproducibility of the method and correlate the shortening velocity of the left ventricular diameter with known contractility index.

Vessel imaging

Echographic and pulsed Doppler systems have been associated to get tomographic sections of vascular lumens. As for a classical echographic instrument, the position of the probe is copied on a CRT screen, and the B-mode is used to display the information. Thus instead of the echoes amplitude a Doppler information "lights the spot" and reveals the presence of flow.

This information is either the velocity itself detected with a classical velocimetric section, or the one derived from specific properties of the Doppler signal 20). The ambiguities problem does not occur here since one only detects the presence of the movement and not its magnitude, but resolution and sensitivity (particularly when atheromatous deposits are present on the wall) are major factors of performances. Fast building of the image is often required for easy investigations. At this time, the full development of this technique is not achieved.

Experimental applications

It is not possible to finish the present survey of the pulsed Doppler systems applications without mentioning the experimental studies 21). The pulsed Doppler method allows precise studies of the flow behavior in vitro (hydraulic models) and in vivo (animal experiments). Velocity distributions within the vascular bed of complex patterns (curves, branchements, valves) can be established, velocity gradients, wall shear forces, instabilities of the blood flow can be estimated in normal and pathological conditions. Some of the methods and results will be certainly extrapolated to the clinical field, during pre-operative or non traumatic examinations.

To conclude, numerous applications of pulsed Doppler systems already exist, but all of the potentialities offered are not yet fully developped probably due to the only recent appearance of such systems in the clinical field. Of course, some progress should be made in order to increase the performances of the instruments, but one can reasonably predict a large increase of pulsed Doppler systems applications in the non-invasive diagnosis field.

References

1) Péronneau P, Deloche A, Bui-Mong-Hung, and Hinglais J: *Débitmétrie sanguine par ultrasons. Développement et applications expérimentales.*
   European Surgical Research 1: 147, 1969.

2) Baker DW: *Pulsed ultrasonic Doppler blood-flow sensing.*
   IEEE Trans. Sonics Ultrason. 17: 170, 1970.

3) Mc Leod FD: *Multichannel pulse techniques.*
   In "Cardiovascular Applications of Ultrasound", R.S. Reneman Ed., North Holl. Publ. Co., Amsterdam, 1974, p. 85.

4) Mc Leod FD, Daigle RE, Miller CW, Moragan JR, and Histand MB: *A digital doppler velocity profile meter.*
   JSABM 312: 55, 1974.

5) Péronneau P, Bournat JP, Bugnon A, Barbet A, and Xhaard M: *Theoretical and practical aspects of pulsed Doppler flowmetry: real-time application to the measure of instantaneous velocity profiles in vitro and in vivo.*
In "Cardiovascular Applications of Ultrasound", R.S. Reneman Ed., North Holl. Publ. Co., Amsterdam, 1974, p. 66.

6) Jethwa CP, Kaveh M, Cooper GR, and Saggio F: *Blood flow measurements using ultrasonic pulsed random signal Doppler system.*
IEEE Trans. Sonics Ultrason. SU-22: 1, 1975.

7) Baker DW, Johnson SL, and Standness DE: *Prospects for quantitation of transcutaneous pulsed Doppler techniques in cardiology and peripheral vascular diseases.*
In "Cardiovascular Applications of Ultrasound", R.S. Reneman Ed., North Holl. Publ. Co., Amsterdam, 1974, p. 108.

8) Morris RL, Histand MB, and Miller ChN: *The resolution of the ultrasound pulsed Doppler blood velocity measurements.*
Journal of Biomechanics 6: 701, 1973.

9) Péronneau P, Sandman W, and Xhaard M: *Blood flow patterns in large arteries.*
In: "Ultrasound in Medicine", D.N. White and R.E. Brown Ed., Plenum Press Publ., New York and London, 1977, vol. 3B, p. 1193.

10) Strandness DE, and Sumner DS: *Clinical applications of continuous wave and pulsed Doppler velocity detectors.*
In "Vélocimétrie Doppler Ultrasonore. Application à l'étude de l'écoulement sanguin dans les gros vaisseaux". Péronneau P, Ed., Publication INSERM 34: 147, 1975.

11) Rutishauser W, Brunner HM, Bollinger A, Brandestini M, Doriot PA, and Anliker M: *Blutflussmessung in arterien aus instantanen Strömungsprofilen mit gepulstem Doppler Ultraschall.*
Verh. Dtsch. Ge. Kreislaufforschg. 40: Seite 149, 1974.

12) Histand MB, Miller CW, and McLeod FD Jr: *Transcutaneous measurement of blood velocity profiles and flow.*
Cardiovascular Research 7: 703, 1973.

13) Péronneau P, Xhaard M, Diebold B, Fiessinger JN, Lévy B, and Bourquelot P: *Débitmétrie transcutanée par vélocimétrie ultrasonore Doppler à émission pulsée.*
La Nouvelle Presse Médicale 5: 2547, 1976.

14) Bourquelot P, Lévy B, Perrey F, and Crosnier J: *Cent carotides bovines modifiées en hémodialyse chronique. Résultats cliniques et hémodynamiques.*
J. Uro-Nephro. (Sous presse).

15) Johnson SL, Baker DW, Lute RA, and Dodge HT: *Doppler echocardiography. The localization of cardiac murmurs.*
Circulation 48: 810, 1973.

16) Angelsen BA, and Brubakk AO: *Transcutaneous measurement of blood flow velocity in the human aorta.*
Cardiovascular Research 10: 368, 1976.

230

17) Diebold B, Guermonprez JL, Péronneau P, Barbet A, Bourassa MG, and Théroux P: *Non-invasive assessment of the patency of aorto-coronary grafts by pulsed Doppler velocimetry. A preliminary study.*
Int. Conf. on Cardiovascular Dynamics, Philadelphia, USA, 3-7 Oct. 1976.

18) Kalmanson D, Veyrat C, Cholot N, and Degroote A: *Non-invasive recording of mitral valve flow velocity patterns using pulsed Doppler echocardiography.*
British Heart Journal (in press).

19) Guglielmi JP, Péronneau P, Diebold B, Lefort JF, and Pernod J: *Real-time Doppler detection of heart wall contraction speed.*
In: "Ultrasound in Medicine", D.N. White and R.E. Brown Ed., Plenum Press Publ., New York and London, 1977, vol. 3B, p. 1213.

20) Bournat JP, Péronneau P, and Barbet A: *Transcutaneous ultrasonic vascular visualization: real-time imaging.*
In "Proc. of Biocapt 75", Int. Conf. on Biomedical Transducers. p. 157, Paris Nov. 1975.

21) Hinglais J: *Applications expérimentales des mesures de profil de vélocité.*
In "Vélocimétrie Doppler ultrasonore. Application à l'étude de l'écoulement sanguin dans les gros vaisseaux". Péronneau P, Ed., Publications INSERM 34: 241, 1975.

Aortic blood velocity measurement by transcutaneous aortovelography and its clinical applications.

by L.H. Light,
Bioengineering Divn, Clinical Research Centre,
Harrow, U.K.

Aortic blood velocity observations complement echocardiography by readily giving information on two important variables which are difficult or impossible to assess echocardiographically: the overall effect of left ventricular contraction and serial changes in left ventricular function.

A technique which maximises convenience and reproducibility in the measurement of mainstream aortic blood velocity has been described 1), 2), 3). In Transcutaneous Aortovelography (T.A.V.), a relatively wide beam of continuous ultrasound is used which is directed from the suprasternal notch towards the transverse aorta (fig. 1). A near-tangential approach to flow is obtained which virtually eliminates the effect

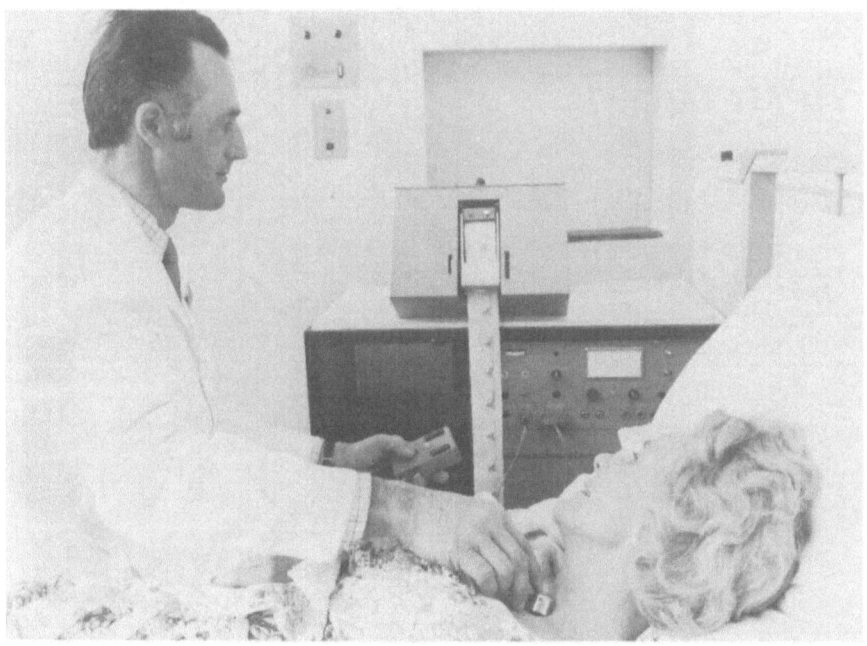

fig. 1. Measurement of aortic blood velocity by transcutaneous aortovelography. Operation of the instrument by doctor, nurse or technician is simple and quickly learnt. There is no discomfort to the patient, who is preferably supine, as this position generally allows a better signal to be obtained.

233

Echocardiology, N. Bom editor, published by Martinus Nijhoff, the Hague 1977.

of the angle term in the Doppler equation 4) (fig. 2). Mainstream blood velocity can thus be calculated, without the need for any calibration, from the highest negative Doppler shift in the signal backscattered at any one time by the red blood corpuscles moving in the arch. The same applies to the signals from the pulmonary artery which may be obtained in children and a minority of adults by the approach "2" in fig. 2a.

Although means exist for displaying this highest Doppler shift in isolation 5), 6), 7), the full spectrum is displayed on-line for the sake of reliability: A sharp outline to the spectrum verifies that mainstream flow has indeed been insonated 8), while the occasional presence of interference from flow in the innominate vein is usually visible in a different shade of grey. Another advantage of spectral analysis is that the spectral outline is visible even for signal-to-noise ratios below unity, so that measurements can be carried out in patients giving poor return signals.

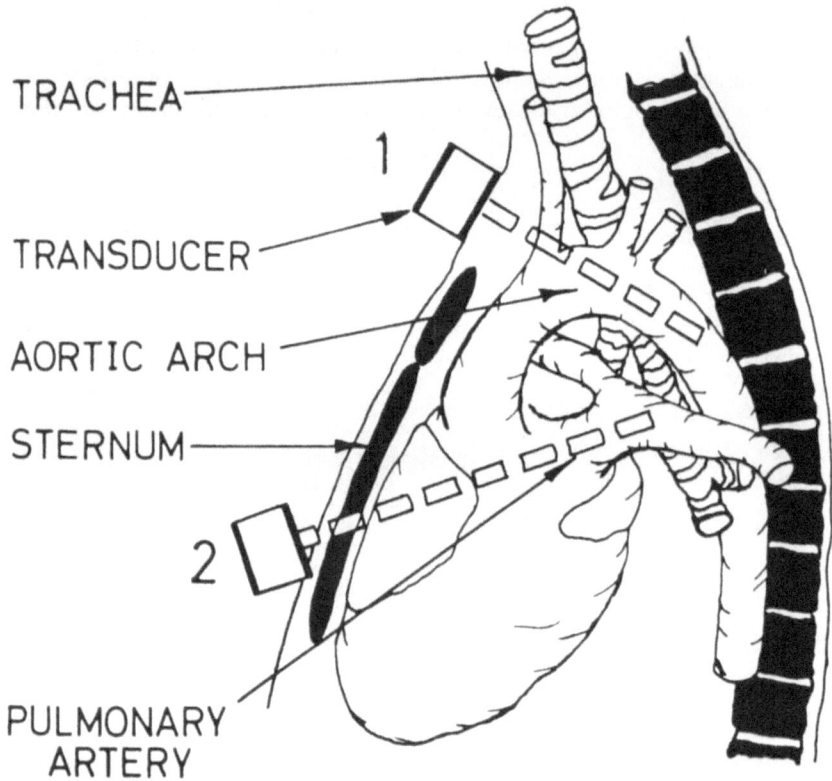

fig. 2a. Lateral view of transducer positions and ultrasonic pathways to aortic arch and pulmonary artery trunk. In each case systolic blood flow is receding and some of the flow is within 26º of the direction of the ultrasound beam, so that reproducible velocity measurements can be obtained *by calculation* from the highest instantaneous negative Doppler shift in the signal backscattered by the red blood cells.

234

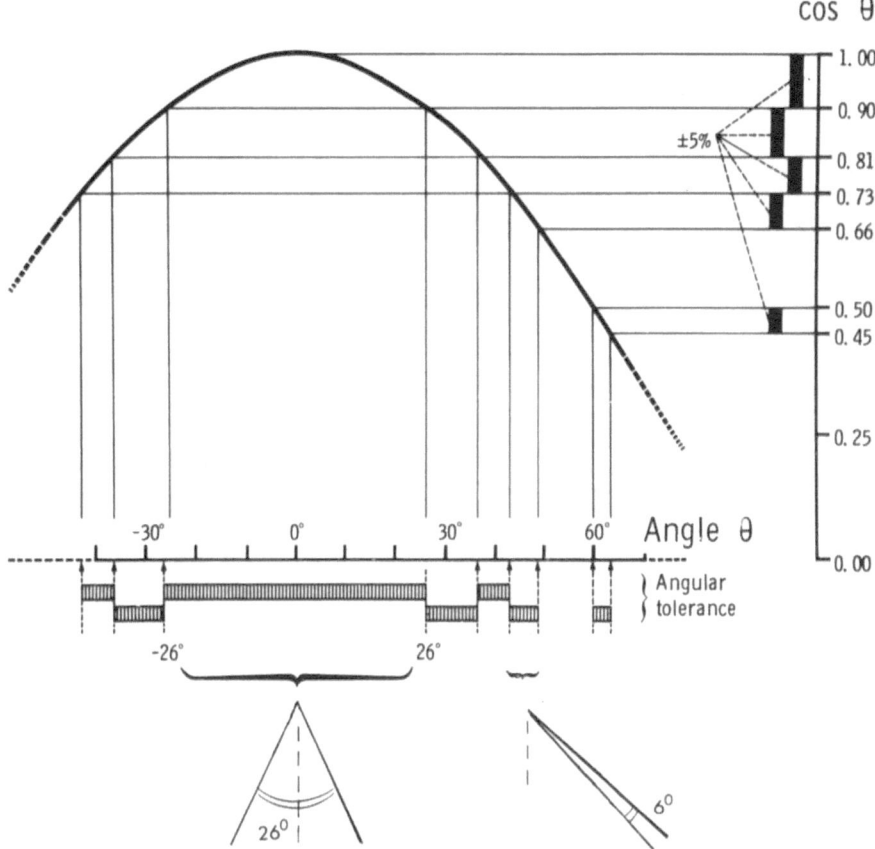

fig. 2b. For quantitative and reproducible Doppler velocity (v) measurements, the angle θ between flow and ultrasound beam must in general be accurately known and exactly reproduced in serial measurements. Exceptionally, for nearly in-line incidence, there is a wide tolerance on the angle (up to ± 26° from exactly in-line for ± 5 percent accuracy). This is a consequence of the cosine-dependence of the Doppler shifts, which are given by $\triangle$ f = 2.55v cos θ for a 2MHz beam. The figure indicates the angular tolerance (shaded bars, bottom) for ± 5 percent measurement reproducibility. Actual angles corresponding to this tolerance are also shown.

The direction-resolving continuous-wave system and a display highlighting the maximum negative Doppler shift, which are used in the instrument, reject most unwanted signals while avoiding the adjustment required to find the appropriate depth which would be required in a range-gated (pulsed) system. Range/velocity ambiguity problems are also avoided.

Verification
Comparisons during diagnostic catherisation with intravascular blood velocity measurements by electromagnetic catheter, (S.E. Labs.) showed good proportionality

235

Figure 3a

Figure 3b

Figure 3c

Figure 3d

Figure 3e

Figure 3f

Figure 3g

Figure 3h

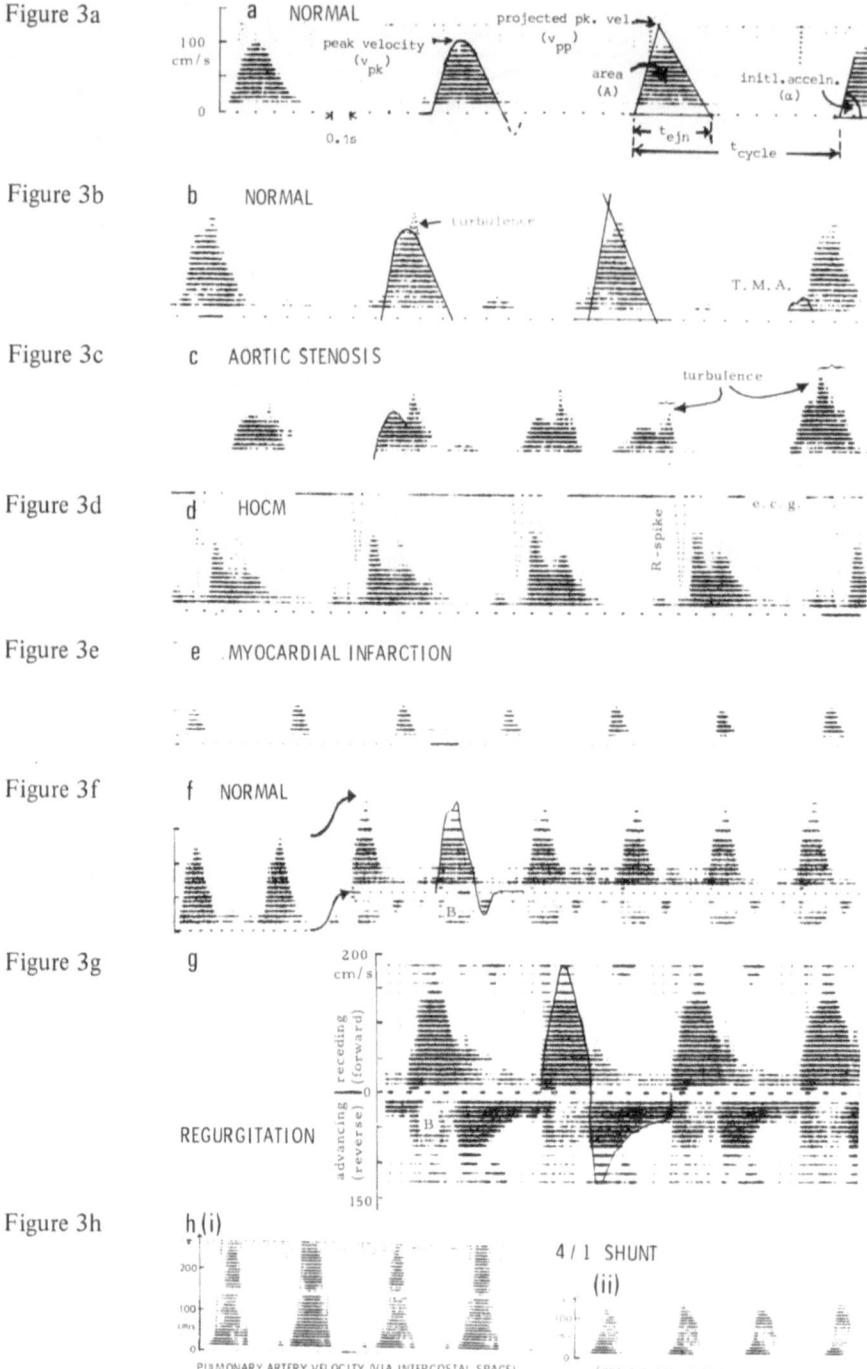

236

fig. 3. Aortic blood velocity measurements. Normally, only negative Doppler shifts (from blood receding from the transducer) are analysed, (a) - (e). A distinct outline to the spectrum (darkened area) indicates the time-course of mainstream flow velocity during systole. The vertical scale is common to traces (a) - (g). Derived variables of haemodynamic interest are shown, as is an approximate form of waveform analysis in which triangles are circumscribed round the systolic complexes. The area of the complex is a measure of stroke volume in any one subject.

a) Normal waveform: a smooth outline indicates laminar flow.

b) Normal waveform: a short spike, indicating minimal flow disturbance, is commonly seen just after the systolic peak in young subjects. (T.M.A. = tissue motion artefact).

c) Sustained irregularity of outline with delayed onset is found when there is an upstream obstruction to flow, as in aortic stenosis.

d) Characteristic double peaks, or a 'shoulder' on the downstroke are found in obstructed beats in hypertrophic obstructive cardiomyopathy. The R-spike from a co-recorded ECG is seen projecting downwards before each complex.

e) Haemodynamic impairment following myocardial infarction is typically signalled by reduced peak velocity and ejection time. Acceleration is not necessarily subnormal during early systole, but is poorly sustained.

f) Aortic backflow (in addition to systolic branch artery flow, "B") is seen below the raised zero line in a bi-directional display. This trace shows the normal brief post-systolic flow reversal.

g) Excess backflow indicates aortic regurgitation, the severity of which can be estimated from the ratio of the systolic and diastolic areas. (Trace (g) was assembled from separate recordings of forward and reverse flow).

h) By the use of an intercostal approach (fig. 2), blood velocity can also be measured in the pulmonary artery (i) of children. This exceeds aortic blood velocity (ii) in cases of severe left to right shunts, as in the 4:1 shunt illustrated.

9) in each of 7 subjects between peak velocities recorded by the two techniques (S.D. = 6 percent), with the degree of agreement on absolute values which might be expected in view of the difficulty of placing the catheter in mainstream flow. Proportionality was also observed between the area of TAV systolic complex and stroke volume as calculated from dye dilution studies (S.D. = 13 percent) 9). It did not, however, prove possible to calculate with adequate accuracy the absolute cardiac output when a single aortic diameter measurement was also available, one probable reason being the non-circularity of the aortic cross-section which has been observed in some individuals. These findings have been confirmed by Mackay & Hechtman 10) using essentially the same technique, and by Huntsman et al 7) using a spectral outline follower.

The negligible angle-dependence of the signal 8) around the optimum and the consistency 11) found in multi-observer reproducibility trials (S.D.= 7 percent) provide circumstantial evidence that the measurement is of actual mainstream blood velocity. Hypodynamic and hyperdynamic conditions can therefore be recognised as deviations from the normal range. Normal peak blood velocities were found to be remarkably independent of age throughout childhood 12) (135 cm/s±18 cm/s S.D.), but to fall gradually with age in the over-thirties.

Quantitation

Quantitation by TAV is thus in terms of blood velocity (peak and mean), expressed in cm/s. Relative blood flow - including the ratio of serial cardiac output values - can also be quantitated by virtue of the close proportionality 9), 13) which exists under most circumstances in any one subject between mean blood velocity and volume blood flow in l/min. A single simultaneous measurement of cardiac output by another technique is required to 'calibrate' the patient when absolute values of cardiac output are essential. However, abnormalities of the absolute level of cardiac output appear to be reflected in abnormalities of the mean aortic blood velocity and usually also in the waveform pattern. It is thus likely that most - if not all - of the clinically useful information on cardiac output presently obtained from invasive measurements is available in TAV recordings, with extra information on the manner of left ventricular ejection being given by the pulsatile waveform.

Applications

Applications fall into two categories, patient assessment, where abnormalities of scale or of wave shape give the required information, and serial monitoring in which the relationship between blood velocity and blood flow allows changes in body perfusion and left heart action to be observed. The results of several reproducibility studies suggest that changes exceeding 10 percent can be detected with greater than 90 percent confidence.

Patient assessment

Abnormalities of scale: abnormally high velocities are seen in thyrotoxicosis and severe anaemia, while low values are found in a variety of hypodynamic conditions, including hypovolaemia. In severe ischaemic heart disease and hypovolaemia, abnormally short flow-time ratios (ejection period divided by cycle period) are also found, (fig. 3e). Back flow in excess of the brief physiological post-systolic flow reversal indicates aortic regurgitation. Backflow is seen (in addition to systolic flow in the branch arteries and occasional venous signals) below the centre-zero line in a bi-directional display. (fig. 3f,g). Quantitation of aortic regurgitation (fig. 3g) appears to be feasible by comparing the area of the forward stroke volume with that of reverse flow velocity 14). This is in spite of the often appreciable variation in aortic cross section and flow profile which exists in this condition between systole and diastole.*

Sustained irregularities of outline, indicating turbulence, are seen in aortic stenosis and other conditions in which the left ventricular outflow tract is partially obstructed (fig. 3c). Quantitation is not possible while an irregular outline indicates that eddies are superimposed on the forward motion of the blood.

---

* Aortic and mitral regurgitation can also be assessed from the non-quantitative aortic velocity waveform which may be obtained from more elementary instrumentation 19), 20). This however, requires expert and relatively time-consuming handling.

In hypertrophic obstructive cardiomyopathy, a characteristic double ejection or a 'plateau' on the down-stroke are seen in obstructed beats, (fig. 3d), which may if necessary be provoked for diagnostic purposes by suitable manoeuvres 14).

Marked respiratory modulation of peak velocity and area of systolic complex may be found in constrictive pericarditis and cardiac tamponade, and is also seen in other circumstances when the circulation is embarrassed. Irregular beat to beat variations of stroke volume are evident in arrythmias, e.g. the ectopic in fig. 3c.

In severe left to right shunts, pulmonary artery velocities have been found to be higher than aortic velocities (fig. 3h). As the cross-sectional areas of the two vessels are not usually comparable in this condition, the ratio of velocities does not necessarily give the volumetric flow ratio. The extent to which such velocity comparisons are useful in the evaluation of shunts is currently being studied 14).

Monitoring applications

Aortic blood velocity is a more direct index of body perfusion and left ventricular function than variables like blood pressure, central venous pressure and left atrial pressure which are commonly used in intensive and coronary care. It, however, also supplements these latter measurements and makes them more readily interpretable. Trends and the patients response to therapy can be seen - the latter is particularly valuable when the therapy involves lowering of the blood pressure. Compared with measurement of limb temperature, aortic velocity observations give much earlier indication of haemodynamic changes.

The product of the area of systolic complexes and the heart rate, or - a direct equivalent - the mean (time-averaged) blood velocity, gives an index of blood flow in any one patient. To a good approximation, the ratio of serial flow values in the descending aorta equals the ratio of observed mean blood velocities 9), 13). Under most circumstances, this also equals the ratio of serial cardiac output values. In very low output conditions, however, when the autoregulation of the cerebral autoregulation is intact, TAV observations become a more sensitive indicator of changes in cardiac output 9). The only known exception to the reliability of serial blood velocity observations as a guide to circulatory changes are conditions in which the proximal aortic tract is progressively compressed. This will affect the otherwise stable transverse velocity profile in the individual subject, so that blood velocity observations over a period of time would no longer be comparable 15).

In addition to changes in mean flow velocity, changes in waveform details are also significant: Peak velocity and often flow-time ratio (ratio of systole to cardiac cycle period) give a good indication of changes in a patient's condition and are readily assessed by inspection.

In addition, systolic acceleration, an index of contractility of the left ventricular myocardium, can be obtained from the recordings, but requires careful interpretation: An increase in acceleration may be the result of improved left ventricular function or of increased sympathetic stimulation, the latter often indicating increased 'stress' and deterioration in severely ill patients 13). These alternatives can however be resolved by attention to other aspects of the waveform, particularly the flow-time ratio.

Compared with invasive methods, TAV has the advantage of being usable from admission - without delay for the placement of catheters - right through to long term follow-up. During the period of active treatment 16), 17), 18), the availability of immediate feed-back on its effect on blood flow widens the range of therapeutic options. Thus blood volume manipulations, the effect of which is difficult to assess a priori, may be undertaken and optimised in the light of the circulatory response.

The effect of lowering the blood pressure can similarly be observed and settings of pacemakers and positive end expiratory pressure in ventilators can be optimised. Drug dosage may be titrated (fig. 4) and the most favourable of alternative agents (e.g. anti-hypertensive, anti-arrthymic) may be chosen in the light of the individual response.

Limitations

With the grey-scale spectral display provided, artefacts are readily recognised and seldom seriously impair the usefulness of the recording. The main limitation of the technique is that a small minority of patients, including those in whom a tracheostomy interferes with transducer placement, give inadequate signals. An oesophageal transducer 21) should offer a modestly invasive alternative when the transcutaneous approach fails.

Other applications of TAV

Other clinical uses exist for the instrumentation, which is in essence a direction-resolving Doppler system with deep penetration and high rejection to tissue movement artefact: Obstructive disease in the aorto-iliac segment can be detected by comparison between the velocity waveforms in the abdominal aorta and femoral arteries, while the nature of flow can be observed in the portal vein and inferior vena cava. From the suprasternal notch, signals can also be obtained from the ascending aorta, but in the absence of range-gating they can be difficult to resolve from the similarly directed branch artery flow. Although the ascending aorta is apparently the vessel of first choice for Doppler observations of cardiac function, this site has a number of practical disadvantages compared with the transverse aorta: the flow pattern tends to be relatively complex (e.g. the vortices in the sinuses of Valsalva), the pressure on the transducer needed to direct the beam behind the sternum is often uncomfortable for the patient, and - perhaps most important - it is not usually possible to obtain the nearly in line approach to flow, which is required for quantitative velocity measurements. Much of the potential of non-invasive blood velocity observations in the deep thoracic and abdominal vessels is still unexplored, and new applications are likely to emerge.

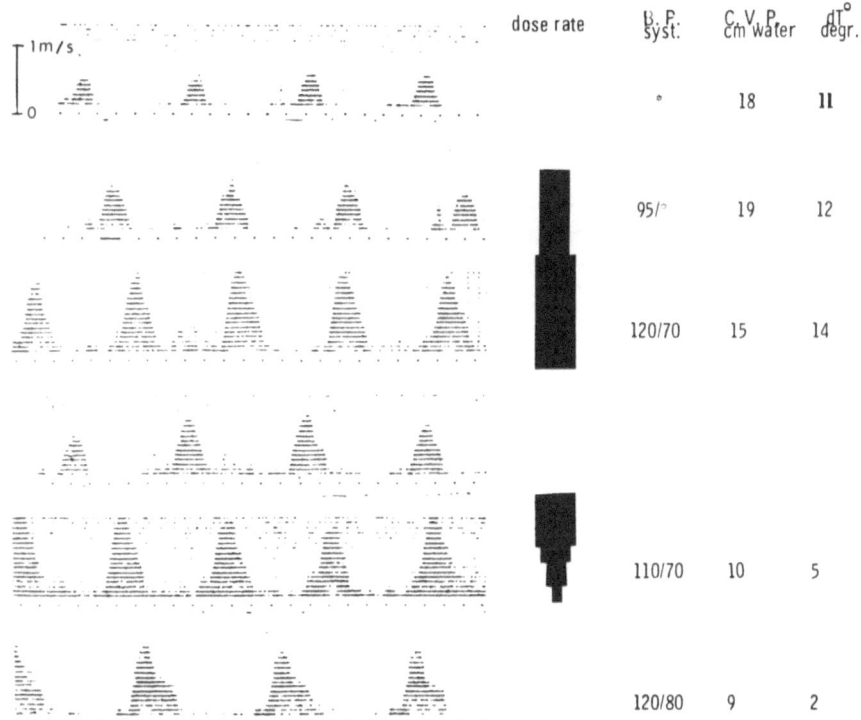

	dose rate	B.P. syst.	C.V.P. cm water	dT° degr.
		°	18	11
		95/°	19	12
		120/70	15	14
		110/70	10	5
		120/80	9	2

fig. 4. TAV in patient management - titration of drug dosage. Serial TAV measurement on a patient admitted in a moribund condition with barbiturate overdose (1st trace). Intensity of therapy (predominantly by isoprenaline) is indicated by the width of the black bar. The infusion was temporarily stopped after 3 hours to determine the degree of circulatory recovery (4th trace). Subsequently the infusion rate was repeatedly adjusted so as to maintain a roughly normal-looking record. Therapy was discontinued after 7 hours when clinical recovery had taken place. The last recording was obtained 30 minutes later. Readings of blood pressure (systolic/diastolic), central venous pressure and temperature difference between toe and rectum taken at the time of the TAV recordings are also shown. The haemodynamic effect of blood volume manipulation, pacemaker or respirator settings can similarly be observed by this non-invasive technique.

Conclusion

A number of trials have shown that TAV offers a quantitative and reproducible non-invasive technique for measuring phasic blood velocity in the aorta. Experimental evidence also supports the theoretical expectation that - in the absence of progressive aortic distortion - such blood velocity measurements give a reliable and reasonably accurate index of body perfusion and left ventricular function. Many forms of malfunction (including hyperdynamic and hypodynamic conditions) and abnormalities of the left ventricular outflow tract are readily detected on inspection of the waveform, while changes give quantitative evidence of disease progression or the effect of therapy. The technique is easily learned and simple to use on the majority of patients. In clinical trials it was found to give information of value in initial patient assessment, in the monitoring of trends and in guiding effective treatment.

Acknowledgements
I am grateful to the many clinicians who have contributed their experience with Transcutaneous Aortovelography, in particular Drs. Gillian Hanson and Anna Buchthal from whose work in Intensive Care fig. 4 is taken, and Dr. R.F. Sequeira who provided some of the pathological waveforms in fig. 3. The help of Geoff Cross has been crucial in the development of the instrumentation.

References

1) Cross G, and Light LH: *Direction-resolving Doppler instrument with improved rejection of tissue artefacts for transcutaneous aortovelography.*
   J. Physiol. 217, 5-7 P, 1971.

2) Light LH, and Cross G: *Cardiovascular data by transcutaneous aortovelography.*
   In Blood Flow Measurement, pp. 60-63. Ed. by C. Roberts, Sector, London, 1972.

3) Cross G, and Light LH: *Non-invasive intrathoracic blood velocity measurement in the assessment of cardiovascular function.*
   Bio-Medical Engineering, 9, 464, 1974.

4) Light LH: *Non-injurious ultrasonic technique for observing flow in the human aorta.*
   Nature 224, 119-1121, 1969.

5) Sainz A, Roberts VC, and Pinardi G: *Phase-locked loop techniques applied to ultrasonic Doppler processing.*
   Ultrasonics 14, 128, 1976.

6) Huntsman LL, Gams E, Johnson CC, and Fairbanks E: *Transcutaneous determination of aortic bloodflow velocities in man.*
   American Heart Journal 89, 605, 1975.

7) Angelsen BAJ: *Analog estimation of the maximum frequency of Doppler spectra in ultrasonic blood velocity measurements.*
   Report 76-21-W, Division of Engineering Cybernetics, Norwegian Institute of Technology, University of Trondheim, 1976.

8) Light LH: *Initial evaluation of transcutaneous aortovelography.*
   Cardiovascular Applications of Ultrasound, p. 325. Ed. by R.S. Reneman, North Holland, Amsterdam, 1974.

242

9) Sequeira RC, Light LH, Cross G, and Raftery EB: *Transcutaneous aortovelography - a quantitative evaluation.*
British Heart Journal 38, 443, 1976.

10) Mackay RS, and Hechtman HB: *Continuous cardiac output measurement: aspects of Doppler frequency analysis.*
Institution of Electrical and Electronic Engineers, Transactions on Biomedical Engineering, BME 22, 346, 1975.

11) Fraser CB, Light LH, Shinebourne EA, Buchthal Anna, Healy MJR, and Beardshaw JA: *Transcutaneous aortovelography-reproducibility in adults and children.*
European Journal of Cardiology, 4, 181, 1976.

12) Beardshaw JA, Shinebourne EA, and Light LH: *Transcutaneous Aortovelography - normal values in children.*
To be published.

13) Light LH: *Transcutaneous aortovelography - a new window on the circulation?*
British Heart Journal, 38, 433, 1976.

14) Sequeira RF, and Watt I: *Assessment of aortic regurgitation by transcutaneous aortovelography,* also: Sequeira RF: *Thesis: Some applications of transcutaneous aortovelography.*
To be published.

15) Light LH: *Non-invasive haemodynamic flow measurement techniques for routine clinical use.*
In Applications of Electronics in Medicine, pp. 21-38. Institution of Electronic and Radio Engineers (Conf. Publication 34), London, 1976.

16) Buchthal A, Hanson GC, and Peisach AR: *Transcutaneous aortovelography - a possible adjunctive technique in the management of the critically ill patient.*
British Heart Journal 38, 451, 1976.

17) Hanson GC, and Buchthal A: *Clinical experience with transcutaneous aortovelography.*
In "Applications of Electronics in Medicine", I.E.R.E., London, 39-48, 1976.

18) Hanson GC, and Buchthal A: *Clinical experience with transcutaneous velography.*
In "Non-invasive clinical measurement". Ed: D.E.M. Taylor, Pitman Medical, London, 32-43, 1977. To be published.

19) Boughner DR: *Assessment of aortic insufficiency by transcutaneous Doppler ultrasound.*
Circulation 52, 874, 1975.

20) Boughner DR, and Nichol PM: *Assessment of mitral regurgitation using Doppler ultrasound.*
Circulation 54, 656, 1976.

21) Duck FA, Hodson CJ, and Tomlin PJ: *An oesophageal Doppler probe for aortic flow velocity monitoring.*
Ultrasound in Medicine and Biology, 1, 233, 1974.

Echo-Doppler systems
Applications for the detection of cardiovascular disorders

by L. Pourcelot, Department of Nuclear Medicine and
Biophysics (Pr. Th. Planiol), Hôpital Bretonneau —
37033 — Tours Cedex (France).

Introduction

The frequency of cardio-vascular illness is well known especially for their effects on the health of mankind. It is necessary to treat patients as quickly as possible and to check their progress regularly during the medical and surgical treatment. Today's methods of internal examination, have the advantage of giving results which are indispensable for both physician and surgeon. But there are still serious risks for the patient, especially if these examinations are used for diagnostic tests or checking the patients state. Non invasive methods, do not at the moment give a sufficiently precise diagnosis.

The need for non invasive examination, which are more precise in diagnoses, has given rise to much research using transcutaneous ultrasonic techniques to study the anatomical and functional modifications in the cardiovascular system of the patients. These methods are used to visualize the arterial walls and cardiac structures by B and M mode displays and to show hemodynamic disturbances by Doppler echography. The sum of these techniques seems to promise a great future in this field of diagnosis if we consider the results obtained recently by researchers.

Doppler arteriography

Doppler examination with a continuous wave (C.W.) apparatus has been used for several years for the diagnosis and monitoring of vascular illness. The development of pulse Doppler systems has made it possible to know with precision the distance between the mobile reflector and the probe. But Doppler examinations are "blind" investigations which set a number of practical problems r.e. manipulation if it is not done with visual aids. This remark is particularly important if we wish to detect the position of the sample volume when using a pulse Doppler system. In addition it is indispensable, in measuring blood flow, to know the cross-sectional area of the artery or of the cardiac orifice, the velocity profile in this section during each cardiac cycle, and the angle of incidence of the ultrasonic beam in relation to the direction of the blood flow.

Echocardiology, N. Bom editor, published by Martinus Nijhoff, the Hague 1977.

In order to develop ultrasonic images using the Doppler shift information, the instrument used is like a B-scanner and consists of a combination of a Doppler detector, with a probe-position resolver and a storage scope. Manual scanning is done by the technician as in normal echography, the probe being slowly displaced at the surface of the skin. The angle of the transducer and its location in the x, y directions are detected by potentiometers. In Doppler arteriography, the modulation of the Wehnelt of the storage scope is produced by the Doppler signal i.e. the image shows only the blood moving in the artery.

C.W. Doppler (fig. 1)

If we use a C.W. Doppler each spot in the screen represents a line of exploration. We get a plane projection of vessels parallel to the skin similar to an oblique view of a contrast arteriogram. During the scan, the Doppler probe remains parallel to itself and inclined in relation to the axis of the arteries to get a correct signal of velocity. The coordinates of the position of the transducer (x, y, Θ) are relayed to the storage scope, and any flow signal greater than a preselected value unblanks the oscilloscope and a spot is stored which corresponds to the line of exploration. A complete scan is gained by a number of monitored parallel lines across the skin of the patient. A complete examination requires a relatively long time: for example a scan for carotid bifurcation takes 5-15 minutes.

Pulsed Doppler (fig. 2)

In case of a pulse transmission, we know the depth of the Doppler detection. Thus it is possible, by moving the probe across the skin, following a line, to get a Doppler tomography, by varying the depth of exploration for each position of the probe This Doppler cross-section corresponds to a right-angle image compared to the arteriography obtained with a C.W. Doppler apparatus. The x-axis corresponds to the displacement of the probe on the skin, while the y-axis corresponds to the depth of the investigated tissue. The advantage of the Doppler tomography is that it shows the arterial lumen, and allows sagittal and transverse cross-sections which are of greatest interest for showing vascular bifurcation. In the future this way of getting a picture would be useful to demonstrate abnormal flow in the cardiac cavities in case of congenital cardiopathies. The Doppler tomography can be produced more quickly if we use a multigated system, allowing the simultaneous storage of a number of separate loci of detected flow.

The ultrasonic arteriography which is the easiest to produce yields a plane projection using a C.W. Doppler. It is difficult though to know the exact plane which crosses, for example, the three carotid arteries when we explore the neck vessels.

Doppler detection

The modulation of the Doppler arteriography can be effected in different ways:
— the operator presses a button for modulation every time he hears a Doppler signal in the headphones. This method is precise, but long and difficult.

246

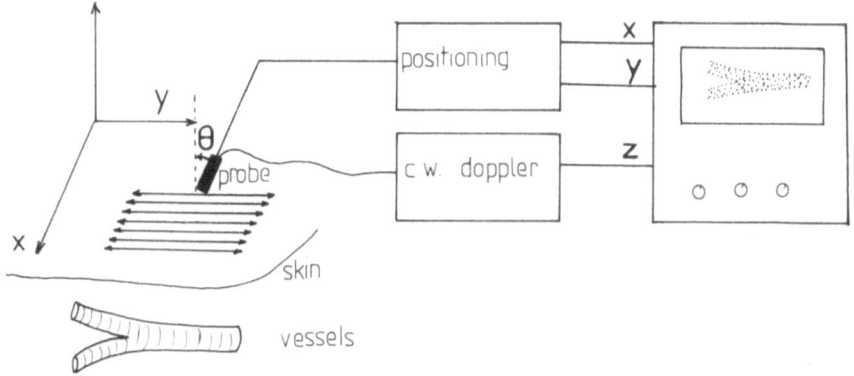

fig. 1. Doppler arteriography: plane projection view of vessels using a continuous wave Doppler system.

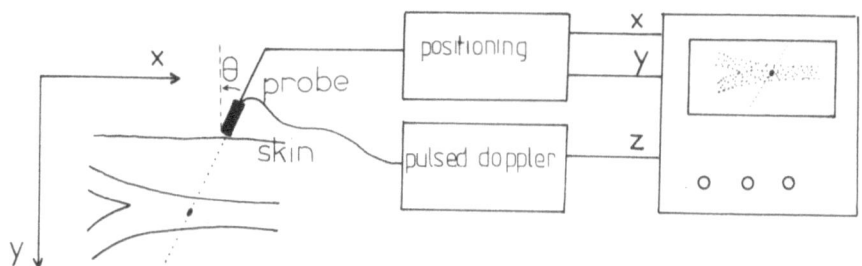

fig. 2. Doppler arteriography: cross-sectional view of vessels using a pulsed Doppler system.

— an electronic circuit detects the Doppler signal and creates a standard pulse of modulation. This method is used in M.T.I. systems.
— an electronic circuit measures the velocity signal and unblanks the oscilloscope each time the preselected velocity threshold is reached. This method is the one most used. It can be wired to a synchronisation system on an E.C.G., so that it will only accept the modulation at certain times in the cardiac cycle.
— in the future the brightness of the arteriogram may be modulated with the velocity signal (if the velocity rises, the spot becomes brighter).

This result can be obtained with the gray scale system of classical B-scanners. If we can produce a lot of Doppler points in a very short time, we can get an instantaneous view of the arteriogram on the screen of the scope showing the velocity modifications with each systole. This functional image of the artery would be of greatest interest for the physician to demonstrate for example the increasing velocities in areas of stenosis, especially if this arteriography is superimposed with a high image rate visualization of reflective tissues.

247

Results (fig. 3 and 4)

Recent research has demonstrated that Doppler arteriography permits non invasive documentation of carotid and femoral occlusive disease. However the presence of arterial wall calcification significantly impairs visualization of the true arterial lumen, by blocking the transmission of the ultrasonic beam. For that reason, Barnes and coll. propose to associate blood velocity analysis with pulsed ultrasonic arteriography. The combined imaging and velocity assessment of carotid artery disease improve the quality of the examination, by studying the blood velocity disturbance associated with proximal stenoses that may not be visualized due to vascular wall calcification. The enlargement of the frequency spectrum can be correlated to the amount of turbulences. This is of great value for assessment of the degree of stenosis.

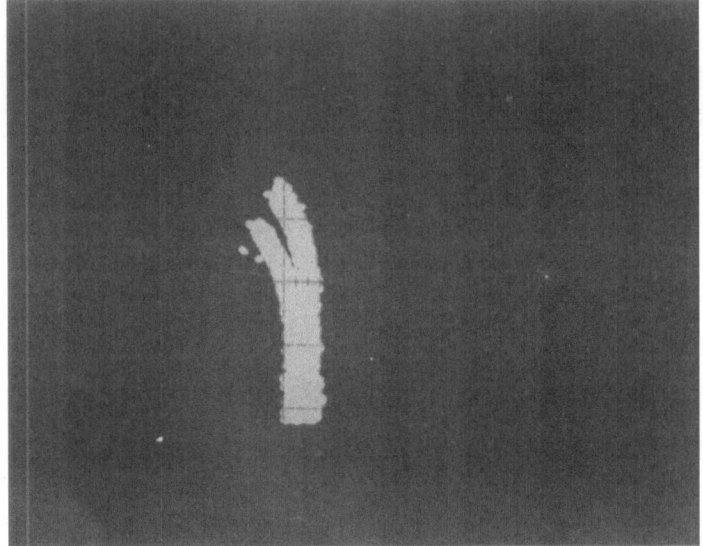

fig. 3. Ultrasonic arteriography: this illustrates a normal right carotid bifurcation (courtesy Dr. D.E. Strandness Jr.).

B-Scan Doppler

The B-scan visualization of the heart and vessels used to be produced by manual scanners. The results were of mediocre quality because of the blurring. The synchronisation of the presentation of the picture on E.C.G. has improved the quality of the image by giving informations at specific moments of the cardiac cycle.

An important breakthrough was recently obtained thanks to the development of rapid scanning machines which work at a frame rate of 15-200 pictures per second.

The rapid change in position of the scanning line can be obtained by a mechanical movement of the probe, either by an electronic commutation of an array of transducers, or by the use of a phased array system. The scanning can be linear or sectorial.

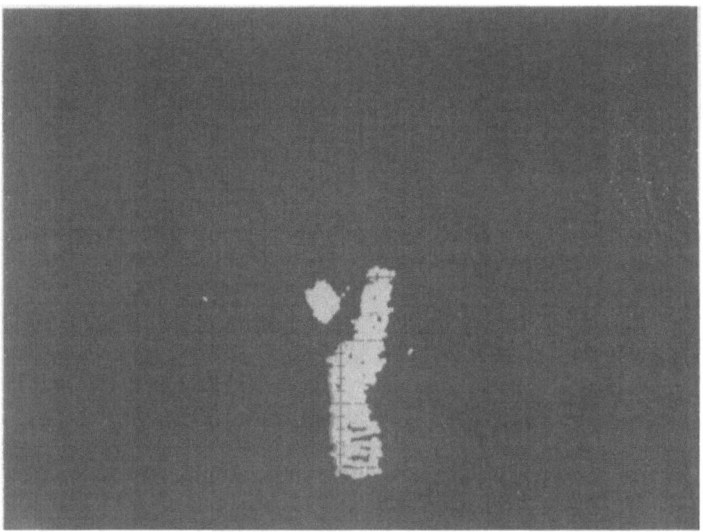

fig. 4. Ultrasonic arteriography. There was a persistant defect in the right common carotid artery just proximal to the origin of the external carotid artery. The origin of the internal carotid artery was sonolucent secondary to calcification. Flow was detected in the internal carotid artery distal to this point but it was abnormal. Flow in the right supraorbital artery disappeared with temporal artery compression. Also, Doppler velocity tracings from the common carotid artery went to zero indicating a high-grade stenosis at the bifurcation. (Courtesy Dr. D.E. Strandness, Jr.).

Because the Doppler arteriography was not obtained at high frame rate, and because the study of anatomical structures is of great importance for the physician, the fusion of B and Doppler scans was indispensable. The machines developed in this way were able to show in cross-sectional views the carotid and femoral arteries and the heart. The Doppler exploration can be effected by a single or a multigated system: the direction and depth of the sample volume (s) are shown in the B dynamic image. So as to avoid interferences between the two methods of detection, we use alternately the Doppler detector and the amplitude detector.
It is usually necessary to use two separate transducers for echo and Doppler investigation. To produce a high resolution image of the cardiac and vascular walls, we must position the echo probe perpendicular to these structures. A Doppler exploration requires, in the other hand, an inclination of the ultrasonic beam with respect to the blood flow vector. These obligations have led the researchers to combine two separate ultrasonic transducers in the scanner head: one to provide for high image

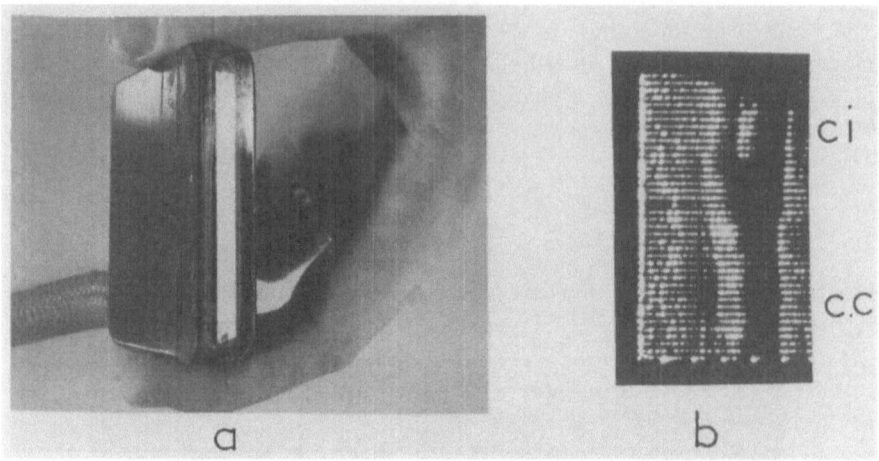

fig. 5. 6 MHz multitransducer probe for vascular imaging (a). Longitudinal view of normal carotid arteries (b): cc = common carotid, ci = internal carotid.

rate visualization of reflective tissues, and one for blood flow study which can be moved in an inclined way related to the lines of B scan.

We hope to develop for easy probe handling an echo-Doppler system with a first linear array of transducers for B-scan and a second parallel array for Doppler investigation. This second array would allow a lateral displacement of the Doppler probe with beam deflection by dephasing.

The advantage of a Duplex echo-Doppler scanning is that it provides an immediate picture which increases the diagnostic potential and reduces the length of the examination. Moreover such a system does not require the patient to stay perfectly stationary, as is the case in the Doppler arteriography. We can superimpose on the B-scan the points of Doppler modulation, or the velocity profile, and record the velocity curves in a spectral or analogical mode. (fig. 6)

The anatomic visualization is very useful in vascular pathology as well as cardiology. In vascular pathology the echo image is used to locate the artery and some atheromateous plaques, and to determine the position of the walls and calcium deposits. The B-scan is then used as a guide to mape out the flow field with Doppler system. Soft atherosclerotic lesions, low in calcium, may produce relatively low backscattering: thus they can appear as relatively sonolucent areas like blood in a B-mode scan. The major interest of the pulsed-Doppler flow detection is to discriminate in this case between the moving blood and the nearly stationary lesions. (fig. 7 and 8)

The slow blood flow velocity near the arterial walls is a problem if one only uses the pulsed Doppler investigation: it makes it difficult to get a precise picture of the vessel, while the B Doppler scanning allows us to distinguish both the walls and the blood flow.

250

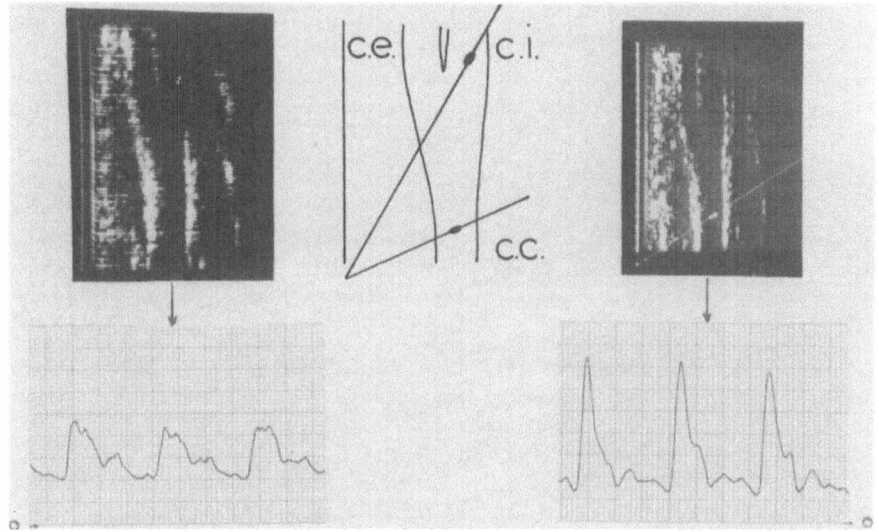

fig. 6. Longitudinal views of normal carotid arteries with a duplex B-Doppler scanner using a multitransducer probe. The line indicates the position of the Doppler beam, with the dot showing the position of the sample gate. Velocity curves of the common carotid (cc) and internal carotid (ci) arteries are recorded.

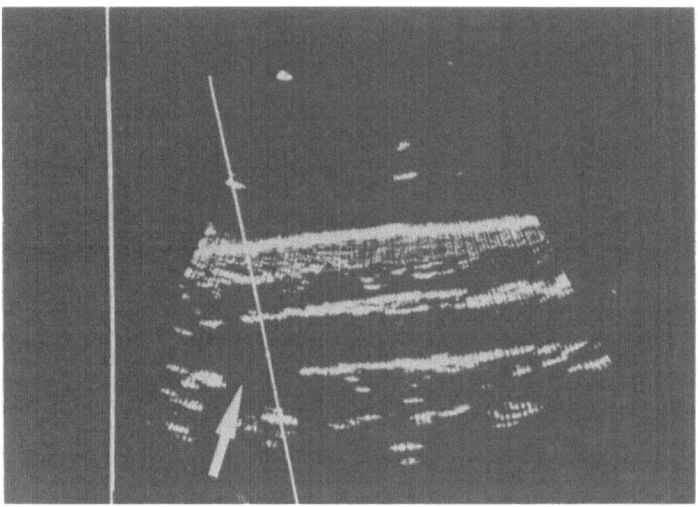

fig. 7. The line indicates the position of the Doppler beam with the dot (in the center of the vessel) showing the position of the sample gate. This is a longitudinal view of the common carotid artery with the carotid bulb to the left. The arrow points to the blank area which signifies acoustical shadowing from calcium within a plaque in the carotid artery. (Courtesy Dr. D.E. Strandness, Jr.).

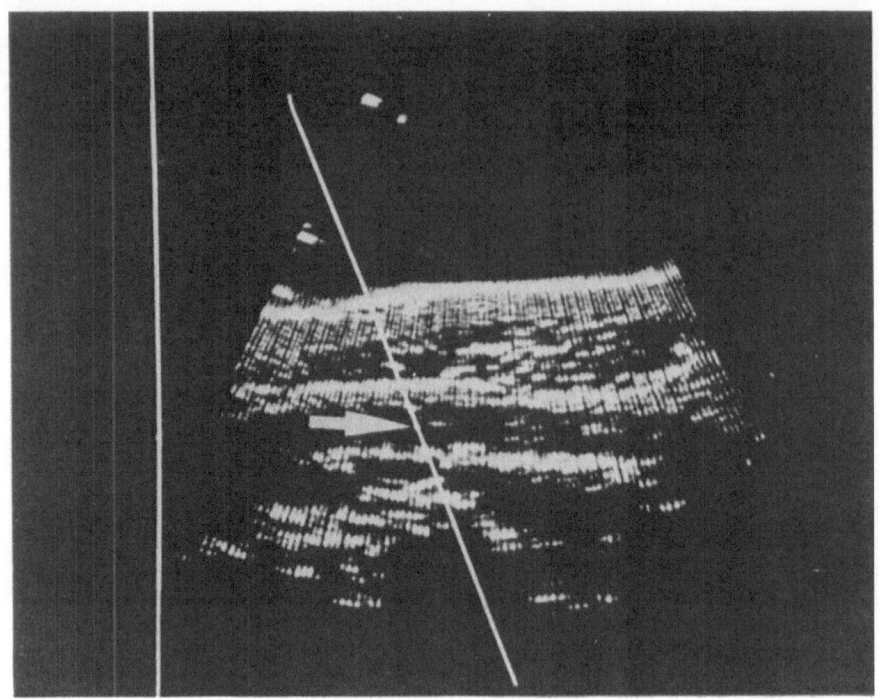

fig. 8. This is a longitudinal scan of a totally occluded common carotid artery. No flow was detected at the point where the sample gate was placed in the mid-portion of the artery. The echoes from within the lumen were arising from the material occluding the artery. (Courtesy Dr. D.E. Strandness, Jr.).

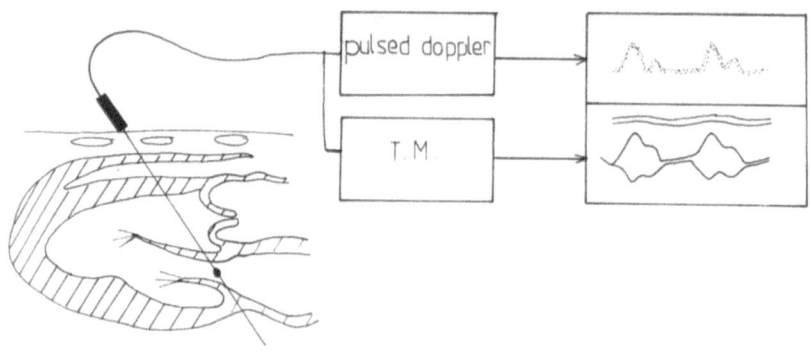

fig. 9. T.M.-Doppler examination: the same probe is used for the detection of the amplitude and Doppler signals.

T.M. - Doppler (fig. 9 and 10)

The study of blood-flow in the cardiac cavities requires absolutely a precise anatomic image to know exactly the position of the Doppler sample volume. This can be
achieved by using a combination of echo-Doppler scanning as previously discussed.
On the other hand, the echographic signal received by a pulsed-Doppler probe can
be partly used to get an amplitude detection, which provides the T.M. signal. With
the same probe it is possible, in this case, to realize simultaneously a Doppler
investigation and a T.M. echography. This principe was used recently to study the
flow in the cardiac cavities. The T.M.-Doppler system is of value for the location of
turbulent zones and for evaluating the degree of stenosis and insuffiency of the
valvular orifices as well as for demonstrating intracardiac shunts.

Real-time Doppler scanning

To obtain   a Doppler echography in real time is an interesting objective for it
would allow instantaneous investigation of the vascular and cardiac hemodynamics.
The problems are difficult to solve because of the relatively long time needed to
produce a map of areas of flow within the cross-section. The detection of amplitude
of an echographic signal requires less than a micro-second while the measure of the
Doppler signal needs a sample time in the order of 100 milliseconds. Thus we only
get 1 point on a Doppler scan when we have produced 1000 to 10,000 points on a
B-scan. As aconsequence if we wish to produce a great number of Doppler points in
a very short time (1/20 second), we need to use a great number of Doppler systems
in parallel. This is technically possible but requires a considerable amount of electronic machinery.

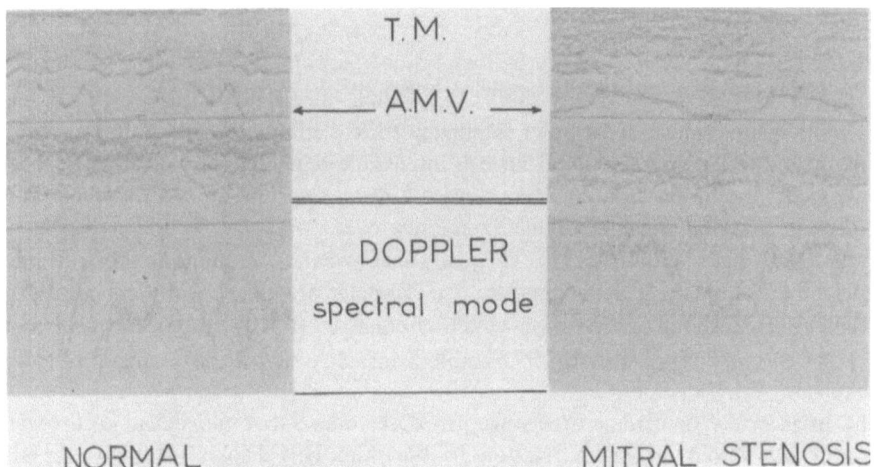

fig. 10. T.M.-Doppler examination: the mitral flow mimics the mitral motion in the normal (left
side). A rapid and constant flow through the mitral orifice is detected during the diastole in
case of moderate mitral stenosis (right side). The horizontal line behind the anterior mitral valve
(A.M.V.) on the T.M. echogram, shows the position of the sample volume.

A clever solution to this problem has been proposed and consists of using a digital conversion of the ultrasonic signal followed by a measurement of the Doppler frequency shift in an electronic memory. We can also get simultaneously a great number of measured points along the axis of the ultrasonic beam. The commutation of one line to the next, as in a fast echographic imaging system, should allow us to get a small Doppler image in a short space of time, and provide an instantaneous picture of the blood flowing in one part of the conventional echographic cross-section. The first results obtained in this way, show great promise for the detection of hemodynamic disturbance in vascular and cardiac pathology. (fig. 11)

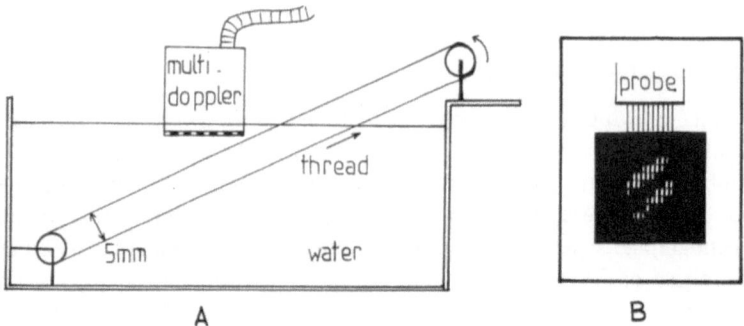

fig. 11. First results of gray scale real-time Doppler imaging at a frame rate of 15 images/second. An array of transducers is used to visualize the moving thread with 10 lines of Doppler scanning. The view is presented on a normal scope (B) and can be direction-sensing if required. This system is presently being tested in vitro.

Particular problems of pulsed Doppler echography

a) The measurement of Doppler frequency shift is limited by the pulse repetition frequency (P.R.F.). Because of this it is impossible to detect certain velocities when we study the blood flow at a considerable distance from the skin surface. Thus there is a systematical error and a relative over estimation of low velocities in relation to high velocities. This is equally true when we explore at short distance the blood flow through a stenosis. The Doppler frequency shift can cross the theoretical treshold of detection which is equal to (P.R.F.)/2. We must raise the rythm of sampling to obtain for example a correct study of the cardiac flow in the adult.

b) In an artery or cardiac orifice we can observe a relative movement of the walls or of the whole orifice in relation to the skin. This displacement gives a false information of flow, which could be important and disturb the measure of the real flow.

c) If the orifice dimensions through which the blood flows become smaller (vascular stenosis, cardiac valvular stenosis or insufficiency), it is often difficult to obtain a correct recording of the velocity curve since this orifice is constantly mobile and moves in relation to the Doppler gate during the cardiac cycle. In this case it is necessary to use a multigated system and to reconstruct the real flow by selecting the gates which are in the best position to detect the blood velocity.

d) In the exploration of intracardiac flow, the amplitude of the valvular echo is very important in relation to the amplitude of the blood echoes. The sample volume is therefore not exactly the same for the blood and for the cardiac structure. Under these conditions there is a greater tendency to record the movement of the valves rather than that of the blood, when the sample volume is near a mobile structure.

Conclusion

Recent research in the field of the combined use of Doppler and 2D visualization have demonstrated the ability to provide safe and rapid informations for direct evaluation of vascular and cardiac disease. The different techniques in development include: C.W. and pulsed Doppler arteriography, duplex B-Doppler scanning, and T.M.-Doppler echography. Although much remains to be done, initial trails with these new modes of investigation of the cardiovascular system have shown great promise for a large reduction of the number of the invasive examination procedures in the near future.

References

1) Baker DW, Johnson SL, Daigle RE, and Olson RF: *Pulsed Doppler cardiac procedures: recording and display techniques.*
   1st Meeting of the W.F.U.M.B., San Francisco, 3-7 August 1976.

2) Barber FE, Baker DW, Nation AWC, Strandness DE Jr., and Reid JM: *Ultrasonic Duplex-Echo-Doppler Scanner.*
   I.E.E.E. Tr. Biomed. Engng., 1974, BME-21, 109.

3) Barber FE, Baker DW, Strandness DE Jr., Ofstad JM, and Mahler GD: *Duplex scanner II: for simultaneous imaging of artery tissues and flow.*
   Ultrasonic Symposium Proceedings I.E.E.E., 1974, Cat R 74, CHO 896-1 SU.

4) Barnes RW, Bone GE, Reinerston JE, Slaymaker EE, Hokanson DE, and Strandness DE Jr.: *Value of blood velocity analysis during pulsed Doppler ultrasonic imaging of carotid artery disease.*
   29th ACEMB, Boston (Massachusetts) 6-10 November 1976.

5) Bournat JP, Peronneau P, and Herment A: *Theoretical and experimental evaluation of a new ultrasonic Doppler method for vascular imaging.*
   1st Meeting of the W.F.U.M.B., San Francisco, 3-7 August 1976.

6) Brandestini M: *Signalverarbeitung in perkutanen ultraschall Doppler Blutfluss Messgeräten.*
   Dissertation I.B.T. Zurich 1976.

7) Fish PJ, Kakkar VV, Corrigan T, and Nicolaides AN: *Arteriography using ultrasound.*
   The Lancet, 10 June 1972, 1269-1270.

8) Fish JP: *Multichannel, direction-resolving Doppler angiography.*
   Proceedings of the Second European Congress on Ultrasonic in Medicine. Munich 12-16
   May 1975.

9) Griffith JM, and Henry WL: *A combined Doppler cross-sectional echocardiographic system
   for measuring cardiac blood flow velocities in man.*
   1st Meeting of the W.F.U.M.B., San Francisco, 3-7 August 1976.

10) Nimura Y, Matsuo H, Kitabatake A, Hayashi T, Asao M, Terao Y, Senda S, Sakakibara H,
    and Abe H: *Studies of intracardiac blood flow with a combined use of the ultrasonic
    pulsed Doppler technique and two-dimensional echocardiography from a transcutaneous
    approach.*
    1st Meeting of the W.F.U.M.B., San Francisco, 3-7 August 1976.

11) Olinger CP: *Ultrasonic carotid echocardiography.*
    Amer. J. Roentgenol. 1969, Vol. CVI, no. 2.

12) Pourcelot L, Pottier JM, Berson M, and Planiol Th: *Multitransducer echoscope (U.S.A.
    B.E.L.). New developments. Applications to vascular visualization.*
    1st Meeting of the W.F.U.M.B., San Francisco, 3-7 August 1976.

13) Ramsey SD Jr., Taenzer JC, Holzemer JF, Suarez JR, and Green PS: *A real time ultrasonic
    B-scan/Doppler artery-imaging system.*
    Ultrasonics Symposium Proceedings I.E.E.E., 1975, Cat ≠ 75, CHO 996-4 SU.

14) Reid JM, and Spencer MP: *Ultrasonic Doppler technique for imaging blood vessels.*
    Science vol. 176, 16 June 1972, p. 1235.

15) Spencer MP, Reid JM, and Paulson PS: *Diagnosis of carotid artery disease and cerebral
    vascular insufficiency with Doppler angiography and ophtalmic artery sonography.*
    Cardiovascular applications of ultrasound. Ch. 21. R.S. Reneman (ed.), Amsterdam, 1974,
    North Holland Publ. Co.

16) Spencer MD, Reid JR, Davis DL, and Brockenb rough:*Cerebrovascular evaluation using
    Doppler C.W. Ultrasound.*
    1st Meeting of the W.F.U.M.B., San Francisco, 3-7 August 1976.

17) Strandness DE Jr., and Sumner DS: *A new approach to arterial visualization.*
    Ch. 19 in Cardiovascular application of Ultrasound. R.S. Reneman (Ed.) Amsterdam,
    North Holland Publ. Co. 1974.

18) Strandness DE Jr., and Sumner DS: *Clinical applications of continuous wave and pulsed
    Doppler velocity detectors. Ultrasonics Doppler Velocimetry.*
    I.N.S.E.R.M., Paris October 1974.

19) Voss DJ, Pedersen PC, Mahler GD, and Barber FE: *A microprocessor – based blood flow
    display for pulsed Doppler systems.*
    1st Meeting of the W.F.U.M.B., San Francisco, 3-7 August 1976.

20) I.N.S.E.R.M. - Grant - A.T.P. 35.76.67.: *Combined use of two ultrasonic techniques
    (Doppler and real-time B-scanning) for the assessment of carotid vascular disease.*

256

A transcutaneous N-channel digital Doppler

by M. Brandestini
Institut für Biomedizinische Technik
der Universität und ETH Zürich

Introduction

The present article analizes the circuitry details of a digitally implemented Doppler flowmeter. The basic ideas of this concept, however, are the contents of earlier papers 1), 2) and will not be exposed in full detail.

The author wishes to forward some design information to the electrical engineer and to complement the previous communications.

Theoretically an unlimited number of possible implementations will yield accept-

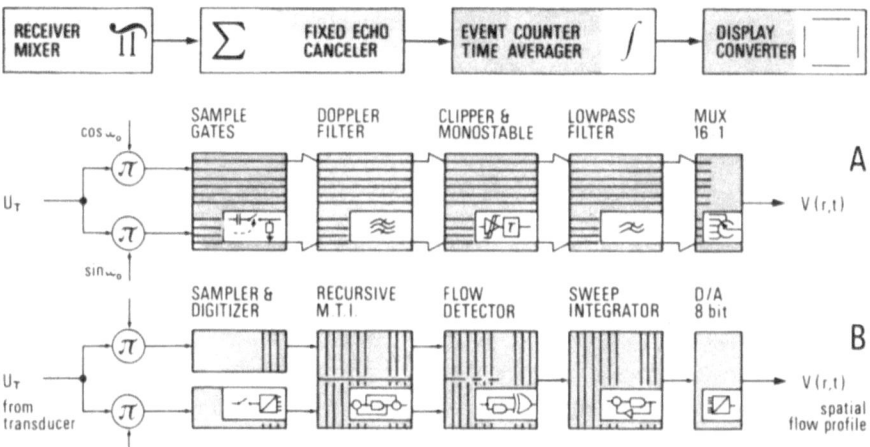

fig. 1. Comparison of conventional multigate (parallel) and digital (sequential) processing scheme.

As a matter of fact the measurement of a spatial velocity distribution by pulsed Doppler techniques calls for a multiplication (π), a subtraction ($\sum$) and an integration ($\int$) in the various observation channels.

Conventionally (A) the output of the demodulator, the so-called video signal, is sampled and distributed into a bank of separate processing channels. Thus all the subsequent circuitry is required n (number of channels) times.

In the digital approach (B) the succesive samples remain discrete time representations and can therefore be processed in sequence. The advantage of this scheme is evident:

A single computational unit can handle any number of channels, provided the information of each range interval is stored in an appropriate memory location.

(Equivalent stages are shown in the same row, e.g. lowpass filter $\triangleq$ sweep integrator).

257

able results. For the realisation of an instrument which is not only subject to pure research, but also to clinical and eventually commercial applications, the expenditure has to remain within a tolerable compass. On the other hand, the apparatus described in the previous articles was just a first attempt to verify the general performance of a digital approach. The clinical results of this pilot model are, however, still inferior to those obtained with established multichannel schemes 3), 4).

The now following section will outline the synthesis of a more elaborate prototype, tailored to the requirements of transcutaneous applications.

Principles of operation

A sideglance to the principle of velocity measurement based on the Doppler effect reveals the three indispensable function blocks we meet in any such system, RADAR, laser, ultrasound etc.. As illustrated in fig. 1 a phasedetector is required to discriminate the motion of the scatterers. The amplified echo signal is therefore mixed with the local oscillator, which supplies a frequency coherent to the transmitted bursts. The following gated high pass filter separates the weak Doppler information from the stationary background. If one is interested in the velocity of more than one range interval, the signal has to be separated into the required number of range bins.

From now on the processing scheme to be described diverges from the classical method as can be seen in fig. 1.

The output of the phase detector is subsequently processed in discrete amplitude portions. But the main difference is the discrete time processing of the different samples which, unlike in the classical system, will never be restored to continuous wavetrains. Finally - to come back to the block diagram - the Doppler shift of each channel is measured and averaged over a certain period. Both methods require a means to convert the result back to an intelligible readout; a multiplexer reconditions the chopped spatial velocity profile - a DAC uncovers the code hidden in binary sequences.

The digital apparatus will simultaneously display the velocity of the full observation range, whereas conventional systems are limited to a small number of channels (e.g. 16), which have to be placed by the operator, according to the vessel diameter and its depth below the skin surface.

The stationary canceler and A/D convertor.

The discrete time representation of the information of every range sample allows to calculate the velocity in all these channels by a single processing unit. On the other hand, the quantitation introduces two major problems:
1) The fast A/D conversion with high resolution,
2) The transformation of the familiar functional blocks into the digital domain.

The suppression of the fixed echoes is achieved by a periodic high pass filter, commonly known as canceler (fig. 2). The necessary sharp roll-off calls for a filter of at least third order. It is adviseable to divide it into two sub-sections. The first is a single delay unit, which takes care of the suppression of the very high but very slow components.

Figure 2 illustrates how this configuration not only performs clutter rejection, but also provides an elegant way of fast, high resolution A/D conversion. The arrangement is set up to digitize the difference between incoming signal and the previously established and D/A retransformed average value. As the Doppler signal lies about 30 ... 40 dB below the clutter, 4 bit has proven to assure proper conversion.

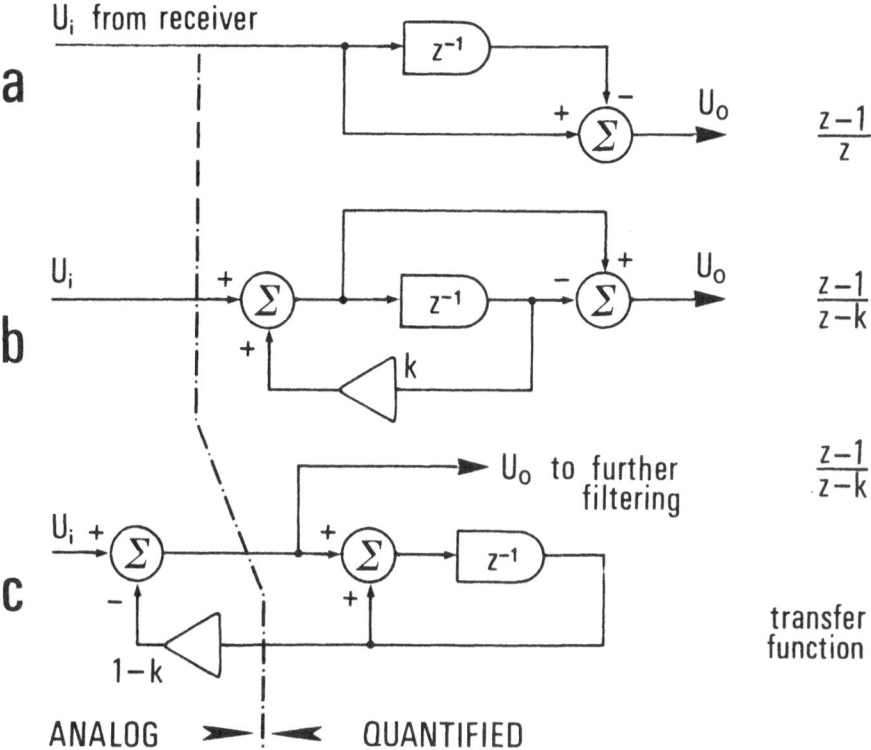

fig. 2. Evolution of stationary canceler.
While the simple canceler (a) doesn't offer any possibility of frequency shaping, the (b) set-up allows to choose the appropriate cut-off point. A closer look at this configuration reveals the familiar sweep integrator (1 > k > 0). If the difference between pre- and post-delay signal is taken, a high pass behaviour is achieved.

The arrangement shown in (c) is the next step and by far the best circuit for our purpose.

As the loops have to be implemented digitally, an A/D conversion has to precede the actual canceler. In the case of (a) and (b) a complete 10 bit conversion at a rate of ≈1 MHz would be inevitable. For (c) only the small difference signal U_0 has to be digitized if the postdelay signal is A/D retransformed.

(Note the identical transfer functions of (b) and (c)).

The modified circuit of figure 3 has still the same frequency response!

Figure 3 shall be accompanied with som design hints:
The fast DAC will be of the current output type. The addition of the two signals is accomplished by an inverting amplifier, which also prevents a "reach-back" to the converter and can be fed-back by clamping diodes to avoid saturation, should "glitches" occur. 4 bit A/D conversion can be implemented with a flash encoder of 15 comparators. Note: the feedback factor k_1 is introduced only after the first summation. The digital adder offers no problems. The memory can be set up as shift register or RAM, the latter offering a more flexible organization at the expense of a more complex adressing scheme.

The loop, which has been realised in the prototype has a k-factor of 15/16, corresponding to a cut-off frequency of 110Hz at a repetition rate of 12kHz. (N.B. 10 bit resolution requires 14 bit word length in the registers!).

The subsequent two delay filter handles a 4 bit input and contributes two more (complex) poles to the entire filter. The feedback factors have been chosen $k_2 = \frac{63}{32}$ and $k_3 = .967$, resulting in a slight peaking around 90Hz. (The corner frequency of the three pole unit is therefore approx. 75Hz.). The odd value of k_3 is implemented with a ROM truth table.

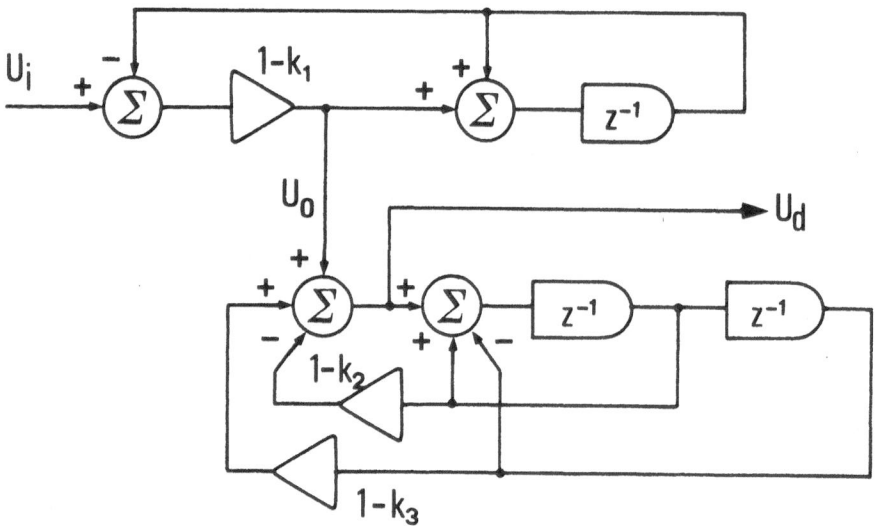

fig. 3. Triple delay stationary canceler.
The drawing shows the division of the filter unit into two sub-sections. The upper single delay loop suppresses the high but slow components. U_0 is reduced to a 4 bit information. The lower dual delay filter adds two more poles to the transfer function. Appropriate values of k_1, k_2 and k_3 (cf. see text) result in an overall cut-off frequency of approx. 75 Hz. The set-up shown here is the result of a computer optimized trade-off between circuit complexity and ideal filter characteristics.

260

The sign of the binary sequence U_d is the hard limited representation of the Doppler frequency in every range cell. The number of sign commutations per time can be counted and averaged as described in the following section.

One word to the problem of hysteresis:

Zero crossers have to provide a certain amount of Schmitt trigger action, in order to eliminate noise detection and consequently yield excessive counts. In our case the hysteresis is 1 LSB i.e. 1 conversion unit of the fast ADC. If this threshold is not crossed, the value stored in the memory will remain unaffected.

Digital frequency meter

Many philosophies exist around the pro's and contra's of the zero crosser as frequency meter. In our case of narrow observation channel spacing and digital (truncated) signals, however, no other element seems more at hand.

In analog systems 5) the clipped Doppler train triggers a monostable, providing a pulse of constant width. These pulses are then averaged by means of a lowpass filter. The digital version combines the hard limited Doppler signal (binary sequence) with its replica, which has been delayed for one interpulse period, in a logic element to detect a change of state and to produce a high output for one period.

The next procedure is to simply count these events for a period long enough to assure enough velocity resolution but still a good response to pulsatile flow (generally 10....20ms). An ideal element is a delay line with n taps and a transversal adder. In practice such symmetric impulse response elements call for an immense memory capacity and are often replaced by recursive integrating elements 6).

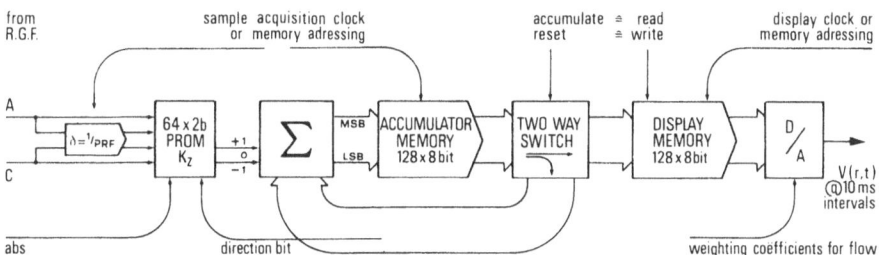

fig. 4. Digital Doppler discriminator.
The two inputs "in quadrature" (A,C) are delayed by one interpulse period. The combinatory element K_z generates an output of + 1, 0, – 1 according to the input state (cf. fig. 6.).
The accumulator adds up these increments and transfers them to the display memory at 10...20 ms intervals. (N.B. for venous flow, i.e. slower and steadier velocities this time can easily be increased). The velocities are stored in a two's complement format, with the DAC wired accordingly.

For our applications the scheme shown in fig. 4 is the best choice. The accumulator counts the zero crossings for a certain period, then shifts its content to the display memory and is reset to integrate over the next 10ms. This approach offers two ad-

vantages over the principle previously used 1):
1) A single 8 bit memory replaces three delay elements and the associated weighting network required to perform a good lowpass function.
2) The stepwise updated values in the display memory allow to write a profile even on a low-cost storage screen and to transfer the high amount of data to other storage or computing devices.

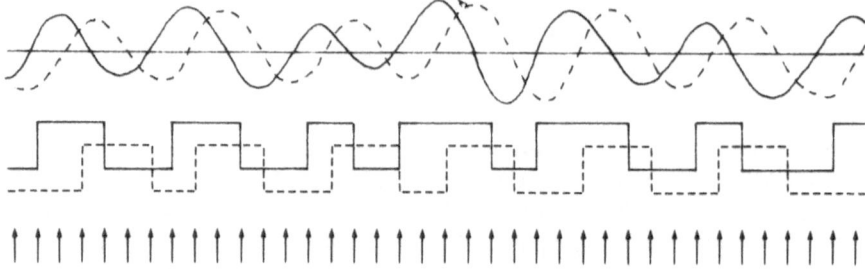

Direction sensing

Figure 5 illustrates, how the inital 90° phase relationship of the two quadrature channels is affected with an uncertainty of one PRF (pulse repetition frequency) interval due to the sampled representation. Direction sensing is consequently only unique up to $\pm 1/4$ PRF. For the remaining two quadrants until $\pm 1/2$ PRF we have to make use of an artifice. A first possibility has been described in previous articles 1), 7).
If we assume, that the velocity in a blood vessel cannot have discontinuities, we can generate a direction bit (cf. fig. 6), as long as we are within the unambiguous range and refer to this additional recursive information whenever needed. The figure also exposes the different combinations of A, Aδ, C, Cδ and D along with the appropriate output of the logic element. If the main flow direction is known (reverse flow stays within 1/4 PRF, the former scheme yields the same velocity; the combinatory gate K_z has therefore been programmed to perform either function.

The possibility of obtaining unique direction information by mixing the echo signal with an offset carrier is not realisable in a digital system. The high clutter amplitude, which is located around DC in the present prototype would be shifted in the region of a few kilohertz and call for a notch filter to be suppressed. But only a linear filter can perform this task without aliasing the frequencies on either side of the midband. Therefore the McLeod method is the only practicable direction sensing scheme in sampled data systems.

262

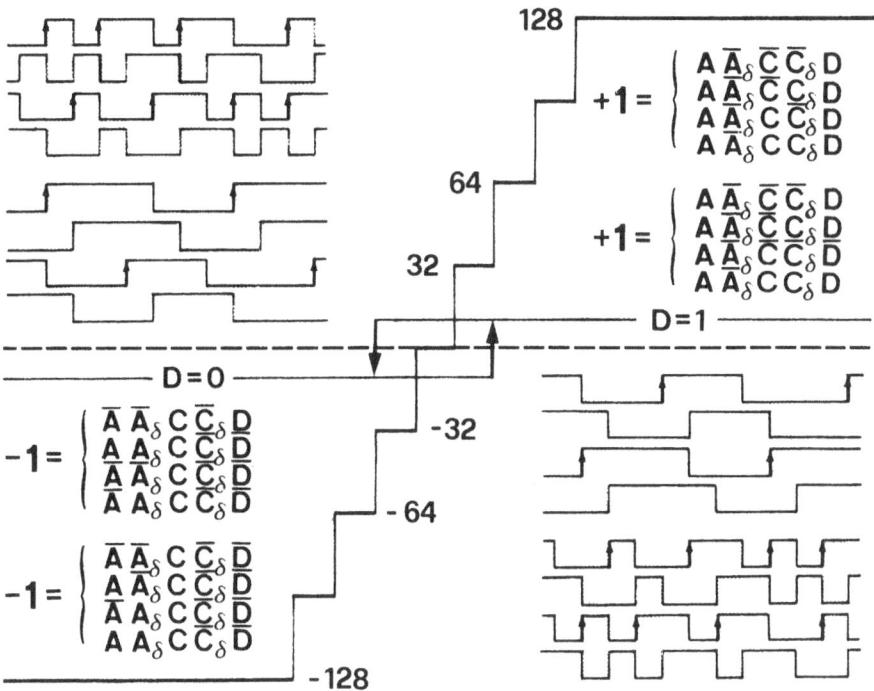

fig. 6. Principle of direction sensitive zero crossing detector.

The input of the combinatory logic element consists of A, Aδ, C, Cδ and D (cf. fig. 4.).

The direction bit is set high if forward flow is detected in a unique way, i.e. the Doppler shift is below 1/4 PRF. D changes its state only if a negative average velocity of 1/8 PRF is accumulated, thus providing a certain amount of hysteresis, as indicated in the diagram.

The Boolean formulas express the corrections with respect to the four possible quadrants. The squarewave trains furtherly illustrate some possible configurations of A, Aδ, C, Cδ (from top to bottom). (Full scale of accumulator is $\pm$128).

Conclusions

Based on a preliminary digital pilot model, which has been tested in a laboratory flow system (in vitro) and in clinical (in vivo) conditions, an advanced processing technique has been evaluated and discussed. The main point of this communication is to suggest an elaborate circuitry to other design engineers involved with Doppler problems.

To conclude, figure 7 discloses the features of the digital n-channel system. Future applications will range from simple profile recording to volume flow computation and arteriographic mapping.

flow in bifurcation

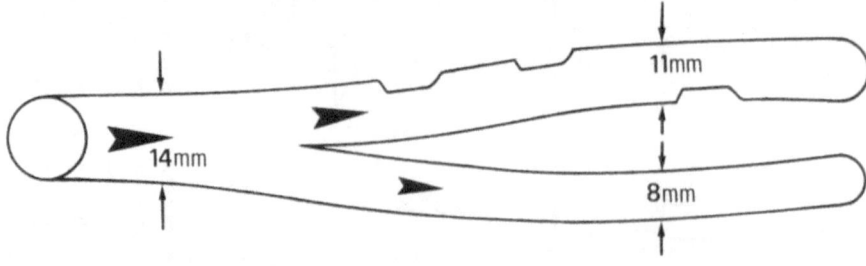

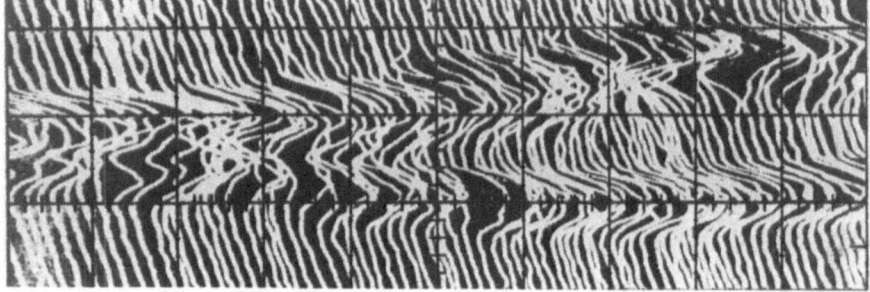

fig. 7. Flow profiles in bifurcation (model).
Velocity profiles recorded along a modelled bifurcation exhibit maximum information about the flow condition.
Note the backflow in the region of the third stenosis in the upper branch.
Such a picture can be recorded in less than one second, with the apparatus requiring only 10ms for a single section. In applications where flow is pulsatile a step-scan device allows to make up to 10 different exposures during the systolic phase and to wait for the next heartbeat to continue the scan.
(velocity: 50 cm/s/div.   slant angle: approx. 70⁰).

References

1) Brandestini M: *Signalverarbeitung in perkutanen Ultraschall Doppler Blutfluss Messgeräten.* Dissertation ETH No. 5711, 1976.

2) Brandestini M: *A Digital 128 Channel Transcutaneous Blood Flowmeter.* Biomed. Techn. proc. of MEDEX, Vol. 21, june 76.

3) Casty M: *Perkutane, atraumatische Flussmessung in grossen hautnahen Gefässen mit einem vielkanaligen gepulsten Ultraschall- Doppler-Gerät.* Dissertation Med. Fak. Universität Zürich, 1976.

4) Keller HM, Meier WE, Anliker M, and Kumpe DA: *Noninvasive Measurement of velocity Profiles and Blood Flow in the Common Carotid Artery by Pulsed Doppler Ultrasound.* Stroke, Vol. 7 No. 4 pp. 370..376 aug. 76.

264

5) McLeod FD: *Multichannel Pulse Doppler Techniques.*
   in Cardiovascular applications of Ultrasound, pp. 85..107, North Holland publ. 1974.

6) Shreve JS: *Digital Signal Processing.*
   in RADAR handbook, p. 35-9, by M.J. Skolnik, McGraw Hill, 1970.

7) Brandestini M: *Topoflow - a Digital Full Range Velocity Meter.*
   submitted to IEEE Trans. Sonics & Ultrasonics, in press.

Chapter 3

TWO-DIMENSIONAL

REAL TIME IMAGING

Real time systems for two dimensional imaging.
General introduction.

by N. Bom and P.G. Hugenholtz
Thorax Center, Erasmus University Rotterdam,
Interuniversity Cardiology Institute, The Netherlands.

Introduction

Diagnostic Ultrasound systems have become increasingly sophisticated and today instruments exist which combine more than just one diagnostic parameter that can be obtained with ultrasound. In figure 1, the four areas of diagnostic information, for which ultrasound is used today are indicated.

ECHOCARDIOGRAPHY

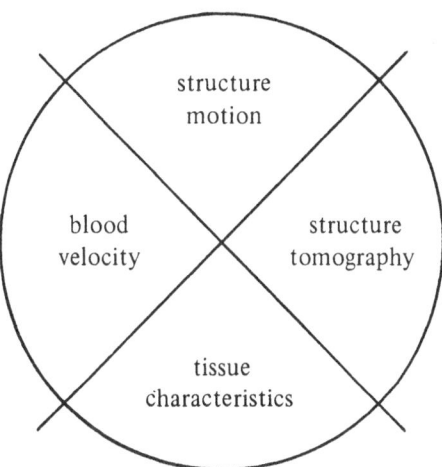

potential diagnostic information

fig. 1. With the use of Ultrasound diagnostic information may be obtained in the indicated four categories.

Although some overlap between the four areas does exist the main diagnostic components of information are:

Structure motion. In 1953 Edler and Hertz 1) introduced the M-mode technique in Lund, Sweden. With their uni-dimensional system the motion pattern of cardiac structures could be studied and most of the presently known echo patterns were first described by them.

269

Echocardiology, N. Bom editor, published by Martinus Nijhoff, the Hague 1977.

Tissue identification. The ultrasound waves must carry information on the micro anatomy of the structure from which they reflect. This information may be present in the angular reflectivity function, in the local attenuation, the spectral content of the echo or some other parameter. Although the heart seems an important object for study only a few centers have given this attention. Obviously the motion of the heart adds to the already existing problems of information detection. Studies so far have been limited to in vitro experiments. An effort to distinguish necrotic from healthy tissue was carried out by Lele et al 2). Another study by Yuhas et al 3) described changes in ultrasonic attenuation indicative of regional myocardial infarction.

Blood Velocity. In 1956 Satomura 4) applied the Doppler effect to evaluate a velocity component of the blood flow. In early applications continuous waves were used and with the first systems no information on the depth of the signal creating structure could be obtained.

Structure tomography. With echo brightness modulation it became possible to build up a two-dimensional echo image or tomogram. It is understandable that at first stationary structures were studied. Imaging of complicated moving structures such as the heart were not mentioned in literature until much later.
The medical application and apparatus acceptance within each of the four zones has been different. Major steps forward were often the result of technological innovations. Without the enormous efforts of both clinically and technically oriented scientists through the last decades the present results would certainly never have been reached.
Recent real time two dimensional (2D) imaging devices present a good example of a powerful diagnostic tool for instantaneous observation of structure motion as well as tomography.

2D evolution

In the early fifties it was realised that the complexity of the sound reflecting structures as viewed with uni-dimensional ultrasound methods would limit the success of ultrasound in medical application. In 1952 Wild and Reid 5) published first results of "a two-dimensional picture such as would be obtained by adding up the information from a series of needle biopsies taken in one plane". They described the principle of a mechanical sectorscan with a crystal pivoting over a sector of 45 degrees. In figure 2 the schematic drawing indicates their sectorwise pivoting crystal construction.

At almost the same time Howry and Bliss 6) reported a simular device which they called a Somascope (see figure 3). Again this was a mechanical sectorscan. Only in a speculation on future application Howry and Bliss do mention the heart. Applications of these systems for cardiac examination have not been reported. A construction of the above quoted mechanical sectorscan particularly designed for viewing the heart was first described by Flaherty 7) in 1965.

270

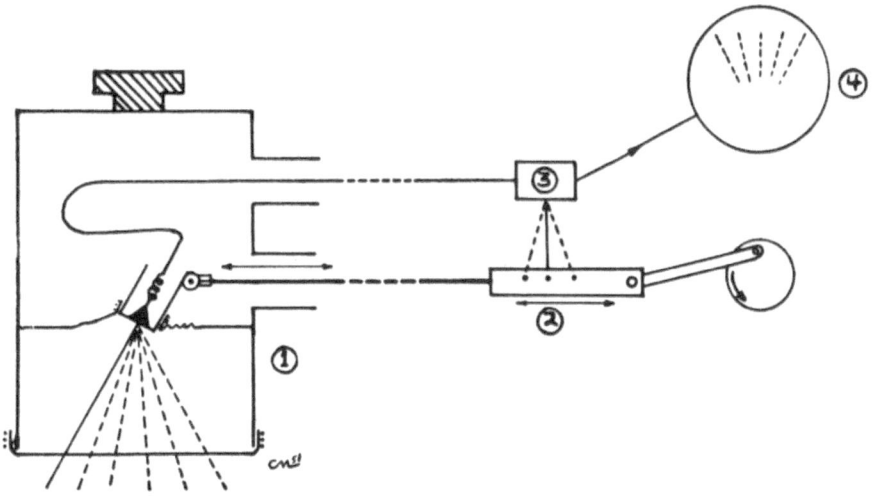

fig. 2. Early publication of the "wobbler" or mechanical sector scanner principle with echo-scope 1; oscillating ram 2; connected with electronic unit 3 and the cathode-ray screen 4.
(From Wild JJ, and Reid JM; ref. 5). Published in Science, Vol. 115, fig. 4. pp 226–228, 29 February 1952; courtesy of the American Association for the Advancement of Science).

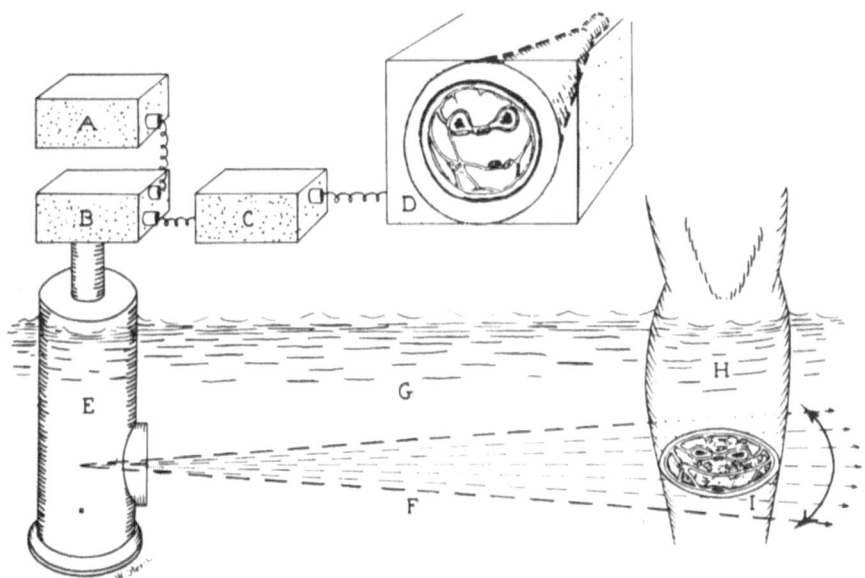

fig. 3. The mechanical sector scan as described by Howry and Bliss. (From Howry DH, and Bliss WR: ref 6)).

In 1958 Donald, MacVicar and Brown 8) described the advantages if a structure were insonified from more than just one angle. They introduced the so called compoundscan where they sought to reproduce a composite cross-sectional view collecting echoes from as many angles as possible. The production of one image did take between 1,5 and 2,5 minutes. Their system was mainly employed for obstetrical work.

Probably the first in vitro attempt to visualize the heart in a 2D image was made in 1957 by Wild, Crawford, and Reid 9). They scanned an excised human heart with a mechanically swept probe. The crystal was linearly swept over a distance of 6.5 cm. They suggested the "stroboscopic" (ECG triggered) imaging method in order to obtain one ultrasound image frame of the living heart. They stated that application to the heart was possible if "the formidable technical difficulties could be overcome".

Even today now and then publications appear whereby a single cardiac 2D image is composed under the control of the ECG. One of the first publications originated in Japan in 1967 by Ebina et al 10). A more recent article was published in 1975 by King et al 11). This technique does not yield real time images and is subject to the limitation caused by irregularity of cardiac rythm and superimposed breathing activity. These limitations probably are the reason for the limited application to date.

The first sequence of 2D cardiac images where structure motion could be followed was published in 1967 in Lund by Åsberg 12) and Hertz 13). They used an equipment which already allowed up to 7 frames/sec. The principle is shown in figure 4 and cardiac cross-sections are shown in figure 5.

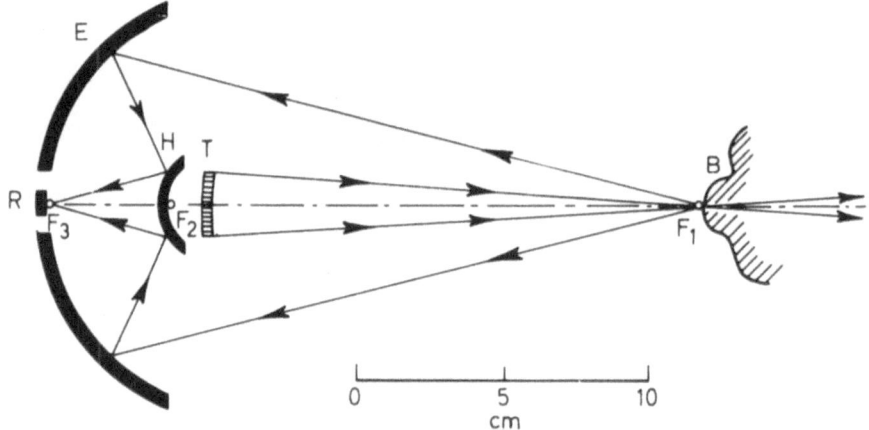

fig. 4. First Ultrasonic mirror system for cardiac observation with transmitter T; receiver R, and mirror E and H. (From Åsberg A: ref 12). Reprint from Ultrasonics, Vol. 5 No. 2 April 1967, published by IPC Science and Technology Press Ltd, Guildford).

The images shown in figure 5 were obtained with waterbath contact. Although the image quality is not bad no further results have been published. A mirror system

272

that did become popular was described by Pätzold 14) in 1970 and comprised a cylindrical parabolic mirror and an ultrasound source mounted on a rotating shaft. The mirror and ultrasound source are accomodated in a housing filled with liquid. This system (Vidoson) did produce 15 frames/sec and was developed for abdominal real time scanning. One of the first applications of this system to the heart was published by Weil 15) in 1973.

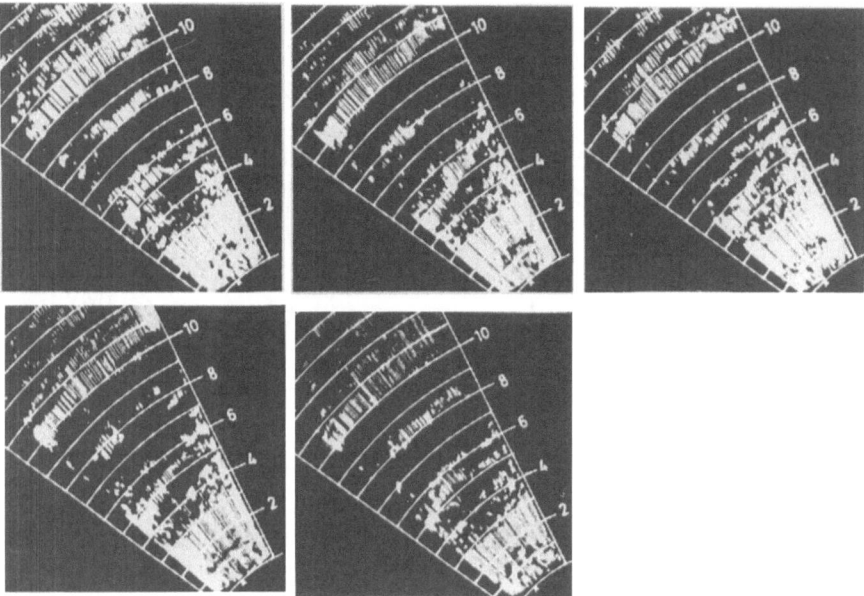

fig. 5. Sequential cardiac cross-sections as obtained in 1967 with the mirror system. The echoes form the chestwall start at 0 cm and the posterior cardiac wall is displayed around 10 cm (From Åsberg A: ref 12). Reprint from Ultrasonics, Vol. 5 No. 2 April 1967, published by IPC Science and Technology Press Ltd, Guildford).

Efforts to build a 2D image without mechanical motion of the transducer were initiated outside cardiology by Buschmann 16) in ophtalmology and Somer 17) for neurology. Prior to 1967 Buschmann forsaw the importance of an integration of echoes into a 2D image by memoscope. However, since no suitable memory tubes were available he introduced electronic switching with elements to yet obtain a 2D picture. The results were not stimulating and he abandoned the method in 1967 when a good memory tube became available. The electronic sectorscan method as first introduced by Somer contained a system whereby all miniature elements acted together and with an electronic phasing a sectorwise beamsteering resulted.

Present real-time 2D methods

With some modifications the electronic sectorscan, together with the mechanical

273

sectorscan introduced by Griffith and Henry 18) and the multiscan introduced by this author 19) form the three realtime 2D methods presently commercially available for routine diagnostic use in cardiology today. The two most important cross-sections that are usually studied with these systems are schematically presented in figure 6.

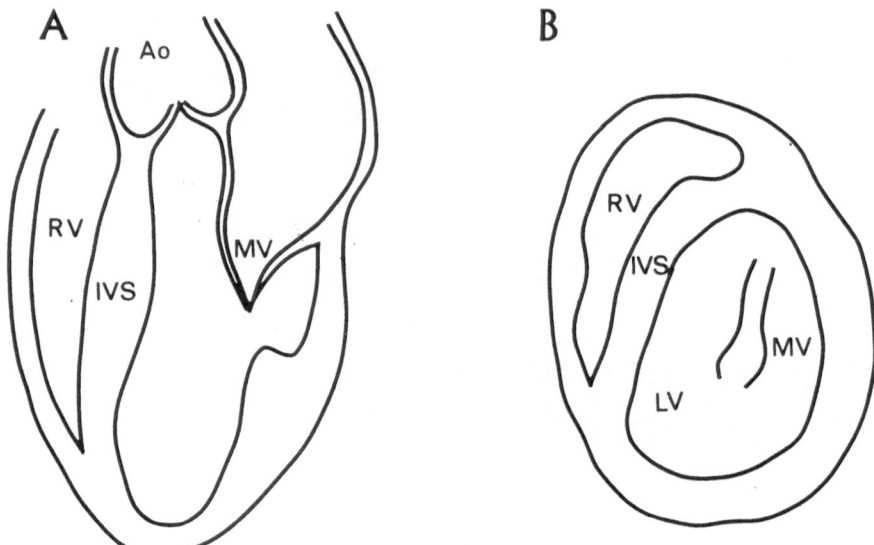

fig. 6. Diagram of cardiac tomogram in the sagittal (A) and horizontal plane (B) with main structures (RV = right ventricle; LV = left ventricle; MV = mitral valve; IVS = interventricular septum; Ao = aorta).

Mechanical sectorscan. The mechanical sectorscan specifically derived for cardiac applications was introduced by Griffith and Henry 18). As indicated in fig. 7 X, the transducer T is continuously reciprocated through an angle. The angular motion is produced by a small motor M via a crank and lever system. The echoes are correspondingly displayed on the monitor. The same figure shows an example of a horizontal cross-section as obtained with their instrument which shows the mitral orifice. These systems yield a sectorial cardiac image.

Phased array sectorscan. In the phased array sectorscan system many small individual elements and for all these elements variable signal delay lines are used to angle the acoustic beam by matching the wave front to the desired direction. In reception for instance (see fig. 7 Y) optimal sensitivity is obtained for the summed signal from all individual elements for beam direction A with equal or no delay introduced.

Optimal sensitivity for echoes from direction B is obtained if the wave front is matched by introduction of a phase shift or delay t_1 to t_n respectively for element 1 to n such that the acoustic beam is "angled" towards direction B (see fig. 7 Y).

274

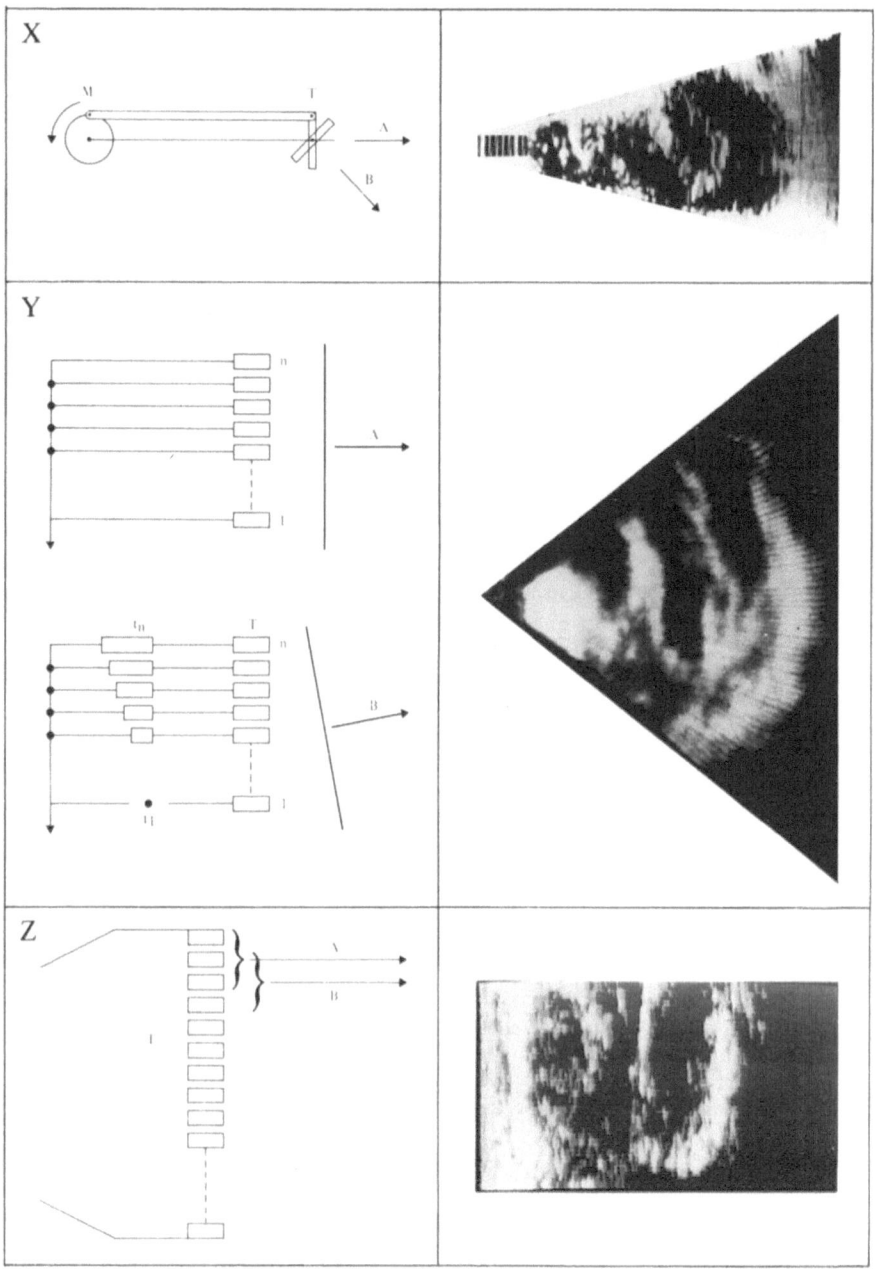

fig. 7. The principle of today's real-time cardiac imaging systems with one clinical example in the horizontal plane obtained with the mechanical sector scanner X (courtesy Jim Griffith), and two sagittal frames obtained with a phased array system Y (courtesy Richard Popp) and with a linear array system Z.

The phased array sectorscan method uses an electronically variable set of delay lines. This allows rapid angling of the beam. No mechanical motion of the probe is necessary and the probe remains relatively small. An example of a sagittal cardiac image as obtained with a phased array system is shown in fig. 7 Y.

Linear array or multiscan method. By rapid electronic switching of one (or a subgroup of) small element(s) in a sequence a number of parallel beams may be formed. Thus in this situation (see fig. 7 Z) a rectangular image may be obtained by subsequent transmission and reception along beam A followed by the same procedure along beam B etc. A sagittal cross-section is shown in fig. 7 Z. This method results in rectangular images obtained without mechanical probe motion.

Lateral resolution of 2D real-time imaging systems

The limitations of diagnostic ultrasound methods are caused by a variety of physical factors. These include the high dynamic range in echo amplitude and as a result difficulties in capturing all important information. Limitations also are imposed by the change in sound velocity and the finite pulse length. Presently the largest source of errors is caused by the (too wide) beam width and secondary lobes (this is the sensitivity of the transducer in directions not equal to the main direction). It is this phenomenon which also in M-mode registration causes some of the known artifacts due to the so called limited lateral resolution.

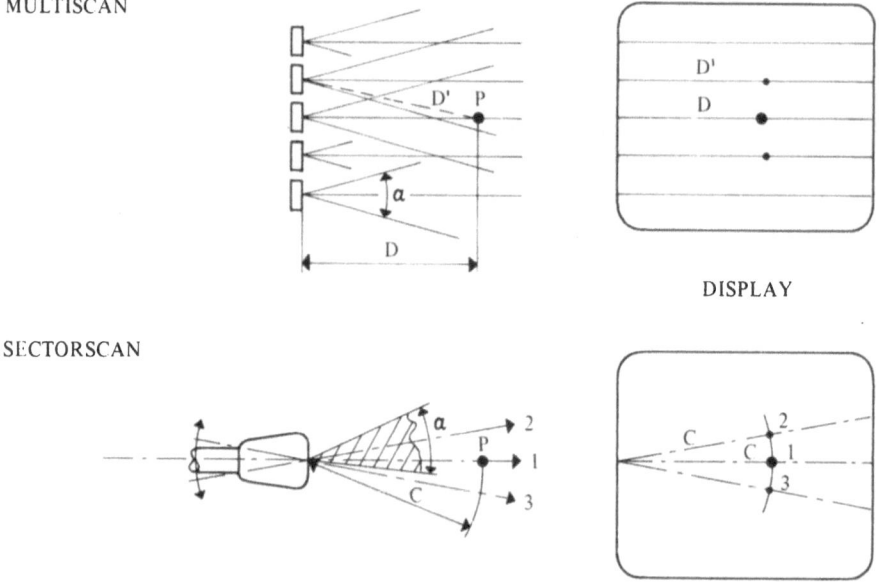

fig. 8. Image deformation due to poor lateral resolution diagramatically indicated for a rectangularly or sectorially formed image.

276

In fig. 8 the spurious echoes are schematically indicated for a linear array system as well as for a (mechanical or phased) sectorscan. Instead of a pencil like narrow main beam all elements have been drawn with an (exaggerated) beam opening of angle a. Thus for the multiscan situation in addition to the correctly presented point reflector P on the display at distance D also adjacent elements will "see" this reflector erroneously at distance D_1.

For the sectorscan the point reflector P is correctly indicated on the display when the probe is aimed in direction 1; in direction 2 however, the reflector is still within angle a and thus detected. Representation will follow on the display in direction 2 etc.

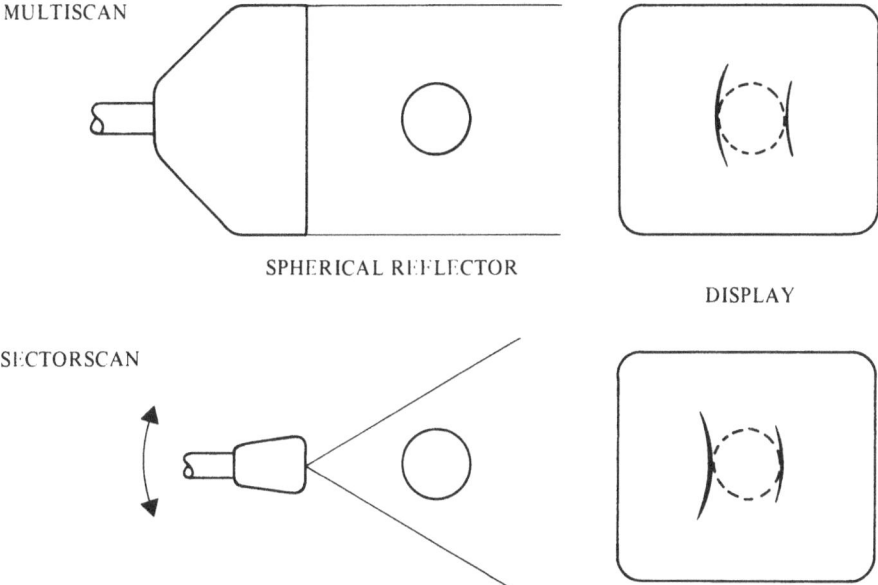

MULTISCAN

SPHERICAL REFLECTOR

DISPLAY

SECTORSCAN

fig. 9. Exaggerated image deformation for highly reflecting spherical object.

In fig. 9 this effect is once more illustrated on a highly reflecting target such as the sphere of a prosthetic ball valve. Apparently the systems have a tendency to deform large echoes in a different way. In practical applications the effect is not as severe as above indicated, but it is nevertheless present and therefore briefly discussed here.

New developments

There is no doubt in authors' mind that the first and most severe problem to be solved concerns the improvement of above discussed lateral resolution. Somehow the beam must be more narrow. This can be achieved by e.g. dynamic focussing. For the mechanical sectorscans this may be accomplished with composite circular ring transducers. In the phased array sectorscan system a dynamic focussing was al-

277

ready introduced and described by Thurstone 20). By way of example a new dynamic focussing multiscan will be briefly described as developed by our group. More details are presented further on in this book. The system operates with 6 focus zones and a transducer of 51 elements. The dynamic focussing is introduced by electronic delay lines which substantially increase the complexity of the apparatus.

In fig. 10 the beamwidth defined as the lateral positions where the sound intensity has dropped to -10 dB as function of depth is shown for the original 20 element system and for the 51 element dynamic focussing system. The gain in lateral reso-

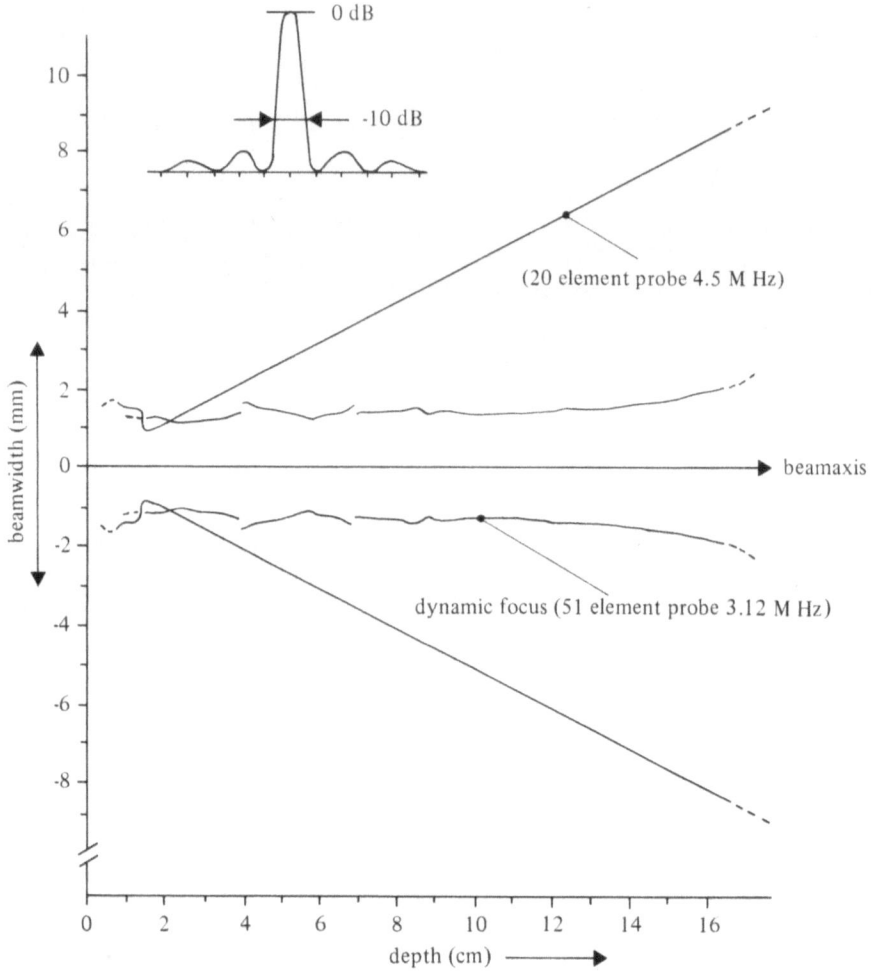

fig. 10. Example of the improvement that may be obtained in lateral resolution with introduction of dynamic focussing. Here the non focussing linear array beamwidth is compared with the beamwidth versus depth for the swept focussing device.

278

lution is substantial, particularly in the deeper areas. From fig. 10 it may be concluded that with such apparatus a reasonably good resolution can be maintained over the entire depth and thus over the entire 2D image. A clinical example of a horizontal cardiac cross-section is shown for the dynamic focussing system in fig. 11. The improved resolving power particularly in septal and endocardial area is obvious.

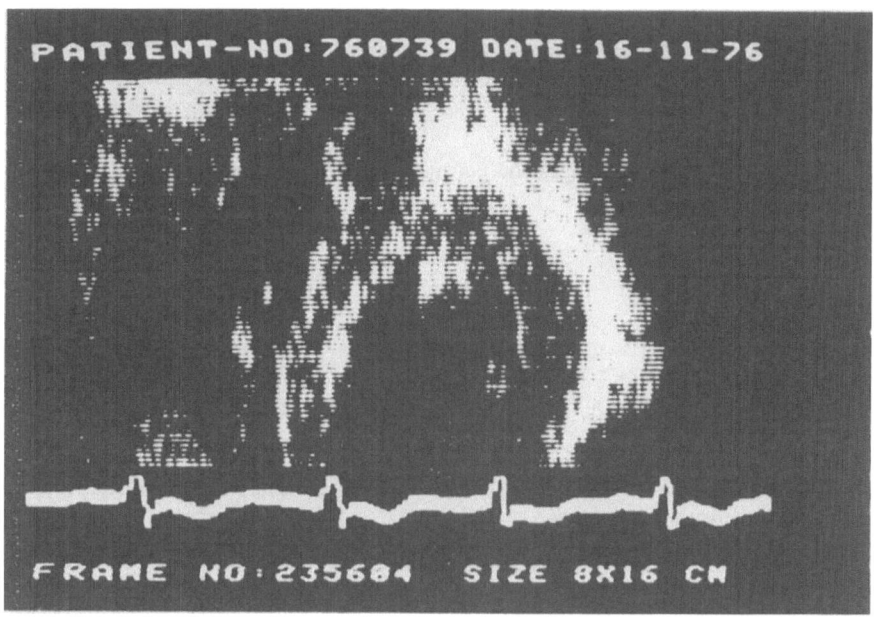

fig. 11. Horizontal cross-section as obtained with the linear swept focus array. Note the improved resolution in the septal and posterior left ventricular area.

Future will tell if in practice the inherent complexity and thus increased cost of such improvements are indeed necessary in the routine use of 2D systems. Probably the improvement will be a step forward again and will carry the applications beyond todays use where only direct observation of gross changes in dynamics and geometry of the heart in motion is made.

The previously discussed 2D imaging has only been one example of the powerful combination of tomography and structure motion as may be obtained with ultrasound. Other area's represented in fig. 1 are presently combined to new and powerful diagnostic methods such as blood velocity measurements and tomography. This is discussed in the chapter on Doppler methods.

Conclusion

Early 2D ultrasound applications presented images of stationary structures only. Today we are capable to visualize the heart in real-time. It is believed that new developments such as swept focussing devices will improve the diagnostic power of these methods yet further. 2D imaging, that is a combination of tomography and motion, has provided a major push forward in diagnostic ultrasound, yet there is much work to be done and we have only just entered the new field of ultrasonic capabilities. The addition of e.g. tissue characteristics will require much research but, as stated by Hertz 21), the electrocardiograph was introduced in 1908 and found its way into hospital only after 1930. Compared to that development the rate of progress in echocardiography seems quite satisfactory.

Acknowledgement

Author gratefully acknowledges the permission to reproduce figure 2, 3, 4 and 5.

References

1) Edler I, and Hertz CH: *The use of the ultrasonic reflectoscope for the continuous recording of movements of heart walls.*
Kungl. Fysiogr. Sällsk. Lund Förhandl 24: 5,1, 1954.

2) Lele PP, and Namery J: *A computer-Based Ultrasonic System for the Detection and Mapping of Myocardial Infarcts.*
Proc. San Diego Biomed. Symp. 13: 121–132, 1974.

3) Yuhas DE, Mimbs JW, Miller JG, Weiss AN, and Sobel BE: *Changes in ultrasonic attenuation indicative of regional myocardial infraction.*
In press.

4) Satomura SS: *Ultrasonic Doppler Method for the Inspection of Cardiac Functions.*
JASA 29, no. 11: 1181-1185, 1957.

5) Wild JJ, and Reid JM: *Application of Echo-Ranging Techniques to the Determination of Structures of Biological Tissues.*
Science 115: 226-228, 1952.

6) Howry DH, and Bliss WR: *Ultrasonic visualization of soft tissue structures of the body.*
Journal of Laboratory and Clinical Medicine 40 no. 4: 579-592, 1952.

7) Flaherty JJ, and Rosauer PJ: *Ultrasonic transducer system.*
United States Patent Office, issued Oct. 1, 1968 No. 3, 403,671. Filed Oct. 24, 1965 Ser. No. 504.346.

8) Donald I, MacVicar J, and Brown TG: *Investigation of abdominal masses by pulsed ultrasound.*
The Lancet: 1188-1195, 1958.

280

9) Wild JJ, Crawford HD, and Reid M: *Visualization of the excised human heart by means of reflected ultrasound or echography.*
Amer. Heart J. December: 903-906, 1957.

10) Ebina T, Oka S, and Tanaka M, et al: *The Ultrasono-tomography for the Heart and Great Vessels in Living Human Subjects by Means of the Ultrasonic Reflection Technique.*
Jap. Heart Journal 8: 331-353, 1967.

11) King DL: *Stop-action imaging.*
Cardiac Ultrasound. The C.V. Mosby Company: 210-227, 1975.

12) Äsberg A: *Ultrasonic cinematography of the living heart.*
Ultrasonics April: 113-117, 1967.

13) Hertz CH: *Ultrasonic Engineering in Heart Diagnosis.*
The American Journal of Cardiology No. 19: 6-17, 1967.

14) Pätzold J, Krause W, Kresse H, and Soldner R: *Present State of an Ultrasonic Cross-Section Procedure with Rapid Image Rate.*
IEE Transaction on Bio-Medical Engineering, July: 263-265, 1970.

15) Weill F, Kraehenbuhl JR, and Becker JC: *Mise en Evidence des épanchements péricardique par tomoéchoscopie et tomoéchographie.*
Coeur de Médicine Interne, Tome XI No. 2: 389-393, 1972.

16) Buschmann W: *Bases, Methods and Reliability of Ultrasonic Diagnosis on the Eye (Review).*
Ultrasonics in Ophtalmology, Symp. Münster, August: 54-75, 1966.

17) Somer JC: *Electronic sector scanning for ultrasonic diagnosis.*
Progress Report Medisch Physisch Instituut August: 37-41, 1968.

18) Griffith JM, and Henry WL: *A Sector Scanner for Real Time Two-Dimensional Echocardiography.*
Circulation, XLIX: 1147-1152, 1974.

19) Bom N, Lancée CT, and Honkoop J et al: *Ultrasonic viewer for cross-sectional analyses of moving cardiac structures.*
Bio-med Engng 6: 500, 1971.

20) Thurstone FL, and Von Ramm OT: *Electronic beam scanning for imaging.*
Ultrasonics in Medicine, Rotterdam, June: 43-48, 1973.

21) Hertz CH: *The interaction of physicians, physicists and industry in the development of echocardiography.*
Ultrasound in Med. & Biol. Vol. 1: 3-11, 1973.

2D imaging versus holography and 3D imaging

by P. Alais,
Institut de Mécanique Théorique et Appliquée,
Université Pierre et Marie Curie, Paris.

Introduction

The first experiments of Langevin in submarine acoustics (1917) were followed relatively rapidly by echographic techniques adapted to industrial applications for non destructive testing. The idea to use acoustical radiation to produce images in a way analogous to the use of optical radiation in the photographic camera is a very old one. The first important attempt was performed by Sokolov who proposed in 1929 the first ultrasonic retina, using a piezoelectric plate in front of a cathodic tube (fig. 1).

Later, echographic techniques and ordinary imaging were developed in parallel but while the sonar techniques met with success in submarine acoustics, non destructive testing, and later in medicine, acoustical imaging in the ordinary optical sense was very unsuccessful. The Sokolov tube was optimized in several different ways but was still lacking the required resolution for good images. On the other hand, acoustical lenses are not so easily built as optical lenses and they produce noise and distorsion in the focused pictures. Then, after thirty five years of quasi stagnation for ultra-

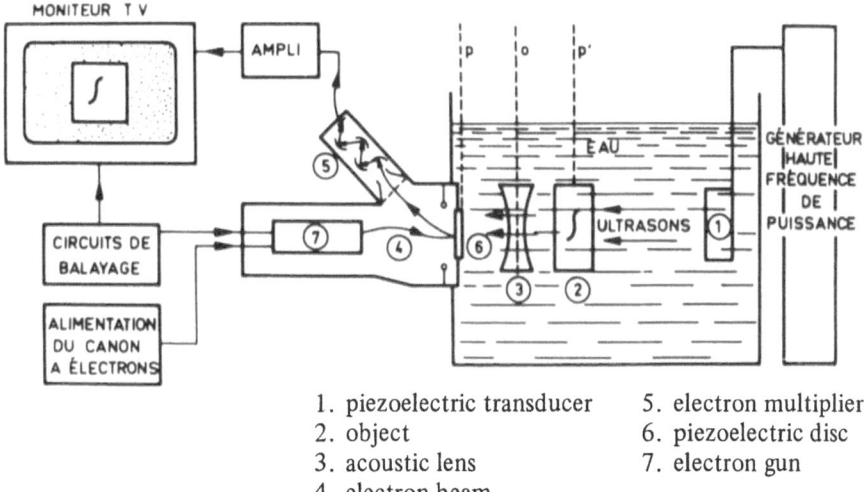

1. piezoelectric transducer
2. object
3. acoustic lens
4. electron beam
5. electron multiplier
6. piezoelectric disc
7. electron gun

fig. 1. Acoustical Imaging with a SOKOLOV Tube (after MARINI, J. thesis LYON 1969)

283

Echocardiology, N. Bom editor, published by Martinus Nijhoff, the Hague 1977.

sonic imaging, the last decade has brought many new and interesting attempts to improve what we may now call, in contrast with 2D B-echographic techniques 3D imaging. After a brief review of these experiments we should like in this paper to examine prospects of 3D imaging in medicine and in cardiology in particular.

Acoustical holography and imaging

The main reason for this revival of acoustical imaging was the discovery of Holography by Gabor and the experimental proof of its efficiency by Leith and Upatnieks (1962) using the coherent laser radiation. All these now classical experiments

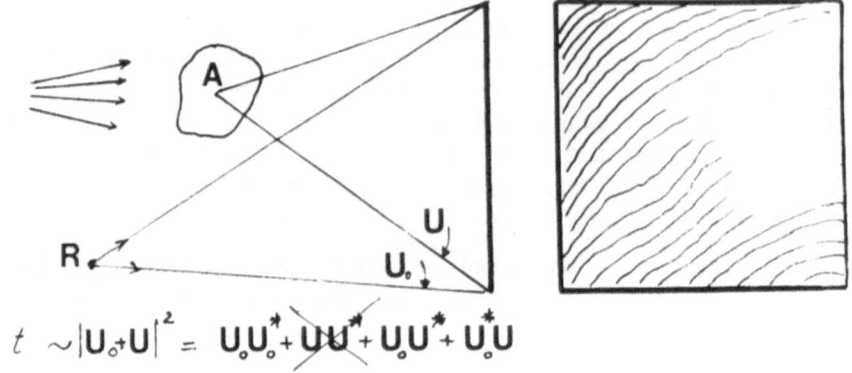

$$t \sim |U_o + U|^2 = U_o U_o^* + UU^* + U_o U^* + U_o^* U$$

fig. 2a. Optical or Acoustical Acquisition of an Hologram.

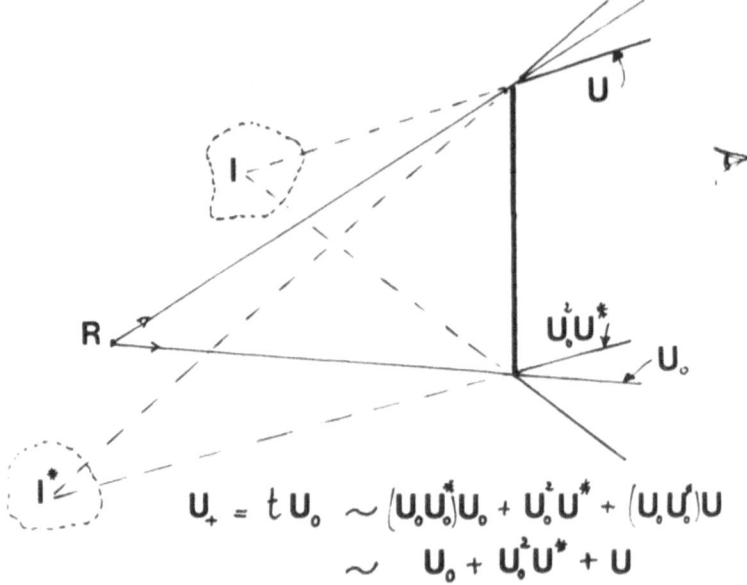

$$U_+ = t\,U_o \sim (U_o U_o^*) U_o + U_o^2 U^* + (UU_o^*) U$$
$$\sim U_o + U_o^2 U^* + U$$

fig. 2b. Optical restitution with the same reference source (in optical holography).

284

with coherent optical radiation and what physicists call "Fourier optics" were in fact delayed by the absence of natural optical coherent radiation, in contrast with ultrasonic radiation for which harmonic coherent waves are the more available ones. Holographic experiments could have been performed in acoustics earlier than in optics. Fig. 2 recalls the principle of holography.

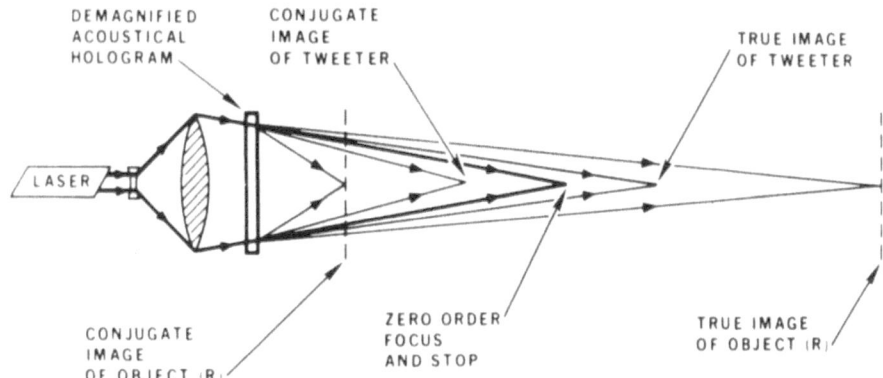

fig. 2c. Optical restitution of an acoustical hologram. (after METHERELL, Acoustical Holography, Vol. 1, p. 203).

The first step consists in storing the hologram i,e, the interference figure of the useful diffracted field carrying information with a field in coherence with the illuminating field. This experiment may be carried out using a coherent acoustical radiation. The second step, the holographic reconstruction is classically performed with a coherent optical laser radiation illuminating the hologram transparency but may also be obtained by numerical computation using a Fresnel transform of the holographic 2D information. In the 1965-1966 years, many physicists were conscious to have been lacking imagination and were anxious to enter this new exciting field: Acoustical holography. The immediate advantages were the perfect coherency of the field and the elimination of need of acoustical lenses. The remaining difficulty was the phonosensitive retina; there seems to be no acoustical equivalent of the photographic emulstion. Among the various solutions offered by many physicists to solve this problem I shall mention the levitation effect of a liquid-gas interface due to the ultrasonic radiation pressure. This technique was first proposed by Mueller and Sheridon 1), 2) and later very successfully used by Brenden 3), (fig. 3) in a semi holographic device: the optical reconstruction performed in real time with the diffraction of a laser beam performed by the levitated interface was in fact a simple demodulation of a focused image of the object obtained with an acoustical lens.

Very beautiful ultrasonic transparencies were obtained in real-time with this technique, which is now available for medical use but in a relatively restricted field of operation due to constraints required for a through imaging operation. It is im-

285

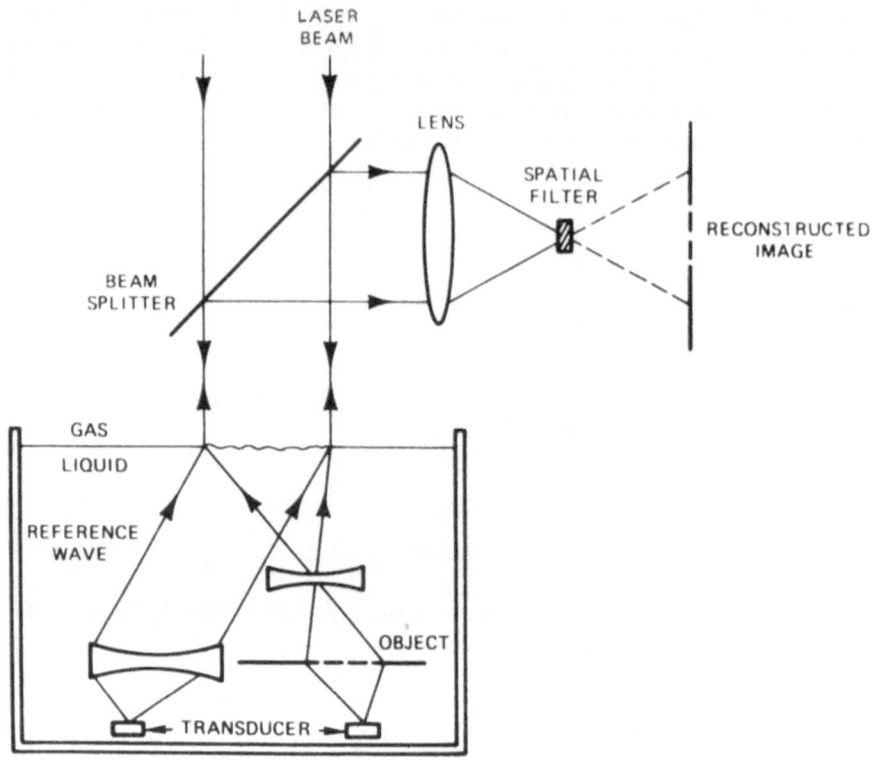

fig. 3. Acoustical imaging with an optical holographic restitution of an acoustical image holo-gram focused at the liquid surface (after BRENDEN 3)).

possible to give here an exhaustive review of all scientists who have developed phonosensitive retinas. To mention a few; the techniques of Metherell 4) and Korpel 5) which detect optically the acoustical oscillations of a liquid-gas or solid-gas inter-face and of Mezrich et al 6) who use instead the oscillations of a thin membrane immersed in the propagating liquid. Other people propose 2D arrays of piezo-elec-tric transducers as the phonosensitive retina. This solution has been seriously in-vestigated by different scientific groups 7). A great difficulty remains at the elec-tronic level where the ultrasonic information must be obtained in real-time. This calls for extensive use of integrated circuit technology, therefore this has limited its application so far. A much simpler technique, using an array of electrostatic trans-ducers built with ordinary printed circuits was proposed in 1972 by us 8). We could in this way perform academic holographic experiments (fig. 4) with, like many other people in the same period, a very limited success in obtaining good images.

The lack of resolution of holographic pictures (fig. 5), obvious when comparing a simple shadowgram obtained from the same object (fig. 6) is still not completely explained. However, the main reason lies in the fact that the resolution required for the reconstructed object is of the order of the wave length i.e. at the level of the theoretical limit unlike in the optical experiments where in general the hologram resolution scale (i.e. the wave length scale $\sim 1\mu$) remains at least 2 orders of magnitude under the object scale resolution required $\sim 100\mu$).

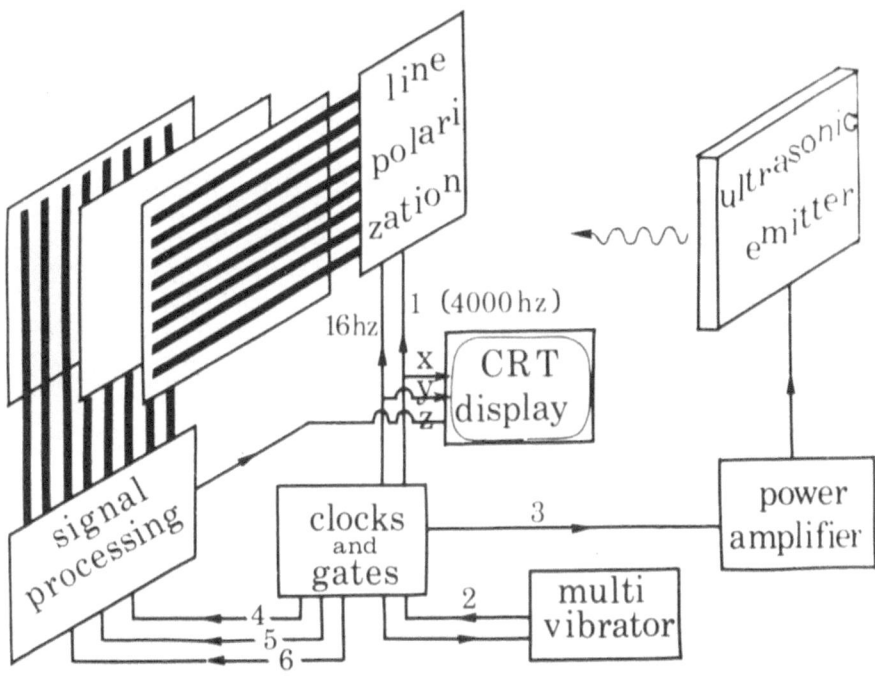

fig. 4. Acoustical imaging or holography with an electrostatic retina using a sequential polarisation of linear electrodes and parallel treatment of the acoustical information delivered by the transducers associated to the polarized, see ref. 8.

This does not mean that good holographic treatment is impossible in acoustics but it requires storing the holographic information with an accuracy much greater than in optics which is not obtained by present experimental techniques. Despite these unsuccessful results of acoustical holography in through imaging, different other attempts have been performed recently in classical imaging with lenses. The most successful one is the Green camera 9) which uses not only a sophisticated acoustical lens but also a system of contra rotative prisms, which permits a fast mechanical scanning of the picture in one direction (10 frames per second) which may be combined with an electronic scanning in the orthogonal direction obtained from a linear array of 192 transducers (fig. 7).

This camera has given excellent transparencies of organs in vitro and very interesting views of the abdomen (fig. 8). However, even in the case of this remarkable realiza-

287

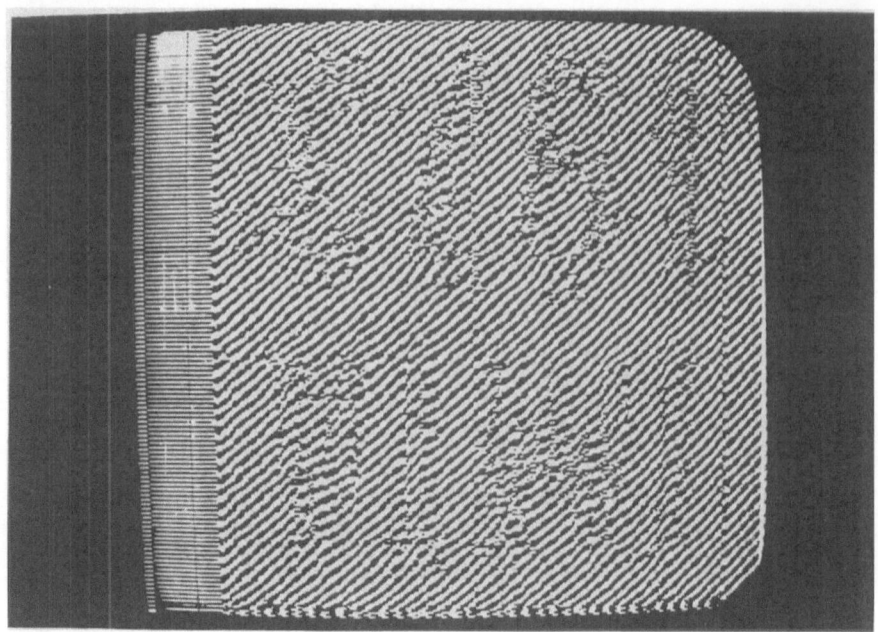

fig. 5a. Hologram obtained from cork letters set at 20 cms from the retina at a frequency of 2 MHz.

fig. 5b. Optical restitution with a He Ne Laser from the preceding hologram demagnified to 5 x 5 mms.

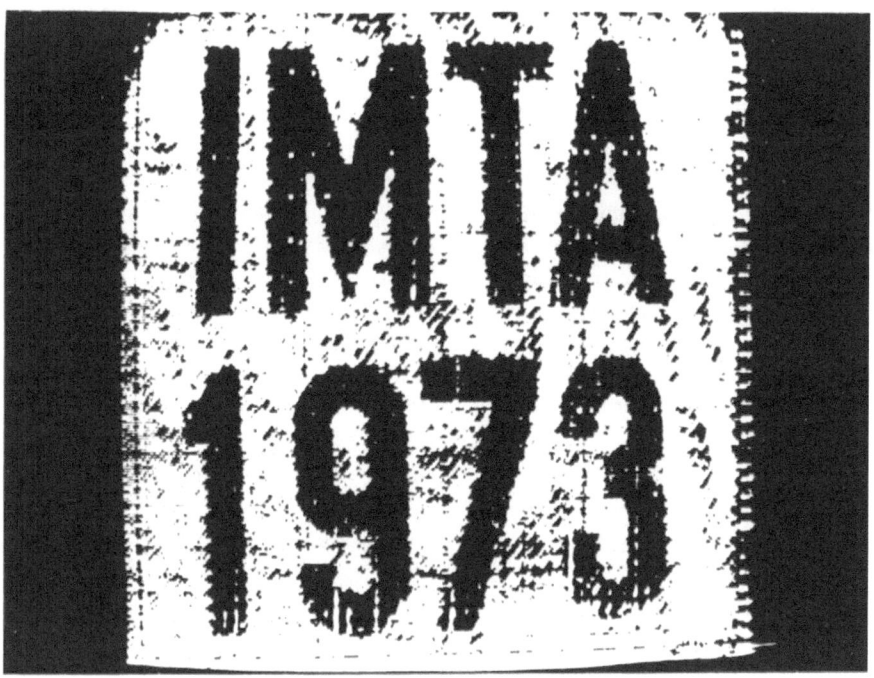

fig. 6. Shadowgram of the same letters set near the retina.

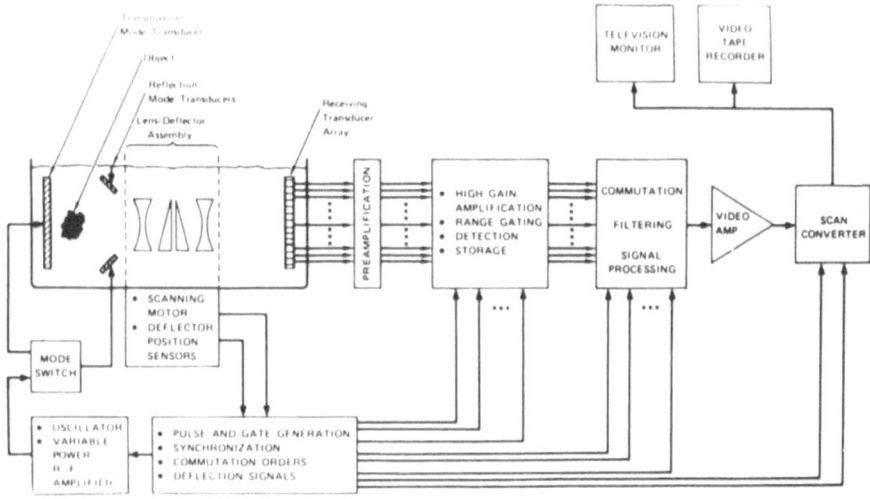

fig. 7. Real time acoustical imaging with a linear array and mechanical scanning of the focused image using contrarotative prisums (after GREEN 9)).

tion, medical applications of through imaging techniques remain restricted for the moment. On the other hand, the scientific contribution of this research must not be forgotten. It has opened the way to new fruitful echographic techniques which will be discussed in the next paragraph.

Large aperture echographic techniques

A- and B-mode echographic techniques were approximately in the same period very successfully developed for medical applications from classical considerations using in general small aperture transducers with restricted focussing. Only recently large aperture devices combined with a fast mechanical scanning or an electronic scanning (θ-scan or X-scan) have appeared. Only a large aperture transducer can give the lateral resolution in both X and Y directions of a scanning plane which is absolutely necessary for 3D investigation. In fact ordinary large aperture transducers may be mechanically scanned in a plane for obtaining 2D information about a plane parallel to the scanning plane, what is commonly called C-echography, or even 3D inform-

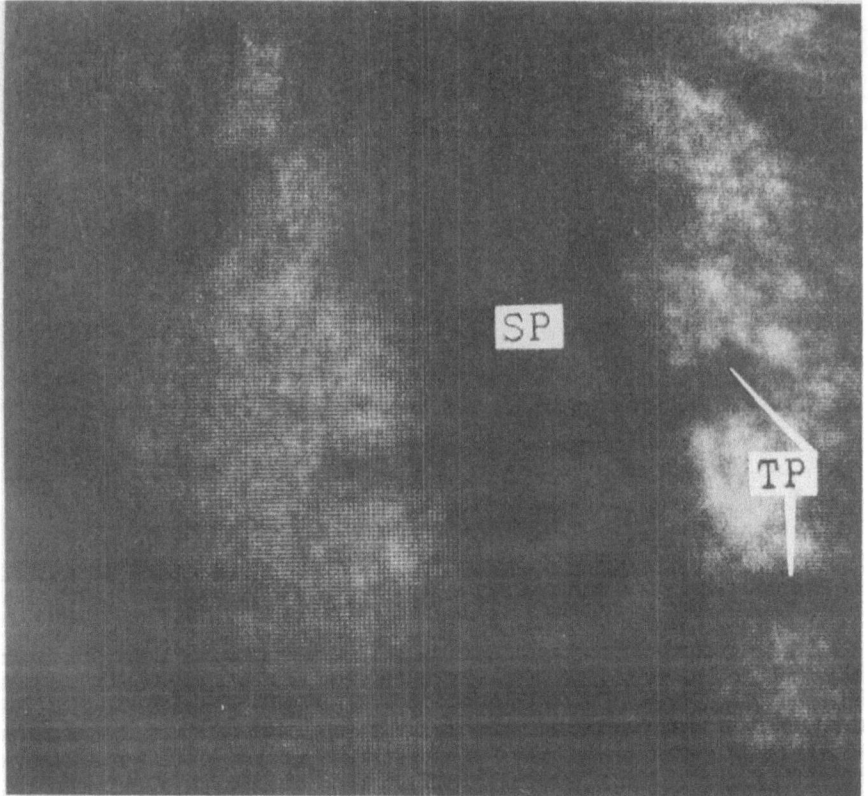

fig. 8a. Anteroposterior projection showing the posterior ribs and the lumbar spine (SP) with the transverse processes (TP) of the vertebras projecting out to each side.

290

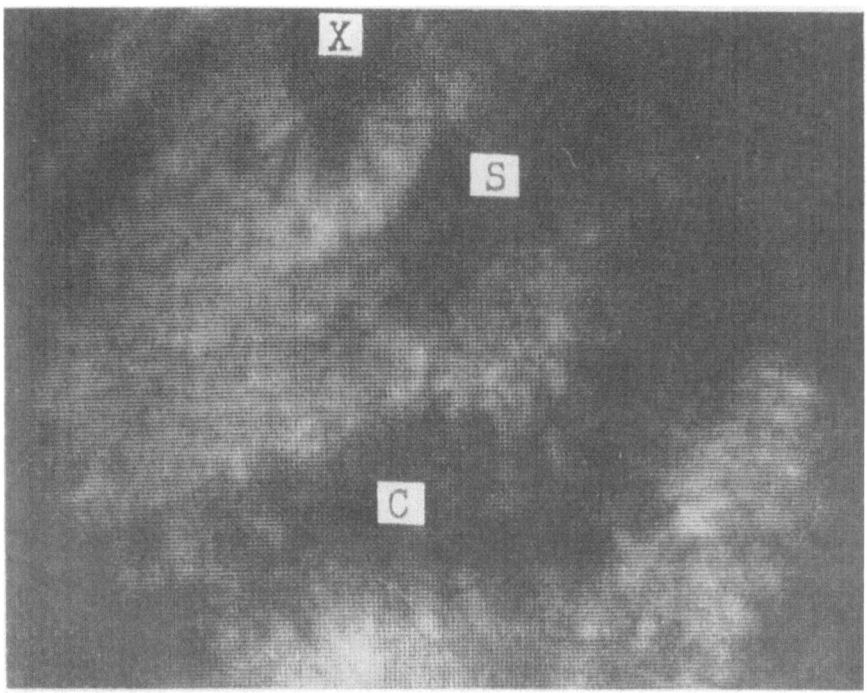

fig. 8b. Posteranterior projection of upper midabdomen. The transverse colon (C) with clear haustral markings runs across the middle of the picture. At the top center the tip of the xiphoid bone (S) appears as a shadow pointing down. Between the colon and the xiphoid there is an oblique broad dark band with lines within it suggesting the pattern of rugae in the stomach (S). (after GREEN 9)).

ation in the neighbourhood of the focal plane 10). This practice is classically used in non destructive testing but is rejected in medecine because of the time required for the entire scan. However, electronic scanning and focusing open new medical perspectives for C or 3D echography. As a first example, we study in our laboratory the medical importance of C-echographies obtained from a linear array of 160 cylindrical transducers (fig. 9). The transducers are naturally focusing in the Y direction with an electronic Fresnel zone focusing in the X direction, obtained from simple commutations of up to 64 transducers, in phase or in antiphase.

A good lateral resolution both in X and Y directions may be achieved in this way (fig. 10) but the sequential acquisition of the image requires about 20s for about 40 000 points obtained from the same number of ultrasonic pulses, corresponding to the maximum echo level obtained from an electronic gate delineating the depth and the thickness of the visualized portion of space. We may also acquire in the same time a sequence of 160 B-echograms at a rate of 12 per second containing information from the volume in the neighbourhood of the focal plane, about 10 cm thick 11).

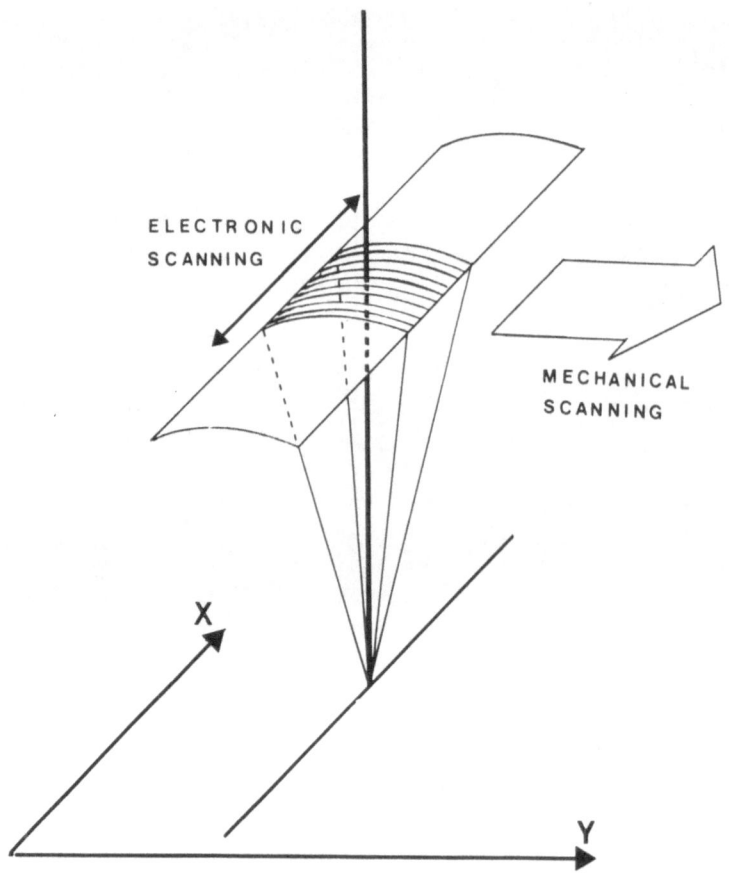

ELECTRONIC
SCANNING

MECHANICAL
SCANNING

X

Y

fig. 9. C or 3 D echographic device using a combination of Y-mechanical and X-electronic scanning, natural focusing in YZ plane and electronic focusing in XZ plane 11).

Different other approaches have been proposed combining X and Y electronic scanning or 2D beam steering and electronic focusing from a large synthetic aperture 12), 13). Anyway this sequential acquisition of data limits the rate of investigation to the same order of magnitude as in our experiment. We shall examine later the possibilities of attaining a real-time 3D acquisition but first would like to emphasize some features of 3D echographic information. For that, we play a game which consists in considering a very simple geometrical model i.e. a spherical interface with a flat piece inside, oriented parallel to the X Y scanning plane (fig. 11).

Due to the dominant specular reflections each X Z B-echogram appears reduced to 2 crescents and a straight segment. The simple superposition of these echograms (perspective view from infinite in Y direction) is quite uninteresting. Even the more sophisticated superposition corresponding to a perspective view from an arbitray direction remains difficult to interpret because there is too much information concentrated in the same image. But a very simple method consists in giving a decreasing visual emphasis to the echograms in function of their Y location. Only the first tomogram is clearly depicted and the following ones just help in locating it in the

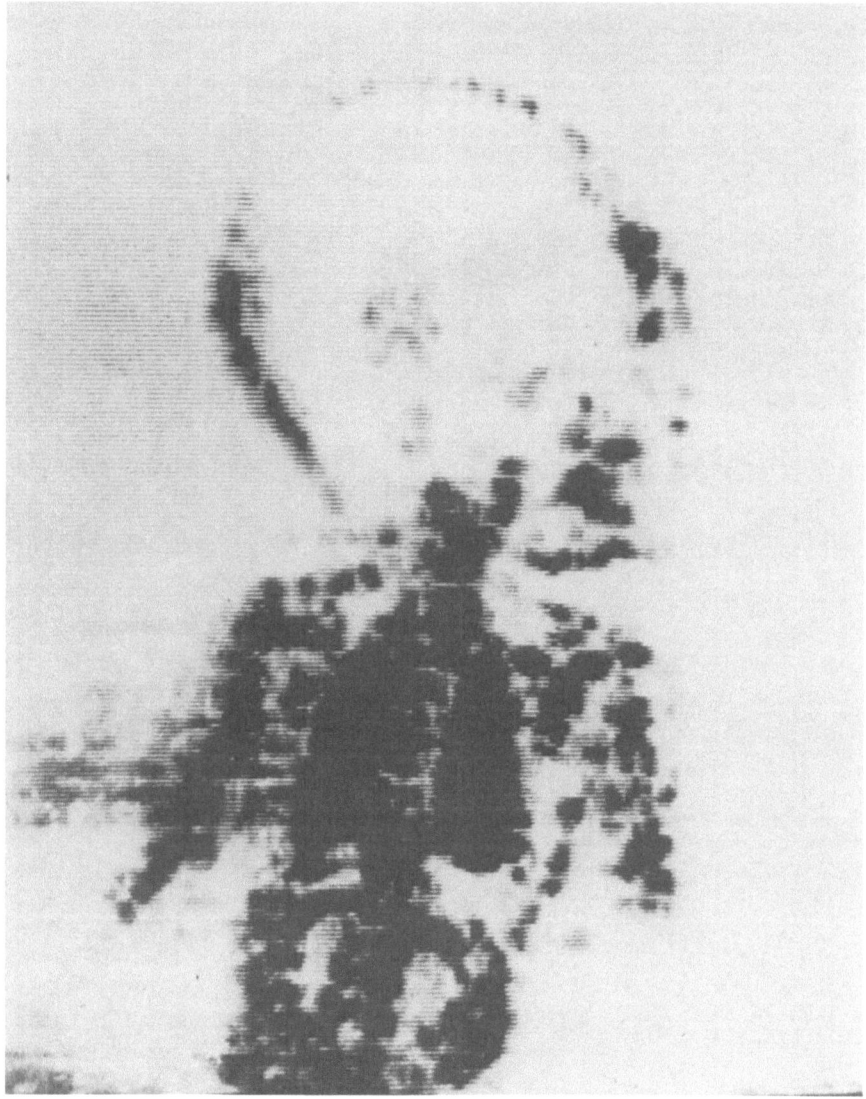

fig. 10. C Echogram of on excised foetus obtained with the device of fig. 9. Spine, lungs and kidneys are visible.

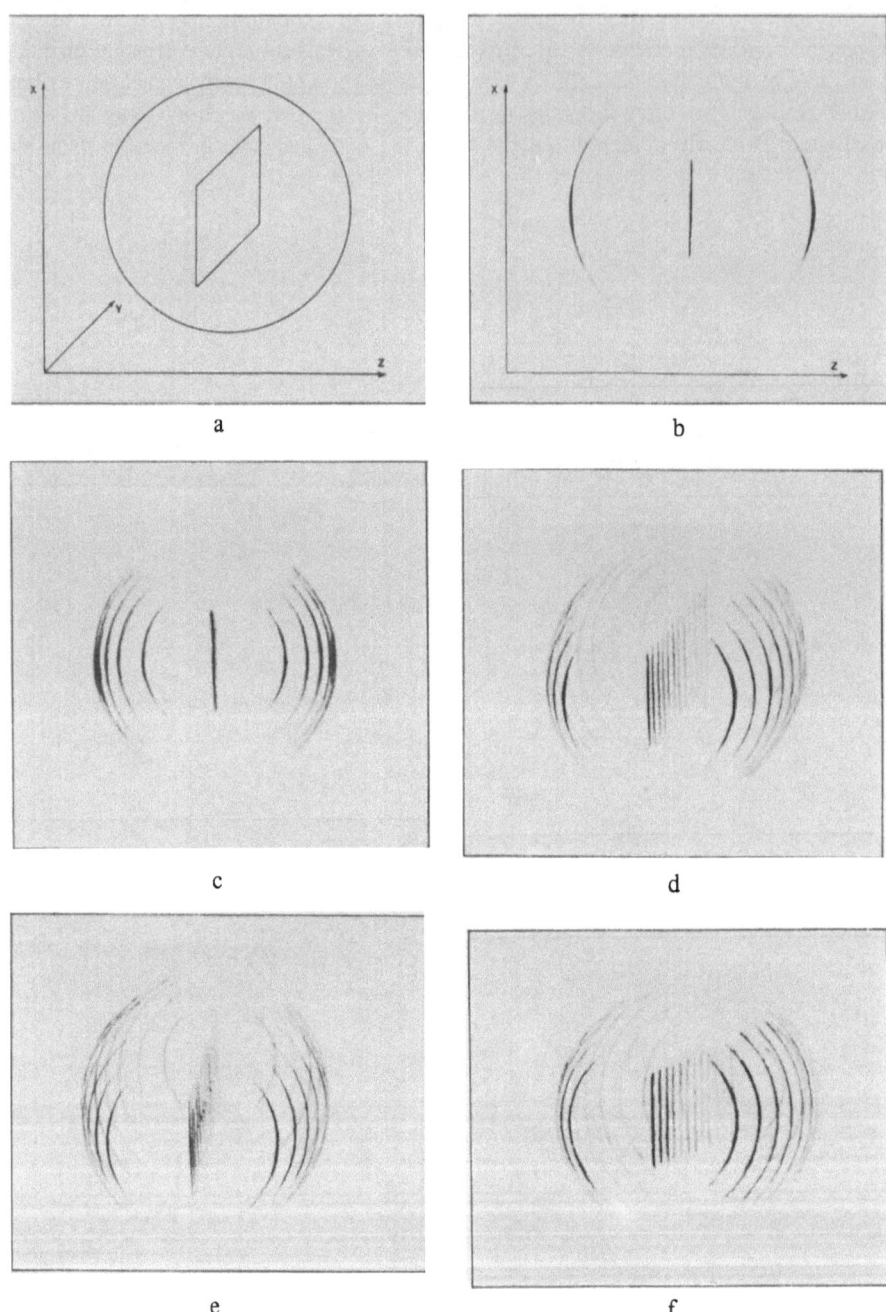

fig. 11. a) A simple geometrical model. b) Typical XZ echogram. c) Simple superposition of echograms. d, e, f) Superposition of XZ echograms obeying to different angles of view with a decreasing ponderation according to the Y direction.

volume. Of course the effects of this trick are greatly enhanced when motion is added by varying continuously the angle viewed. Varying the parameters of superposition creates to some extent parallax effects. This could be theoretically done from our data using a huge electronic memory with a very fast access. On the other hand it might be done in a much simpler way with a real-time 3D acquisition device which could interest cardiologists. This device does not exist but we may try to see how it might work, taking into account the conditions that Nature offers us.

Prospects of 3D real-time medical ultrasonic echographic investigation

Investigating 3 dimensions in real-time with ultrasound requires necessarily parallel acquisition of data in at least one direction. The holographic acquisition of the Brenden through-imaging technique is an example of parallel acquisition in X, Y, Z directions, where, at least theoretically, acquisition may be obtained in the time of a few acoustical oscillations i.e. in a few microseconds. Using an echographic technique imposes a sequential acquisition in the Z direction in a time of the order of 200 μs (in medical applications). An analog retina like the Mueller Brenden one, used in an echographic technique could permit X-Y-parallel acquisition of inform-

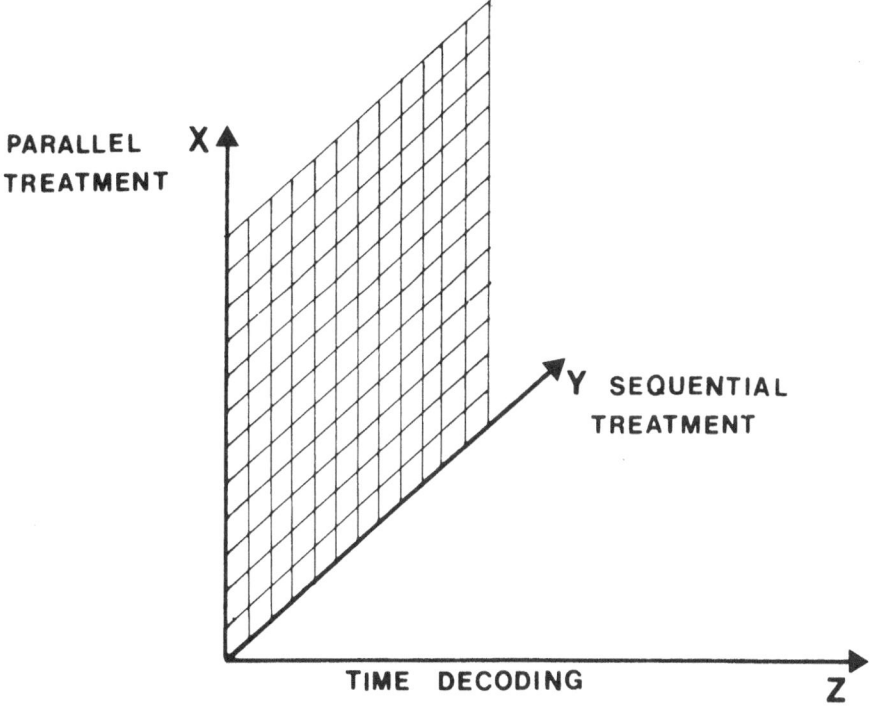

fig. 12. Prospect of a real time 3 D echographic device.

ation delivered sequentially from planes parallel to the X-Y reference plane. The holographic decoding is then limited at each time to a 2D information and more easy to carry than the 3D decoding of ordinary holography. This fact is an essential key of the success obtained with echographic technique, i.e. the natural decoding of information versus time in the Z direction. Although theoretically achievable, an X-Y-parallel, Z-sequential technique does not seem to be the best approach, except for ultra fast acquisition. It is possible to obtain an acquisition in 20 ms (50 pictures per second) using a sequence of 100 ultrasonic pulses combined with an electronic scanning in the Y direction. The parallel decoding is then restricted to the X direction, equivalent to the holographic restitution of a 1 dimensional object form a 1 dimensional hologram, i.e. a 1 dimensional Fresnel Transform which may be performed through an analogical process or through a specific computer. Data should then be acquired via an ultrafast multiplexing at frequencies of 100 MHz giving a video signal scanning the X direction in a time of the order of 1 µs (fig. 12). It must be emphasized that such real-time 3D acquisition should be much easier to display in the way suggested earlier according to fig. 10. The superposition of a large number of X-Z echograms is then possible in real-time with classical means i.e. a fast scanning oscilloscope.

Conclusion

The deceiving results of Acoustical Holography should prevent us from excessiveley optimistic comments about the future of 3D imaging. It seems reasonable to say that through-imaging techniques remain interesting for specific applications and should be developed with classical focusing lenses. On the other hand, echographic devices have proved their greater versatility specially after the development of the dynamic B-echography. These devices have already largely benefited from holographic or synthetic aperture concepts to improve the quality of imaging and their lateral resolution particularly. Extension of B-echography to 3D imaging is still limited by the rate of data acquisition with a classical sequential process, which is too low for many medical applications such as for cardiology. A real-time 3D device needs at least parallel treatment of information according to one direction of space and requires for any subsequent signal treatment an ultrafast multiplexing. Such techniques appear feasible in the next years and would have the great advantage of avoiding the enormous storage of data which is required by slow techniques experimented with today. Current use of 2D imaging greatly facilitates optimal structure selection for proper registration of M-modes. 3D imaging may similarly provide an excellent method to the selection of a diagnostically important tomogram.

References

1) Mueller RK, and Sheridon HK: *Sound Holograms and Optical Reconstruction.*
   Appl. Phys. Lett. 9, 328, 1966.

2) Mueller RK, and Keating PN: *The liquid-Gaz Interface as a Recording Medium for Acoustical Holography.*
   Acoust. Holg. 1, 49-56, 1969.

3) Smith RB, and Brenden BB: *Refinements and Variations in Liquid Surface and Scanned Ultrasound Holography.*
   I.E.E.E., Trans Sonics Ultras. SV 16, 29, 1969.

4) Metherell AF, Spinak S, and Pisa EJ: *Temporal Reference Acoustical Holography.*
   Acoust. Holog. 2, 69-85, 1970.

5) Korpel A, and Desmares P: *Rapid Sampling of Acoustical Holograms by Laser Scanning Techniques.*
   J. Opt. Soc. Amer. 45, 881, 1969.

6) Mezrich R, Etzold K, and Vilkomerson D: *Ultrasonovision.*
   Communication VI, Congrès Acoustical Holog. and Imaging San Diego Fév. 1975.

7) Erikson KR, and Zuleeg R: *"Integrated Acoustic Array".*
   7th International Symposium of Acoustical Imaging and Holography. To be published in "Acoustical Holograph", Vol. 7.

8) Alais P: *Real Time Acoustical Imaging with a 256 x 256 Matrix of Electrostatic Transducers.*
   Acoust. Holog. 5, 671-684, 1974.

9) Green PS, Schaefer LF, Jones PD, and Suarez JR: *A New High Performance Ultrasonic camera.*
   Acoust. Holog. 5, 493-503, 1974.

10) Green PS, Schaefer LF, and Macovski A: *Considerations for Diagnostic Ultrasonic Imaging.*
    Acoust. Holog. 4, 97-111, 1972.

11) Alais P, Fink M, and Perrin J: *Acoustic Imaging with an Electronically Focused and Scanned Array.*
    Communication Congres "Ultrasonics in Medicine", Mai 1975, Munich.

12) Havlice JF, Kind GS, Kofol JS, and Quate CF: *An Electronically Focused Acoustic Imaging Device.*
    Acoust. Holog. 5, 317-333, 1974.

13) Thurstone FL, and Ramm OT: *A New Ultrasound Imaging Technique Employing two dimensional Electronic Beam steering.*
    Acoust. Holog. 5, 249-259, 1974.

Acoustical image reconstruction devices

by R. Torguet, C. Bruneel, E. Bridoux and J.M. Rouvaen,
Centre Universitaire de Valenciennes 59326, Valenciennes.

An improved use of ultrasound in the medical and non destructive testing areas is made nowadays. The very first ultrasonic apparatuses were performing in the A-scan mode, that is to say that a pulsed ultrasonic wavetrain was launched and the position in time of the echoes, which were reflected by the obstacles, were observed. In such a way, the motion of a moving obstacle (like a cardiac valve) may be studied or the defects (like scratches in a metal piece) may be detected. These informations are truly interesting, but a growing interest has evolved among the uses towards the visualization of the obstacles. A number of acoustic imaging apparatuses have been built for this purpose and the actual studies are directed towards the following two directions: first the amelioration of the image quality and second the extension of the application field for these apparatuses.

The need for an image reconstruction

The majority of the acoustic imaging devices are working in the B-scan mode, that is to say, like for the A-scan mode, the propagation delay of the ultrasonic reflected pulses is used for differentiating obstacles lying at different depths, giving the first dimension in the image. The second one is obtained by mechanically translating an hand-held probe, or by using the electronic commutation 1) of an assembly of probes. In these devices, the spatial resolution is diffraction limited and the image rate is very low. Focusing techniques are now devised in order to circumvent the resolution problem 2), 3), but that of low image rating stays, a feature which is especially undesirable in the cardiologic field, owing to the very fast motions of the cardiac valves. It is thus necessary to perform a global imaging process, unlike the actual apparatuses, where a line by line reconstruction scheme is used. The reconstruction of a true image is therefore necessary, since diffraction effects produce only a shadow of the object: it is very similar to take a picture, in the classical optical sense, with a camera whose objective lens is taken off or is misfocused. A true image (fig. 1) is obtained when a small region, say a point, of the image contains informations only on a small region, say the resolution element, of the object.

Image reconstruction schemes

Several techniques are available for image reconstruction, but in all cases phase and amplitude informations are both needed. The technique may be distinguished between numerical techniques performing an inverse Fresnel transform on a computer and analogical ones, which perform the same operation by purely physical means. Only the last techniques will be considered here.

Echocardiology, N. Bom editor, published by Martinus Nijhoff, the Hague 1977.

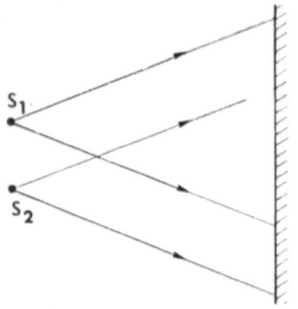 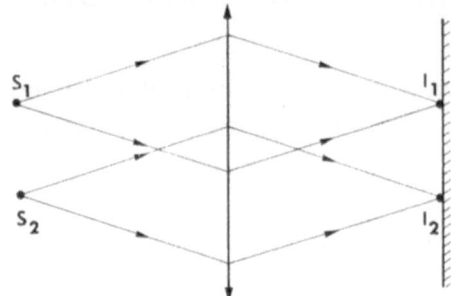

fig. 1. Shadow and true image.

Acoustic lens

The less involved technique for image reconstruction is to use an acoustic lens, that is to say, a material with a special shape and an acoustic velocity differing from that of the surrounding propagation medium, between the object and image planes. The influence of this lens may be studied from two alternative view points using either the classical refraction laws or the inversion of the relative phases of the acoustic rays.

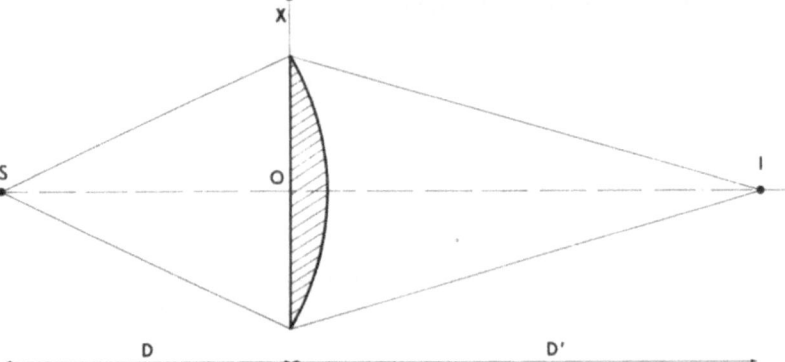

fig. 2. Image reconstruction by an acoustic lens device.

On the object side of the lens, the phase distribution is given by (see fig. 2):

$$\psi(x) = -\frac{\pi x^2}{\lambda_1 D}$$

Where λ_1 is the wavelength.
On the image side, the phase distribution is now:

$$\psi'(x) = \frac{\pi x^2}{\lambda_1 D'}$$

These relations are easily established assuming that the equiphase surfaces are spheres centered respectively at the source and image points. The inversion of the

300

relative phases is simply produced by the variable delay induced by the lens:

$$\Delta\psi = \frac{\pi X^2}{\lambda_1} \frac{(n-1)}{R} \qquad n = \frac{v_1}{v_2} = \frac{\lambda_1}{\lambda_2}$$

Where R is the radius of curvature of the lens. The calculations are valid in the paraxial approximation.

In the B-scan mode echography, the distance to the object is varying very fast. A speedy variable focal length is thus needed, a feature which may not be accomplished using a classical lens. Alternative solutions have therefore been searched for.

Optical processing 4)
Acoustical waves produce a moving diffraction grating, with alternate compression and dilation zones, which scatters an optical beam. The calculations show that the first (plus and minus) diffracted orders are phase and amplitude modulated by the acoustic wave. Using optical lenses, a true image of an insonified object may then be obtained. The focal length variation is provided by scanning the light beam in front of a conical lens.

Acoustic processing: acoustoelectronic lens 5)
The behaviour of a lens may be described, as it has previously been said, in terms of the inversion of the relative phases of rays emerging from a point source. This phase inversion may be obtained by purely electronic means. The acoustic field, after reflection on the obstacles, is sampled using an array of piezoelectric receivers and transformed into electrical signals, which are then mixed with a higher frequency reference (local oscillator) signal. Let $A \cos(\omega t + \psi)$ be the initial signal and $B \cos(\Omega t)$ the reference one. After mixing in a ring modulation, we get:

$$A\,B\,\cos(\omega t + \psi)\cos\Omega t = \frac{AB}{2}\cos\left[(\Omega - \omega)t - \psi\right] + \frac{AB}{2}\cos\left[(\Omega + \omega)t + \psi\right]$$

The signal at the higher $(\omega + \Omega)$ frequency is filtered out and a signal is thus obtained whose amplitude is proportional to that of the acoustic field, but whose phase is inverted. These last electrical signals are then converted into acoustical ones using a reemitting array of piezoelectric transducers, order to perform exactly the same operation as with an acoustic lens. A true real image is then obtained, with the interesting capacity of varying the focal length very easily: this distance is a function of the reemitted signal wavelength which may be adjusted via the reference signal frequency.

Practical implementation: optical processing system

Principle of the method
The acoustic pulses, with a time duration of 1 or 2 microseconds, are launched by a small aperture rectangular transducer. After some elapsed time, the echoes carry

informations about a line parallel to the transducer. This allows the exploration of a tomography whose width is equal to the acoustic beam aperture, length is equal to that of the transducer and depth is equal to, say, 15 centimeters in living tissues (this figure is limited by ultrasound absorption). The echoes are allowed to interact with a light beam, which therefore carries information about line objects lying at growing depths as time goes. These informations are spatially separated by using a rotating galvanometric mirror whose oscillations are synchronous with ultrasound emission (see fig. 3). A conical lens, set behing the mirror, is used for correcting the variation in object distance and obtaining a well focused image, which is picked up by a T.V. or cinematographic camera (fig. 4).

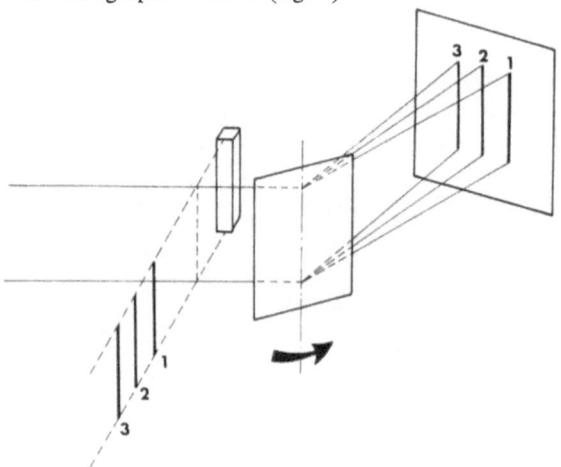

fig. 3. Principle of the 2^d dimension restitution.

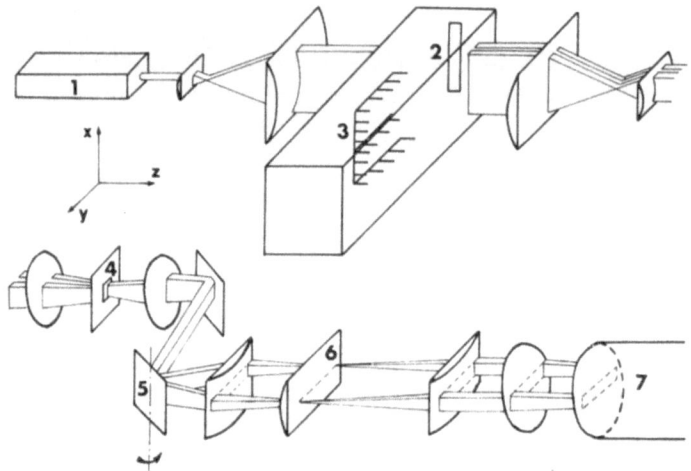

fig. 4. Diagram of the imaging system.
1: laser, 2: transducer, 3: object, 4: spatialfilter, 5: galvanometric mirror, 6: conical lens, 7: vidicon-tube.

302

Matching to biomedical applications

The direct interaction system is not well suited for medical applications owing to its poor sensitivity and to the impractical use of a water bath. An alternative system is therefore used in which the reflected acoustic field is sampled by an array of transducers. The received signals are amplified in parallel and converted back to acoustic signals by a second array of transducers: the acoustic field is thus reconstructed inside a separated medium with a high acousto-optic figure of merit.

Results

The reconstruction technique allows to obtain very high image rates, higher than 1000 images per second in the B-scan mode. The optimal resolution is nearly equal to 2 mm for an ultrasonic frequency of 3 MHz, that is to say a 0,5 mm wavelength in biologic media. Such a resolution is analog to that given by moving focus systems. The actual prototype has 20 acoustic channels, the image of an human heart, taken with a 5 cm length acoustic probe is shown in fig. 5, where the resolution is seen to be nearly equal to 3 mm. Studies are now in progress for designing a fast camera system with magnetic recording capacility in order to resolve the fast movements of the cardiac valves.

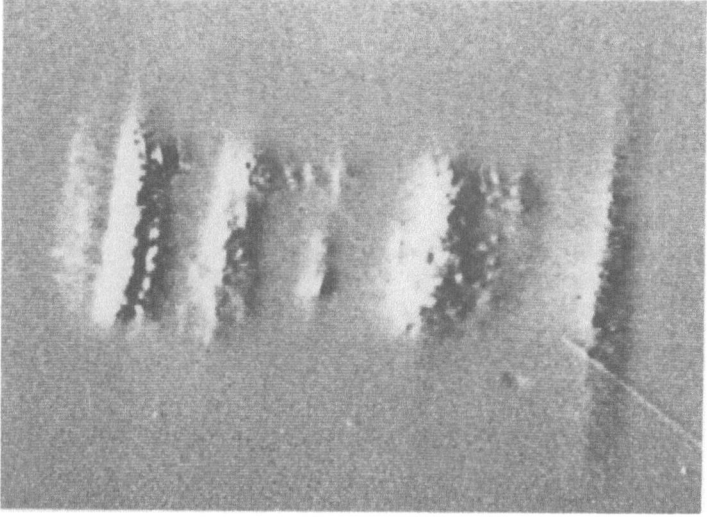

fig. 5. Tomography of the heart using the biomedical imaging system.

References

1) Bom N, Lancée CT, Honkoop J and Hugenholtz PG: *Ultrasonic viewer for cross sectional analyses of moving cardiac structures.*
Biomedical Engineering November, 1971.

2) Thurstone FL, and Von Ramm OT: *A new ultrasound technique employing two dimensional electronic beam steering.*
Acoustical holography vol. 5, P.S. Green, Editor, Plenum Press, 1974 P. 249-259.

3) Alais P and Fink M: *Fresnel zone focussing of linear arrays applied to B. and C. echography.*
7th International Symposium of Acoustical Imaging and Holography (Chicago, August 1976).

4) Bruneel C, Torguet R, Rouvaen JM, Bridoux E and Nongaillard B: *Ultrafast Echotomographic system using optical processing of ultrasonics signals.*
7th International Symposium of Acoustical Imaging and Holography (Chicago, August 1976).

5) Bruneel C, Nongaillard B, Torguet R, Bridoux E and Rouvaen JM: *Reconstruction of an acoustical image using an "acousto-electronic" lens device.*
Submitted to Applied Phys Letters.

304

Mechanical sector scanners

by A. Shaw,
West of Scotland Health Boards,
Department of Clinical Physics and Bio-Engineering,
Glasgow, United Kingdom.

Mechanical sector scanners

Mechanical sector scanners are characterised by the use of an electric motor to move the ultrasonic transducer and when the transducer sweeps over the area of interest the returning echoes are displayed as a series of single line B scans. If the transducer is moved at a frequency several times faster than the rate at which the heart is beating then real time pictures of 2 dimensional sections through the heart are produced. There are two basic ways in which the transducer can be moved (fig. 1). It can be either rotated in one direction 1) or oscillated like a pendulum 2). Our own development was concerned with optimising the design of a hand-held instrument employing an oscillating transducer which pivoted about its front face 3).

The scanning head

Some fundamental requirements for a practical system are illustrated in fig. 2. All moving parts should be enclosed; the drive mechanism should produce little vibration and should operate reliably. A fairly large transducer should be employed,

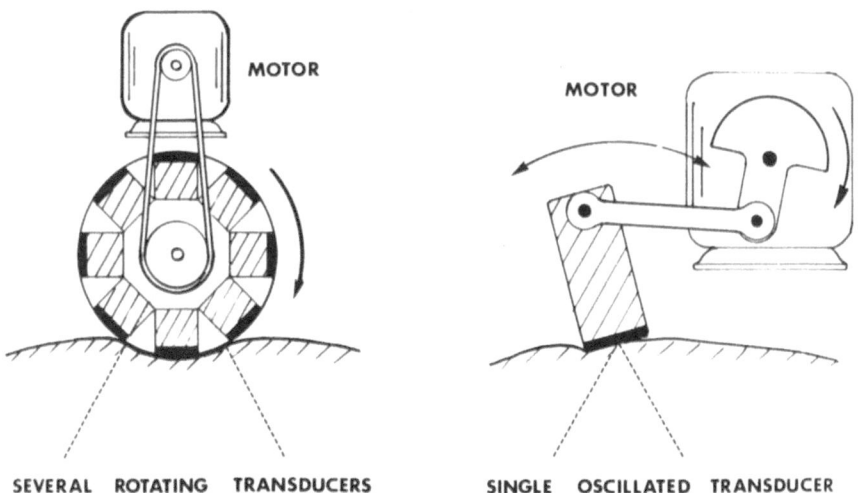

SEVERAL ROTATING TRANSDUCERS   SINGLE OSCILLATED TRANSDUCER

fig. 1. The basic types of high speed mechanical scanners.

305

for transducer size has a direct bearing on overall performance. For a transducer operating at a frequency of 2.5 MHz a crystal diameter of about 12 mm is needed; for a 5 MHz transducer the crystal diameter has to be about 6 mm diameter. The transducer should be interchangeable in the scanning head so that the appropriate frequency and amount of focussing can be selected for each application. There should be a built-in fluid coupling between the moving transducer and the front of the scanning head, the fluid being maintained in position by a rigid membrane of appropriate acoustic impedance. This minimises patient discomfort and ensures good coupling is maintained as the transducer sweeps across the field of view, particularly at the extreme edges of the scan. The surface area of the membrane in contact with the patient's skin should be kept reasonably small so that the scanning head can be tilted to a substantial angle before an air gap (and therefore a loss of picture) occurs between the patient and the scanning head. In our experience this ability to display sectors at oblique angles can make the difference between obtaining the correct view for diagnosis or otherwise. Another advantage of a limited area of contact is that the scanner can be aimed through intercostal spaces, limiting masking by ribs.

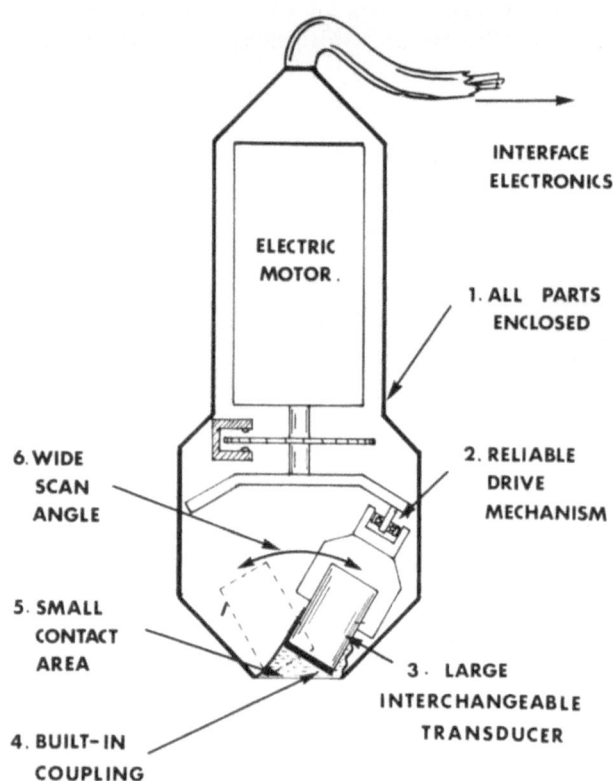

fig. 2. Practical requirements for applications in cardiology.

306

The transducer should sweep through an angle of at least 60 degrees, because smaller angles are too restrictive for many developing diagnostic applications e.g., in studying congenital abnormalities by means of a transverse scan. Fig. 3 illustrates the problems which arise if the scanning angle is restricted to 30 degrees. It is often not possible to include the main pulmonary artery, the tricuspid valve cusps and right ventricular outflow on a single 30º view.

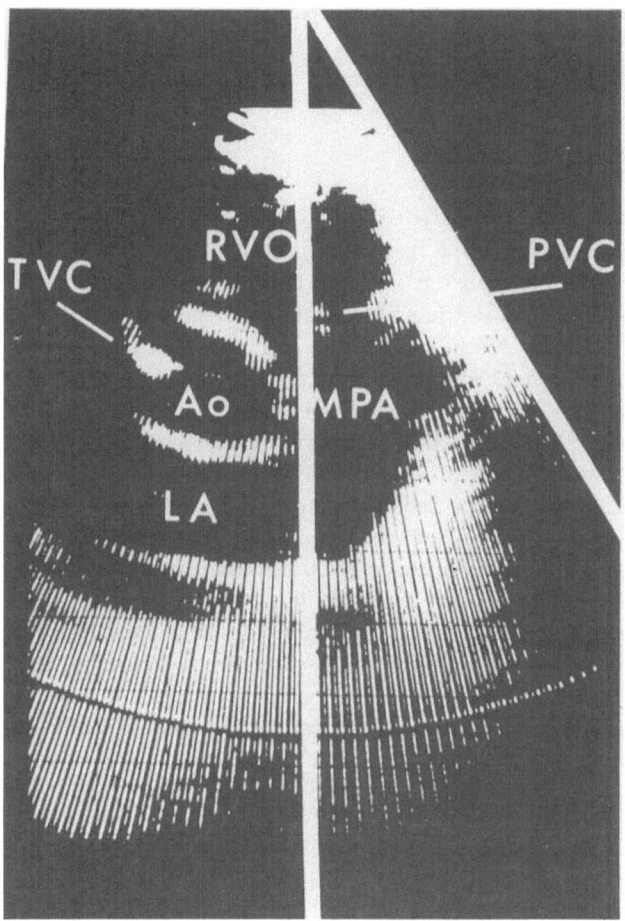

fig. 3. A transverse view through the heart. The angle subtended by the two thick white lines overlaid on the scan is 30º. The diagram illustrates the need to have a scanning angle of about 60º to show clearly the relationship between cardiac structures. RVO - right ventricular outflow; PVC - pulmonary valve cusps; MPA - main pulmonary artery; LA - Left atrium; Ao - aorta; TVC - tricuspid valve cusps.

307

Image presentation

A video recording system is desirable for it has the advantage that diagnosis can be made without the patient's presence. Recent improvements in video systems will lead to increased use being made of disc recorders with their attendant improvement in image quality, particularly on slow speed replay. However, as an alternative to video recording, we have found useful a rather specialised form of ECG gating. It operates by synchronising a single swept display of the transducer to the ECG triggered signal. A static frame for each part of the heart's cycle can be written out and stored on the oscilloscope. The appropriate image is preselected by setting a suitable time delay from the Q.R.S. complex. A digital readout on the display indicates the actual delay period selected. A large number of consecutive still frames through the heart's cycle can be obtained and the appropriate views used for diagnosis.

Limitations and advantages

The main limitations on the performance of mechanical sector scanners are the maximum speed at which the transducer is oscillated and the pulse repetition frequency of ultrasound generated at the crystal. Most rotational and oscillating mechanical scanners are restricted to a transducer speed of about 15 cycles/second i.e., 30 frames/second for an oscillating transducer. If 100 lines per frame are displayed, then the average pulse repetition frequency will need to be 30 x 100 i.e., 3000 pulses/second. But since oscillating transducers will move faster in the middle of the scan than at the edges, then to maintain an even increment between each line of display the maximum pulse repetition frequency needs to be about 4000 per second. This is close to the maximum rate which can be achieved because of the velocity of ultrasound in tissue. Interspacing additional lines of the same information on each frame of the display 4) will not improve the diagnostic value, giving only a superficial impression of improved image quality.

In our experience the restriction of mechanical speed of oscillation does not appear to be a serious constraint. Consider one of the most demanding applications, the rapidly beating heart of the newborn. Good quality diagnostic images can be readily obtained (fig. 4). The transducer speed was 26 frames/second and 128 lines are displayed on the single frame illustrated.

The important application of diagnosing cardiac problems in infancy also illustrates some of the technical problems associated with other 2 dimensional imaging systems e.g., the problem of achieving good resolution in the near field using phased array devices. Fig. 4 shows that the areas of clinical interest are within a few centimetres of the transducer, yet it has proven impossible to obtain images closer than about 4 cm from the transducer with at least one phased array system 5). This problem was attributed to ring down artifacts.

Whether the patient is a child or an adult another factor which must be considered is the resolution of the ultrasonic beam in the plane at right angles to the sector dis-

308

played. Beam divergence in this plane will introduce artifacts on the display. Von Ramm and Thurstone 5) have suggested that the closest resolution in this direction is about 8 mm with their phased array system. This dimensional inaccuracy is almost identical to the total diameter of the ascending aorta (8.2 mm) which can be clearly seen in our illustration fig. 4. Mechanical sector scanners are capable of imaging appropriate fine slices through the heart without introducing artifacts due to the curvature of the vessels.

However, this can only be achieved by using a transducer which is large enough to achieve the right amount of focussing at relevant penetrations and this is incompatible with say 100 lines of real information per frame using a linear array system. Each element in the linear array is too small to focus the beam accurately. Electronic timing of several elements helps improve the resolution in the plane of the image, but not at right angles to it 6). Because a large symmetrical transducer is employed with some mechanical systems, good beam control is achieved in all 3 dimensions.

Applications

Real time 2 dimensional scanning offers direct visualisation of the anatomical structures of the heart and their spatial relationship throughout the cardiac cycle.

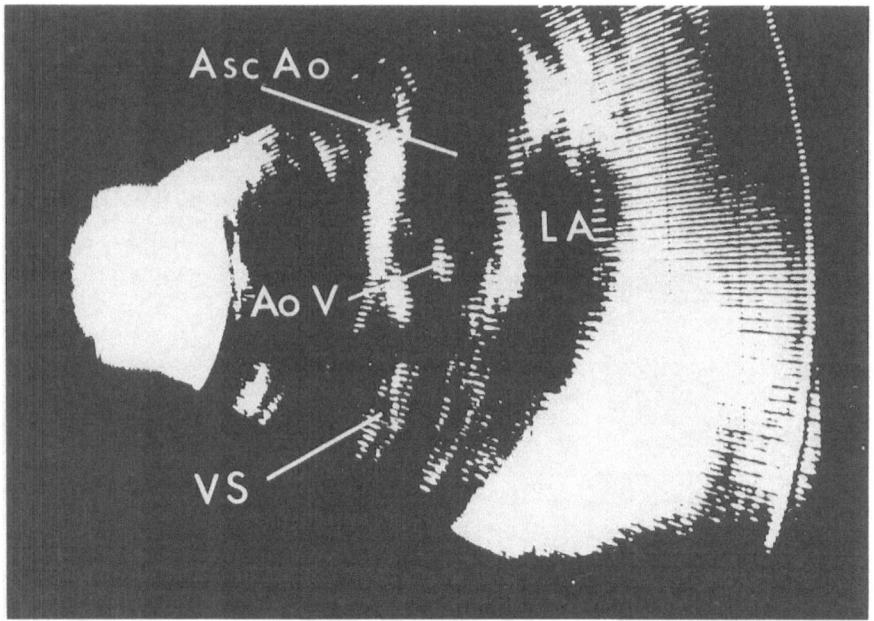

fig. 4. A longitudinal scan through the heart of a healthy neonate weighing 2.6 kg. The total depth of the heart is about 3.2 cm and the heart rate was about 148 beats/minute. Asc Ao - ascending aorta, Ao V - aortic valve, VS - ventricular septum.

309

It assists the optimisation of image position for presenting time-position (T-P or M-mode) displays e.g., in locating the tip of the mitral valve. Provided suitable electronic processing is incorporated it is possible to produce time-position echo-cardiographs directly from the 2 dimensional real time display. Obviously time-position scans can be selected from various levels of the heart. Used in this way it enhances diagnosis and reduces investigative time.

As a technique in its own right it offers considerable diagnostic potential in both congenital and acquired heart disease. Mechanical sector scanners have been applied to the diagnosis of left ventricular aneurysms, in the examination of the interatrial septum and in the rupture of the sinus of valsalva 7)-9).

Amongst other applications, we have applied this technique to the diagnosis of heart disease in childhood. In particular, for examining transpositions of the great arteries, tetralogy of Fallot, double outlet right ventricles and persistent truncus arteriosus. Fig. 5 illustrates one application and is a longitudinal scan taken from an infant with transposed great arteries. If we compare this display with a normal heart (fig. 4), we can see that in the normal anatomy there is a characteristic upward course to the ascending aorta above the cusps of the aortic valve. In fig. 5 the aorta is positioned anterior to the ventricular septum with the aortic valve cusps clearly distinguishable. The posterior great vessel is the main pulmonary artery and the dis-

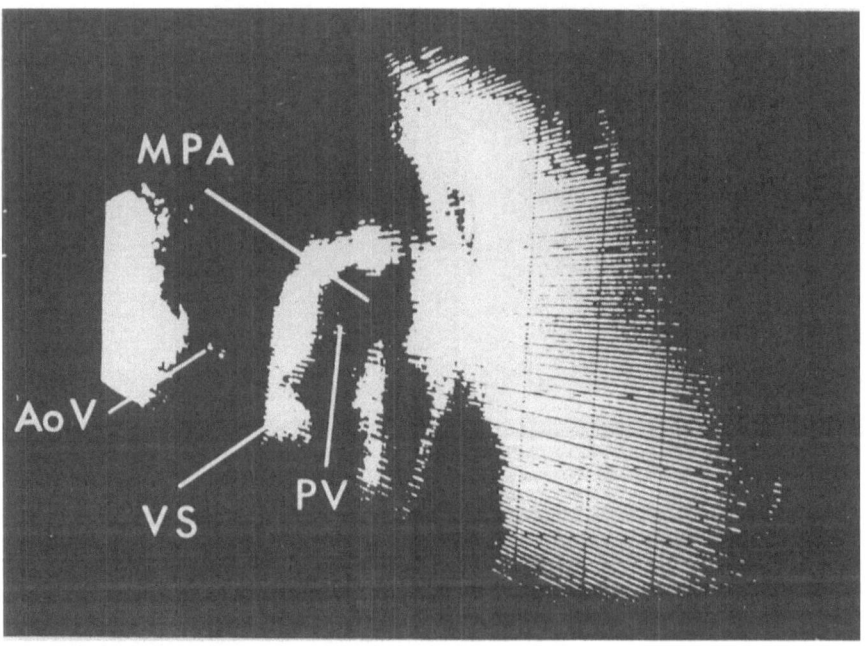

fig. 5. A longitudinal scan of a patient with transposition of the great arteries. MPA - main pulmonary artery, PV - pulmonary valve.

play is differentiated from that of the normal anatomy by the clearly defined posterior sweep of this vessel (to the right in fig. 5) close above the level of aortic and pulmonary valve cusps.

In conclusion, real time 2 dimensional scanning makes possible ultrasonic imaging of the heart in its true anatomical relationship and is rapidly becoming a viable alternative to angiography. It is a sensitive method which will improve our understanding of cardiac function in the various stages of disease. Because of its non-invasive nature it can be repeated with little inconvenience to the patient.

Mechanical sector scanners can produce good quality information at modest cost and will play an important part in the continuing development of 2 dimensional real time systems in echocardiography.

References

1) Holm HH, Kristensen JK, Pedersen JF, Hanche S, and Northeved A: *A new mechanical real time ultrasonic contact scanner.*
   Ultrasound in Medicine and Biology 2: 19, 1975.

2) Griffith JM, and Henry WL: *A sector scanner for real time two dimensional echocardiography.*
   Circulation 49: 1147, 1974.

3) Shaw A, Paton JS, Gregory NL, and Wheatley DJ: *A real time 2-dimensional ultrasonic scanner for clinical use.*
   Ultrasonics 14: 35, 1976.

4) Kloster FE, Roelandt J, ten Cate FJ, Bom N, and Hugenholtz PG: *Multiscan echocardiography II. Technique and initial clinical results.*
   Circulation 48: 1075, 1973.

5) Von Ramm OT, and Thurstone FL: *Cardiac imaging using a phased array ultrasound system. I. System design.*
   Circulation 53: 258, 1975.

6) Whittingham TA: *A hand-held electronically switched array for rapid ultrasonic scanning.*
   Ultrasonics 14, 19, 1976.

7) Weyman AE, Peskoe SM, Williams ES, Dillon JC, and Feigenbaum H: *Detection of left ventricular aneurysms by cross-sectional echocardiography.*
   Circulation 54: 936, 1976.

8) Dillon JC, Weyman AE, Feigenbaum H, Eggleton RC, and Johnston K: *Cross-sectional echocardiographic examination of the interatrial septum.*
   Circulation 55: 115, 1977.

9) Nishimura K, Hibi N, Kato T, Fikui Y, Arakowa T, Tatematsu H, Miwa A, Tada H, Kambe T, Nakagawa K, and Takemura Y: *Real time observation of cardiac movement and structures in congenital and acquired heart diseases employing high-speed ultrasoncardiotomography.*
   American Heart Journal: 92, 340, 1976.

311

A dynamically focused multiscan system

by C.M. Ligtvoet, J. Ridder, C.T. Lancée,
F. Hagemeijer and W.B. Vletter,
Thoraxcenter, Erasmus University, Rotterdam, Netherlands.
W.J. Gussenhoven, Interuniversitair Cardiologisch Instituut.

Introduction

Clinical ultrasound instruments with a linear array transducer are nowadays one of the methods which can be used to obtain real time two dimension cardiac images 1), 2), 3). Unlike mechanical sector scanners 4) and phased array sector scanners 5), linear array systems produce a rectangular cross-sectional image of the moving heart. A rectangular picture ensures a complete imaging of structures in the vicinity of the transducer as well as of structures deep inside the body.

As with all two dimensional real time instruments, the image of a linear array system may show a limited number of lines on the display. With linear array systems, this is related to the number of acoustic beams formed by the multi element transducer and the short time, available for one complete frame. Recently introduced processing techniques effectively eliminate this disadvantage for a linear array system 6). With this processing, the echo data is digitized and temporarily stored in a memory. Additional lines are calculated from the available echo information and added to the existing lines, to produce an image with a high line density.

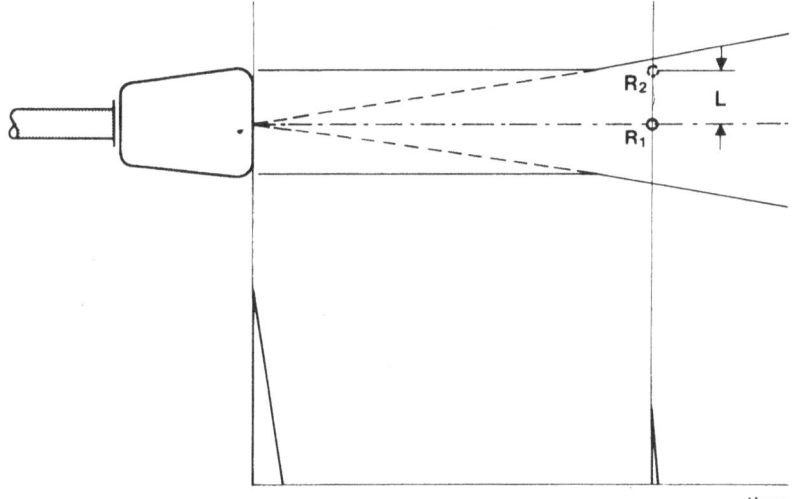

fig. 1. Diagram demonstrating the display in the A-mode of two structures lying within the soundbeam of a transducer. A reflector positioned at R_1 or R_2 would result in the same echo, suggesting one structure on the main axis.

313

Echocardiology, N. Bom editor, published by Martinus Nijhoff, the Hague 1977.

Another limiting factor of clinical ultrasound systems is the limited lateral resolution, resulting from the finite beam width of the transducer. Off-axis structures in the sound beam of the transducer are "seen" and erroneously displayed on the main axis (see fig. 1). The shape of the sound beam depends on transducer frequency and geometry.

For a good lateral resolution a small beam width is required. As a first step towards a better lateral resolution, transducers were constructed with an acoustical lens, which resulted in a fixed focal point. Transducers with a fixed focal point however, offer only a solution to the problem in the direct vicinity of the focal point. In diagnostic ultrasound the target is a continuous object and an optimal solution calls for focusing over the entire field of view. This requires a continuous focus.

In this paper a linear array system will be described, where for each scan a sub-array of 12 elements is used in transmission and reception. In transmission an axicon focus is applied. During the reception period the focal point is adjusted, corresponding to the position in the body where the echoes originate at that particular moment.

The physical background of this focus technique will be discussed as well as the electronic set-up of the system. The clinical evaluation of this system has been performed in our clinic and some results will be shown.

System design

Familiar methods of focusing in ultrasound systems are focusing with a curved transducer, an acoustical lens and a phased array. The first two methods give a focal point at a fixed distance from the transducer. A good lateral resolution only appears in and at short distances from the focal point. Outside the vicinity of the focal point, transducers with a fixed focal point behave like unfocussed transducers. With a transducer array consisting of a large number of small acoustical elements it is possible to vary the distance between the transducer and the focal point by means of phasing methods. Such a "phased array" transducer gives the opportunity to maintain a good lateral resolution over the entire scan depth.

A phased array transducer can be included in a linear array transducer and a so called linear phased array transducer is formed. For each scan of the linear phased array, a sub-set of elements is used as a phased array. The next scan is performed with a new sub-array, consisting of n-1 elements of the previous scan and one new adjacent element. Part of a linear phased array is schematically shown in fig. 2. This linear phased array technique is the basis for a dynamically focused ultrasound system.

In this system two different focus techniques have been incorporated, one in transmission and one in reception. In the transmission period of a scan, an axicon focus is applied. Contrary to the more common point focus, this type of focusing has no focal point, but a focal line. Fig. 3 illustrates a phased array with a point focus and one with an axicon focus. Due to the distribution of the focus over a line, the

314

axicon focus is weaker than the point focus. In transmission, axicon focusing is accomplished by activating the individual elements of the phased array at short time intervals. The outer elements are excited first, the elements in the middle of the array last.

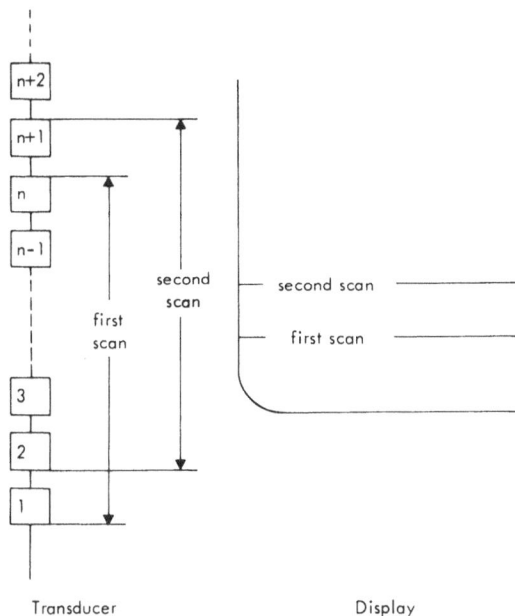

fig. 2. Schematic representation of linear phased array principle. The first scan is formed with the elements 1 up to n, the second scan is done with the elements 2 up to n +1. Each scan is performed with n-1 elements of the previous scan and an extra adjacent element 9).

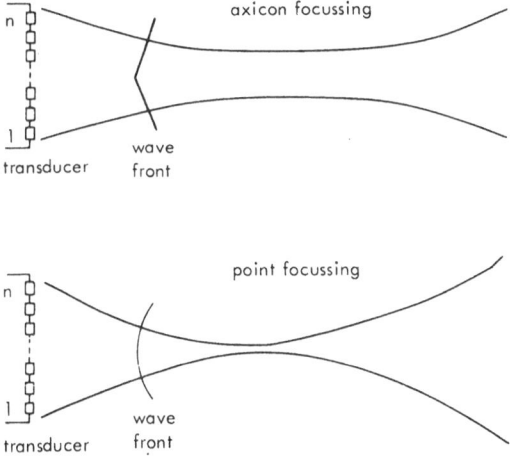

fig. 3. Illustration of two focusing methods, axicon focus and point focus, shown for a phased sub-array of n elements.

Directly following the transmission pulse, the system is switched to reception. Since echoes from nearby structures arrive first, the phased array is focused at structures a short distance away from the transducer. This is accomplished by a compensation for the time differences between the reception moments of the echoes by the various elements of the phased array. During the reception period, six adjacent focal zones are used. The system adjusts the time compensation when a new focal zone is entered. Each focal zone contains one focal point. Fig. 4 shows a multi-element transducer with six sequential focal zones.

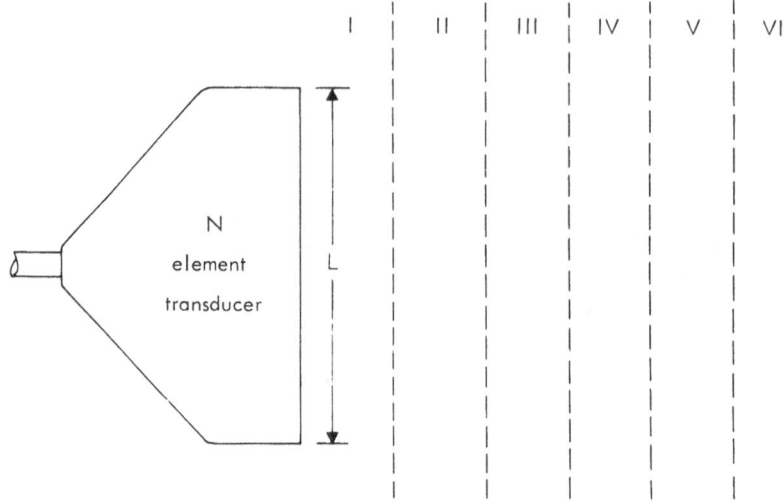

fig. 4. Multi-element transducer with six sequential focal zones. During the reception period the system focuses with a subset of n elements in one of the six zones. When a focal zone boundary is crossed, the system switches to the focal point of the new zone 9).

For optimal transducer design a number of parameters had to be considered. These include for the sub-set of elements, used to form one scan, the aperture as well as the number of individual elements and their size and frequency. Preferably no redundancy may occur between two adjacent scans. The lateral resolution determines the lateral distance between adjacent scans in the body. The optimalisation of the array was performed with a computer model. Calculation showed, that for an effective focusing over 16 cm scan depth, and with a given fundamental transducer frequency of 3.12 MHz, an aperture of 24 mm is needed. The array is divided into 12 elements of 2 mm width each. This results in a lateral spacing of 2 mm between two adjacent scans. Fig. 5 shows a comparison between measured and calculated beam width as a function of axial distance. The measurements with the 12 element phased array transducer were made in a water tank. The -10dB beam width is defined as the lateral displacement of a thin wire reflector from the main axis to both sides where the echo amplitude has the defined value, relative to the echo strength on the main axis.

316

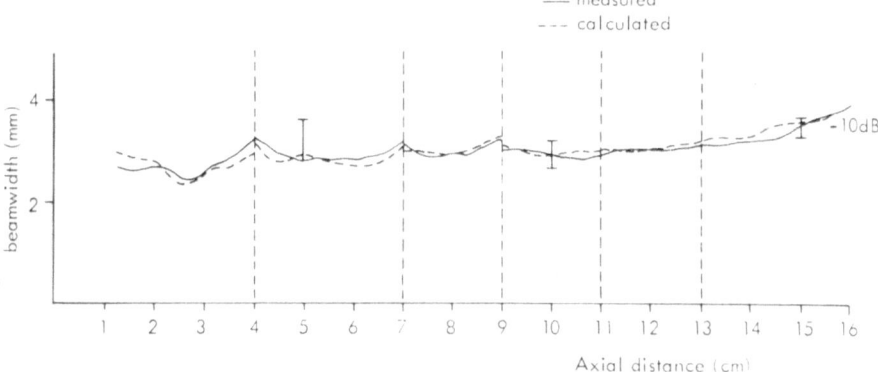

fig. 5. Calculated and measured beam width as a function of axial distance at the -10dB level of a reflection diagram. The vertical dashed lines give the boundaries of the focal zones 9).

A total number of 40 scans was chosen, which results in 51 elements in the linear phased array transducer and an overall length of 10.2 cm. The dimensions of the rectangular two dimensional image, which can be composed with this transducer is 8 x 16 cm.

Each element of the transducer is connected to the main frame of the system by means of a thin coaxial cable. For easy handling of the transducer, a special cable was constructed consisting of 51 coaxial cables with a total diameter of only 1 cm. A low mechanical Q is achieved by using heavy backing. The backing material is a mixture of araldite and tungsten powder.

As mentioned before, twelve elements are activated for a single scan. To each element three periods of 3.12 MHz are applied, resulting in a transmission pulse of about 1 usec. The axicon in transmission is achieved with digital delay lines. One complete frame is built up from 40 scans. A reproducible axicon focus over the 40 scans can only be achieved if the transmitters are closely matched in time. Therefore, no thyristors were used in the transmit circuit, but a transmitter consisting of transistors was designed. The overall inaccuracy of the timing of the transmission circuit was established at 5 nsec $\pm$ 5 percent of the delay from the digital delay lines.

In the reception period of one scan, the same twelve elements are used as in the transmission period. The echoes received by these elements are conducted to twelve pre-amplifiers. Analog multiplexers connect the outputs of these pre-amplifiers to the delay lines. The delay lines pass the echo information with different delay for each element and compensate for the differences in distance between a target on the main axis and the various elements of the array. Due to the symmetric configuration of the 12 elements in the phased array, only six analog delay lines are needed. Each focal zone uses an unique tap configuration from the six delay lines. The echo information is summed for each zone, so that at any moment the echo

317

data is available for each zone. The computer model, used for the evaluation of the transducer configuration, showed that a reduction of the sidelobe level was possible by summing the high frequency echo information of different zones.

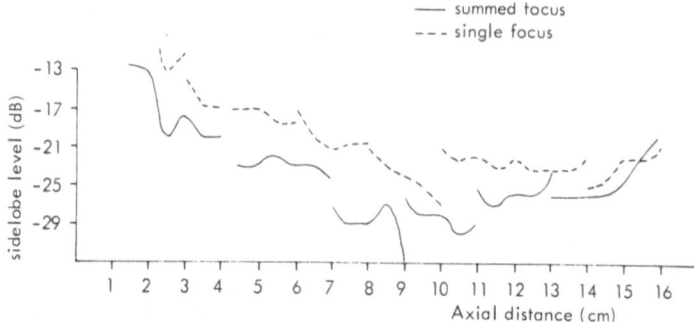

fig. 6. Measured beam width and side lobe levels as function of axial distance for single focal zones and for high frequency summated focal zones 9).

In fig. 6 a comparison of side lobe levels is made for the situation of the single focal zones and the situation where sequentially the high frequency signals from two or three focal zones are summated. Besides, the beam width is not notably changed. Simultaneous processing of 12 analog signals for 40 different scans requires special attention for the tolerances in the electronic components. The analog circuits were designed with a maximum amplitude error of ± 1,5 dB and a maximum time error of 20 nsec. The analog delay lines introduce a time inaccuracy of 5 percent of the time delay.

To determine the influence of the inaccuracies in the transmitter and reception circuits on the beam width a computer program was developed. In this program a routine was used to imitate the random distribution of the errors over the electronic circuits in the system. Fig. 7 gives the results of this calculation and shows that for worst cases, only a slight influence on the beam width can be observed.

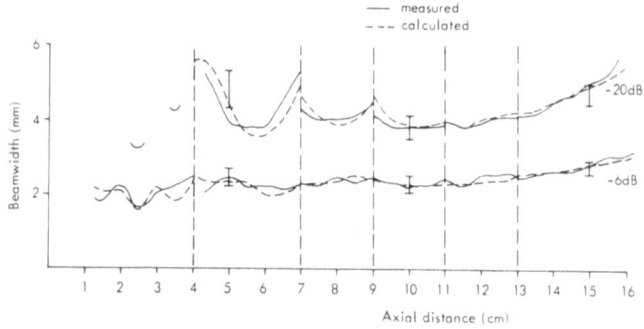

fig. 7. Calculated and measured beam width as a function of axial distance at the -6dB and -20dB level. The six vertical solid lines represent the possible variation of the beam width due to the inaccuracy of the electronic components 9).

318

Six fast analog switches, one for each focal zone, select the correct zone. The switching is controlled by a digital timing circuit started at the beginning of a scan. To preserve the high dynamic range of the echo signals, a switch design was used minimizing the cross talk between digital control signals and echo signals. Fig. 8 shows the block diagram of the focused system, with the focusing in transmission and in reception.

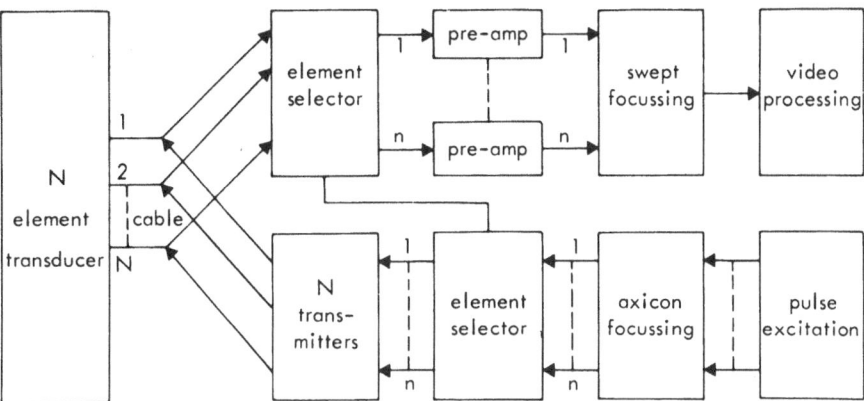

fig. 8. Block diagram of the dynamically focused linear array system. The lower part of the diagram shows the processing during transmission schematically, the upper part gives the signal handling during reception 9).

The signal from the switches is processed in the time gain amplifier and detected. The detected signal is displayed on the screen of a television monitor. The echo information is electronically processed to video speed with a line converter. This converter doubles the line number by means of an electronic interpolation technique. A detailed description of this converter has been published 6).

Clinical results

Clinical evaluation of the focused multiscan system was performed in our laboratory for clinical echocardiography which did have experience with an unfocused multiscan system 7). Standardized transducer positions were used; the first following the long axis of the left ventricle; the other perpendicular to the first one.

During the clinical evaluation, it became clear that the focused multiscan system does yield a better outlined display of the cardiac structures. Especially deep lying structures, such as the anterior mitral valve leaflet and the left ventricular posterior wall are better seen than with an unfocused multiscan system. This is in complete agreement with theory, which states that the lateral resolution of unfocused systems decreases with increasing axial distance. The focused system maintains a good lateral resolution, over the entire depth. As a first example of the focused multiscan system, fig. 9 shows a longitudinal cross-sectional image of a patient with a subaorta membrane. In this picture, a visualization of the deep lying structures is obtained. A transverse cross-sectional image can be observed in fig. 10. The interventricular septum as well as the left ventricular posterior wall are both seen.

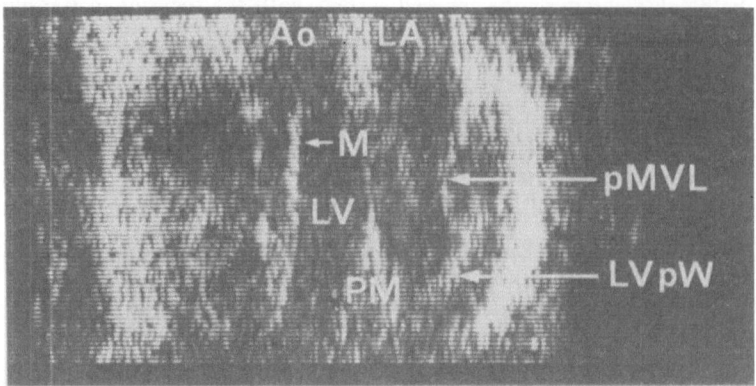

fig. 9. Long-axis cardiac cross section obtained from a patient with a sub-valvular membranous aortic stenosis. Ao = Aorta; LA = Left Atrium; M = Sub-valvular Membrane; pMVL = posterior Mitral Valve Leaflet; LV = Left Ventricle; LVpW = Left Ventricular posterior Wall; PM = Papillary Muscle.

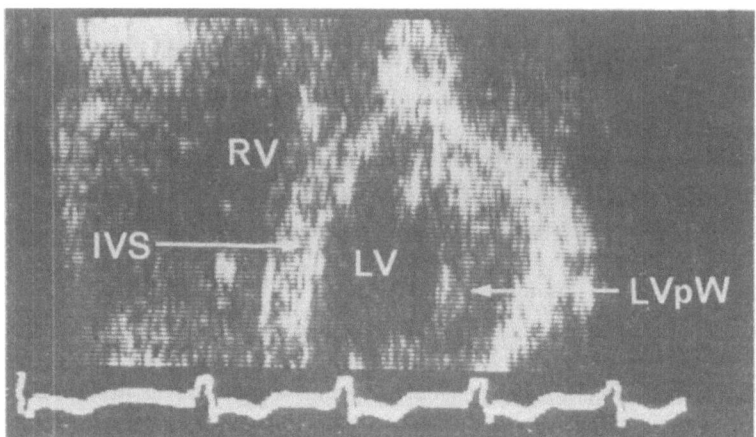

fig. 10. Short-axis cardiac cross section of a patient with an enlarged right ventricle. RV=Right Ventricle; IVS = Interventricular Septum; LV = Left Ventricle; LVpW = Left Ventricular posterior Wall.

Roelandt et al 8) stated that an unfocused system displays the anterior mitral valve leaflet in systole as a combination of vertical lines. This distortion is caused by the overlap of echo data over different scans. The focused system, where each scan con-

320

tains unique echo information, displays the mitral valve leaflets as a curved structure (fig. 11). As a last example of clinical observations, fig. 12 illustrates a left atrial myxoma. A longitudinal cross-section is shown, and the good lateral resolution of the focused system strikingly outlines the myxoma boundaries; surgery showed that the size of the myxoma had been accurately measured by this echocardiological technique.

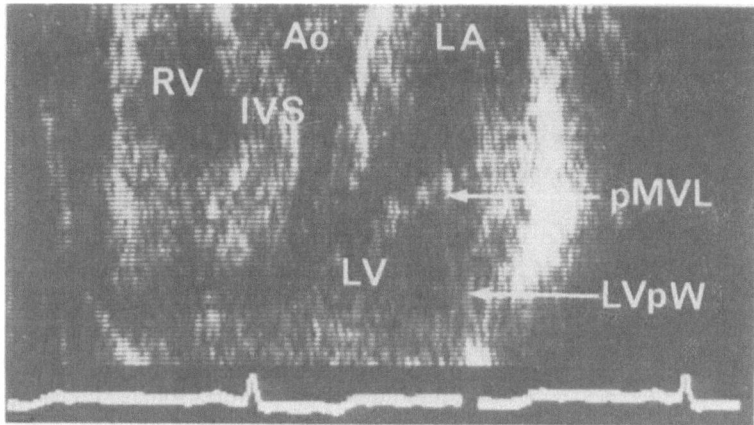

fig. 11. Long-axis cross section of a heart of a patient with a thickened septum. The posterior mitral valve leaflet is visualized without the vertical distortion sometimes noticed in unfocussed linear array systems. Ao = Aorta; LA = Left Atrium; RV = Right Ventricle; IVS = Interventricular Septum; LV = Left Ventricle; pMVL = posterior Mitral Valve Leaflet; LVpW = Left Ventricular posterior Wall.

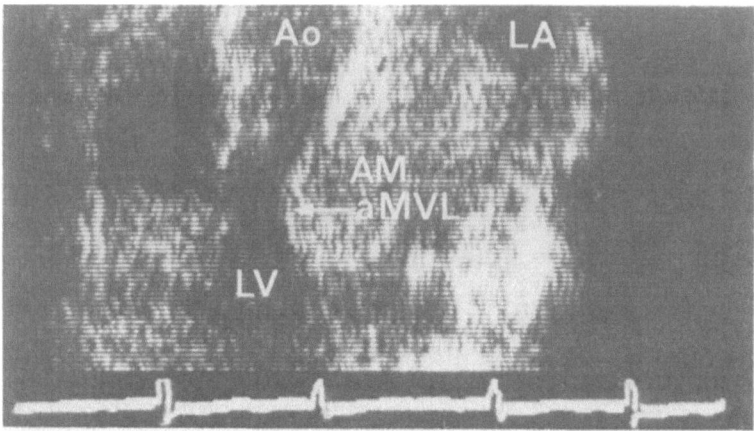

fig. 12. Long-axis cross section obtained from a patient with an atrial myxoma. Ao = Aorta; LA = Left Atrium; LV = Left Ventricle; aMVL = anterior Mitral Valve Leaflet; AM = Atrial Myxoma.

Discussion

The quality of the cross-sectional images obtained with the described dynamically focused linear array system shows a remarkable improvement over the results of unfocused linear array systems. In a few patients however, the signal to noise ratio in the two dimensional image was degradated compared to the images obtained with an unfocused multiscan system. A careful investigation showed that this degradation was not caused by the electronic processing of the echo signals. We believe that the loss in signal to noise ratio is caused by side lobe levels at -35dB or less, under wide angles. When strong reflectors are in the direction of these side lobes, ambiguous echoes may arise and these echoes are displayed on the main axis. Attempts are made to reduce these side lobes.

The quality of the images produced by the focused system is due to the excellent lateral resolution. This resolution is only guaranteed when the electronic circuits are not overloaded by strong echo signals. An incorrect time gain compensation setting can easily overload the time gain amplifier. Therefore, the time gain compensation mechanism must be carefully adjusted during clinical examination.

Incidentally, the time gain compensation only operates in one direction of the two dimensional image. In the other direction, parallel to the multi-element transducer, a considerable divergence of echo amplitudes may occur. In some cases, an optimal image over the entire scan plane necessitates a local overloading of the system. A solution to this problem would be a compression of the echo amplitudes before time gain compensation. A compression of the signal after the delay lines however, results in a severe degradation in beam width with increasing side lobe level. Computer calculations and water tank experiments have shown that a compression before the delay lines only slightly affects the beam width and side lobe level. We believe that prephasing compression may further enhance the quality of the images in future.

Acknowledgement

The authors wish to thank Dr. N. Bom, head of the Thorax center Technology group, for his valuable suggestions during the construction and the clinical evaluation of the system.

References

1) King DL: *Cardiac ultrasonography: cross-sectional ultrasonic imaging of the heart.*
   Circulation 47: 843-847, 1973.

2) Bom N, Lancée CT, Van Zwieten G, Kloster FE and Roelandt JRT: *Multiscan echocardiography I. Technical description.*
   Circulation 48: 1066-1047, 1973.

3) Whittingham TA: *A hand-held electronically switched array for rapid ultrasonic scanning.*
Ultrasonics 4 no. 1: 29—33, 1976.

4) Griffith JM, and Henry WL: *A sector scanner for real time two-dimensional echocardio-graphy.*
Circulation 49: 1147-1152, 1974.

5) Von Ramm OT, and Thurstone FL: *Cardiac imaging using a phased array ultrasound system I. System design.*
Circulation 53: 258-262, 1976.

6) Ligtvoet CM, Vogel JA, van Egmond FC, and Vletter WB: *Direct conversion of real-time two-dimensional echocardiographic images.*
Ultrasonics 15: 89-92, 1977.

7) Kloster FE, Roelandt J, Ten Cate FJ, Bom N, and Hugenholtz PG: *Multiscan echocardio-graphy II. Technique and initial clinical results.*
Circulation 48: 1075-1084, 1973.

8) Roelandt J, van Dorp WG, Bom N, Laird JD, and Hugenholtz PG: *Resolution problems in echocardiology: a source of interpretation errors.*
The American Journal of Cardiology 37: 256-262, 1976.

9) Figures 2, 4, 5, 6, 7 and 8 from J. Ridder, ontwerp van een ultra-sonoor systeem voor real-time twee dimensionale weergave met een groot oplossend vermogen, doctoral thesis, Technical University Delft, oktober 1975.

Phased array systems

by J.C. Somer
Rijksuniversiteit Limburg Maastricht.

Introduction

Phased arrays serve the same purpose as multi-element switched arrays, and that is
electronical fast scanning, with ultrasound.
There is, however, a fundamental difference between the two systems.
The first case is based on the principle of beam-steering, whereas in the latter beam-
position is varied by activating several transducers sequentially.
Another way of expressing this is that phased arrays enable electronic sector scanning and switched arrays accomplish electronic linear (or B) scanning.
From this it may be clear that phased arrays are small and comparable in size with
conventional single transducers, whereas switched arrays have dimensions determined by the width of the field of scanning.

Principle of electronic sector scanning

The principle of the electronic sector scanning method has already been described
elsewhere 1), 2), 3). Therefore, only a brief outline will be given here.

Electroscan
The Electroscan is a system developed by Somer 4), 5) at the Institute of Medical
Physics TNO. It is based on an array transducer, which in this case consists of 21
elements spaced half a wavelength apart (ca. 0.5 mm).

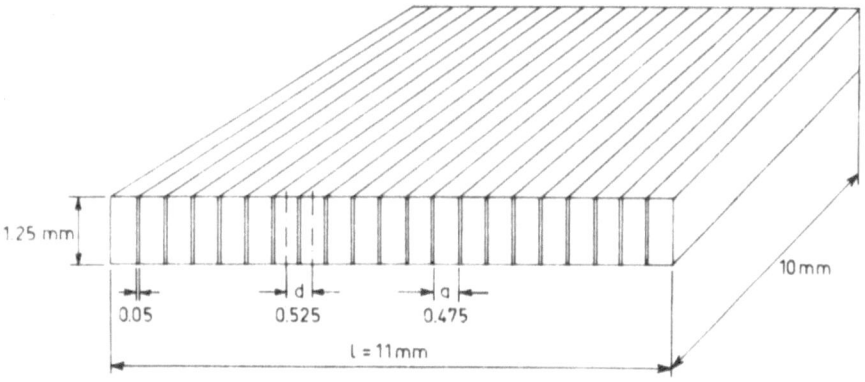

fig. 1a. Array construction.

325

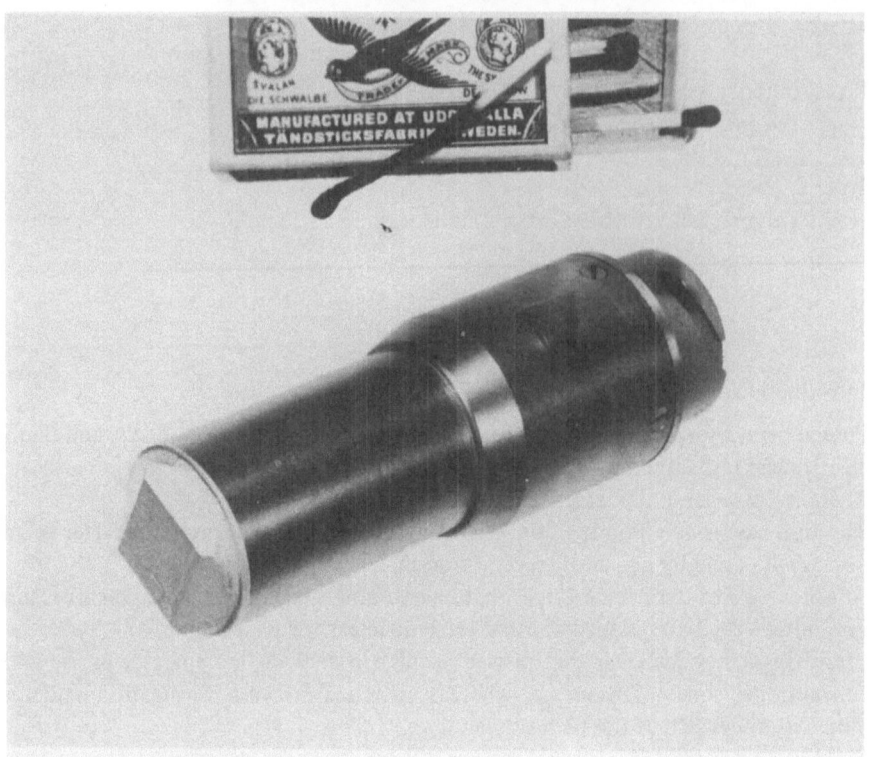

fig. 1b. Actual probe, size compared to match-box.

Figure 1a shows the construction of the array, whereas in figure 1b the size of the actual probe is compared to a matchbox, emphasizing that its overall dimensions are similar to those of conventional transducers.

Each element can be excited individually by means of its own local short-pulse oscillator and will then emit a practically circular wave front, because of its small width of ca. $\lambda/2$ (fig. 2).

According to Huygens' law interference will occur. Provided that the local oscillators generate delays with equal increments, as shown in figure 2, a resulting flat wave front will be achieved. The angle between this wave front and the array surface, which is also the direction off-axis of the produced beam, depends only on the delay-increments mentioned above.

Changing these delay intervals electronically for every transmitted pulse results in different angles of the beams.

One will appreciate that these delay intervals are virtually small and serve to create phase differences between the frequency components of the pulses. The maximum delay between the excitations of two adjacent elements will occur at the widest possible deflection angle of 45 degrees and amounts about 0.25 microseconds. This

326

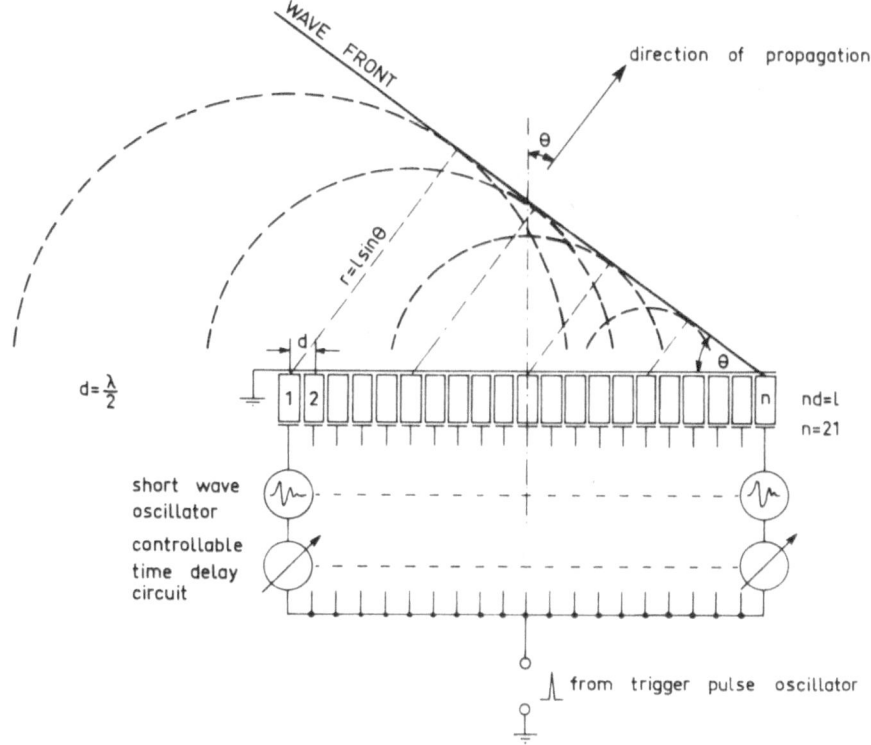

fig. 2. Principle of beam-steering at transmission.

is only one third of the period of the center frequency of 1.3 MHz. As a result all elements contribute by their individual wave fronts to the resulting transmitted pulses in any direction. The delay differences can be generated by electrically controllable time delay circuits, for instance by means of a control voltage, so that direction can be varied very fast.

Figures 3a and 3b show Schlieren pictures of the transmitted beams in two different directions.

Modern technology makes it also possible to have all steering information programmed in digital form.

Reception is performed in a reversed way. Differences in arrival times of echoes at the array elements are dependent on the direction in which a pulse was just transmitted. Therefore, the control voltage is also used for steering a delayline system (fig. 4) so that for each particular direction of transmission there is compensated for the delay differences between the outputs of subsequent elements. For this direction output is maximum since all individual signals add in phase.

Figure 3a

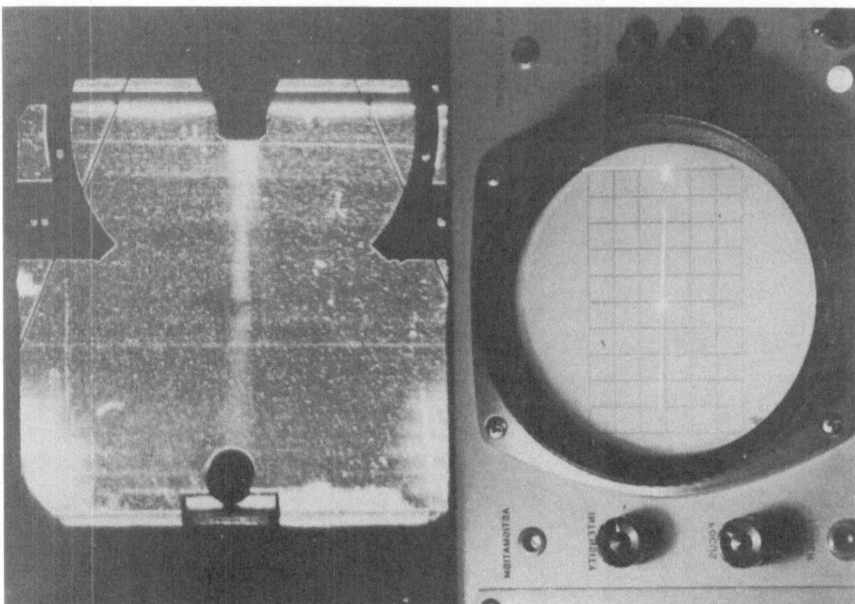

Figure 3b

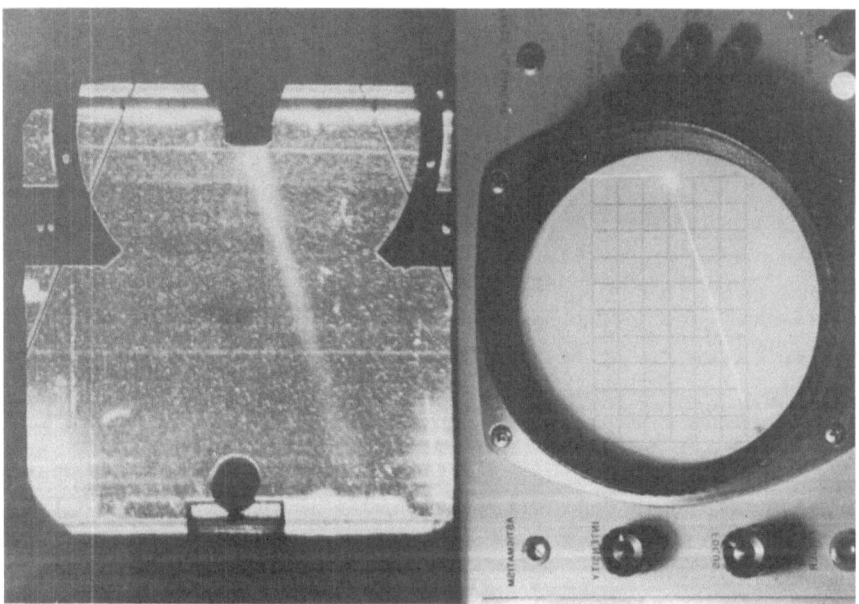

fig. 3a. Schlieren-picture of non-deflected beam. Echo from target displayed on the oscilloscope screen.
fig. 3b. Schlieren-picture of deflected beam.

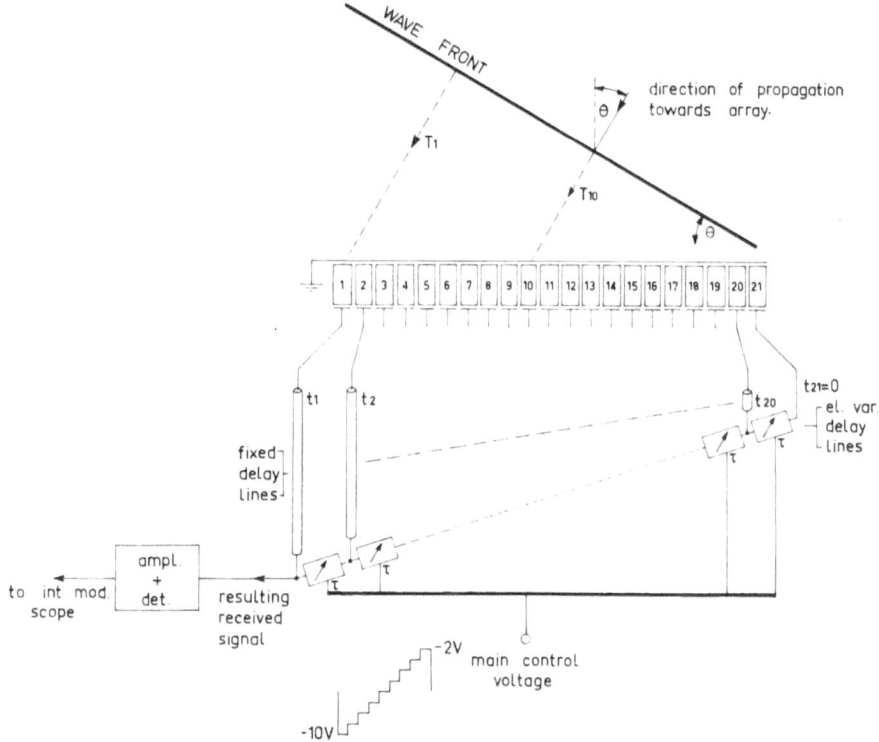

fig. 4. Principle of beam-steering at reception.

Echoes are to be displayed in the B-mode on the screen at positions according to the sites of the actual reflecting structures. Directional information of the beam is therefore also used for supplying proper voltages to the deflection inputs of the display system. Figure 3a shows how the echo of a target (a metal bar at the bottom of the tank), is displayed as a bright spot on the oscilloscope screen.

The first prototype 4), Electroscan I, provided only the facility of choosing between either 32 or 128 directions, both covering a sector of 90 degrees.

Due to the used pulse rate of 1000 pulses per second the sector of 32 directions is scanned about 30 times per second. In the case of 128 lines the actual situation is that four successive sectors of 32 lines are slightly displaced with respect to another. This means that although each line is written on the screen about eight times per second in the latter case, no excessive flicker is present on the screen.

The easiness of accomplishing these two possibilities is due to the fact that only one control voltage regulates the whole system as fas as directionality is concerned. More profit of this situation was taken in the design of the second prototype, Electroscan II. This unit has been in use for clinical routine work for more than five years in the Neurological Department of the University of Freiburg 5).

In addition to the above mentioned facilities, a choice can also be made here in sector width. Either 90 or 30 degrees can be chosen. The latter provides with 32 lines an image with seemingly as good a resolution as a sector of 90 degrees and 128 lines but with high scanning rate. This is of particular advantage in observing pulsating structures, because of the proved relationship between frequency of pulsation, persistence of the screen and the required scanning rate.

As an extra feature the sector of 30 degrees can be rotated as well within the sector of 90 degrees.

A most profitable facility of Electroscan II is the display of echoes of two independently variable directions in the A-mode on a separate screen. For making a preselection, the whole sector and these two A-scan directions can be displayed simultaneously on the main screen, the latter as brighter lines. Then the A-scan directions can be adjusted in order to display the echoes of a particular moving structure. After this adjustment the sector can be switched off, which provides the maximum repetition rate of 500 Hz for each A-scan pattern. This may be useful for time motion recording or for moving target indication methods (MTI).

This electronic sector scan system has now become commercially available. Compared to the original two prototypes several new features have been incorporated in the system, particularly with a view to cardiological applications.

The present cardiological version is operating at a frequency of 2.5 MHz, being twice that of the prototypes, with the same array-dimensions, which doubles the near field range to about 50 mm. This makes it possible to realize to some extent fixed focusing at transmission and variable focusing at reception.

The latter implies that non-linear timing functions have to be superimposed on the linear ones that are needed for the beam deflection. All data required for all directional functions and display modes are stored in digital form.

Figure 5 shows a tomographic image of the human heart obtained by this version of the Electroscan, now called Echostat. Several cardiac structures are shown. For a realistic idea of the actual performance, however, one has to observe the real time capability by video tape or movie.

Thaumascan

Another system of electronic sector scanning has been described in the literature, called Thaumascan 6), 7), 8). This device differs in several respects from the Electroscan and Echostat respectively.

The primary difference is the size of the array itself, expressed both in mm and in wavelengths.

The Electroscan array is about 11 x 10 mm, consists of 21 elements of each $\lambda/2$ width, which gives the whole aperture a width of 10λ, at the frequency of 1.3 MHz

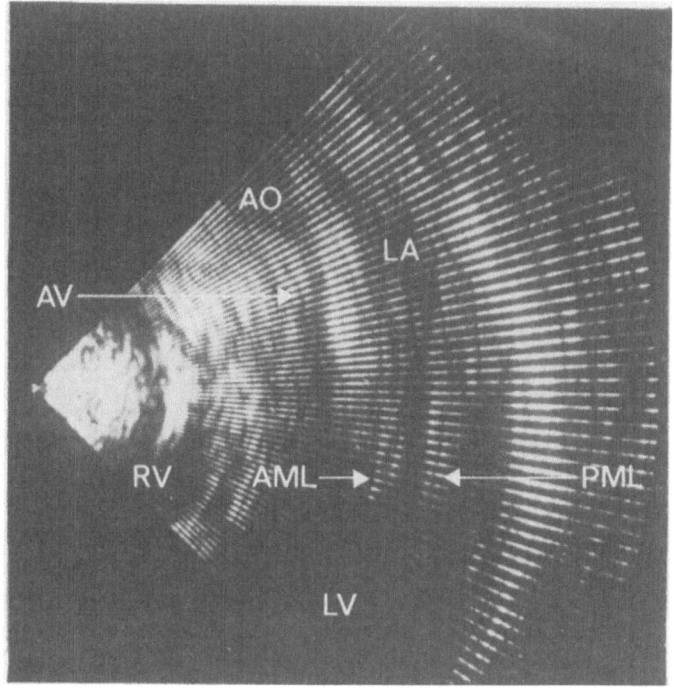

fig. 5. Longitudinal scan of the heart. AO = aorta, AV = aortic valve, LA = left atrium, AML = anterior mitral leaflet, PML = posterior mitral leaflet, LV = left ventricle, RV = right ventricle.

(or 18 λ when a frequency of 2.5 MHz is used in the case of Echostat).

The Thaumascan array is 24 x 16 mm and has 16 elements of 1.5 mm or 2λ each, which makes the whole aperture 32λ at the frequency of 2 MHz, used in this system. The Thaumascan near field range is ca. 190 mm. This means that the latter operates essentially in the near field.

This has the advantage of the realizability of effective focusing of the beam over the whole depth of scanning.

A consequence of the relatively wide elements of the Thaumascan (2λ), is that not as wide an angle can be scanned as with the Electroscan (elements of $\lambda/2$).

Figure 6 shows a longitudinal sectorscan through the heart obtained by the Thaumascan. The scanned angle is 60 degrees, whereas the Electroscan is able to generate sectorscans up to 90 degrees (fig. 5).

Further characteristics of the Thaumascan are the computer control of beam steering and the non-linear processing of the received signals.

The timings of the excitations of the elements at transmission as well as the generation of the proper delays for each receiver channel are all provided by a computer. Here each delay line consists of 6 binary coded switchable lumped constant analog

331

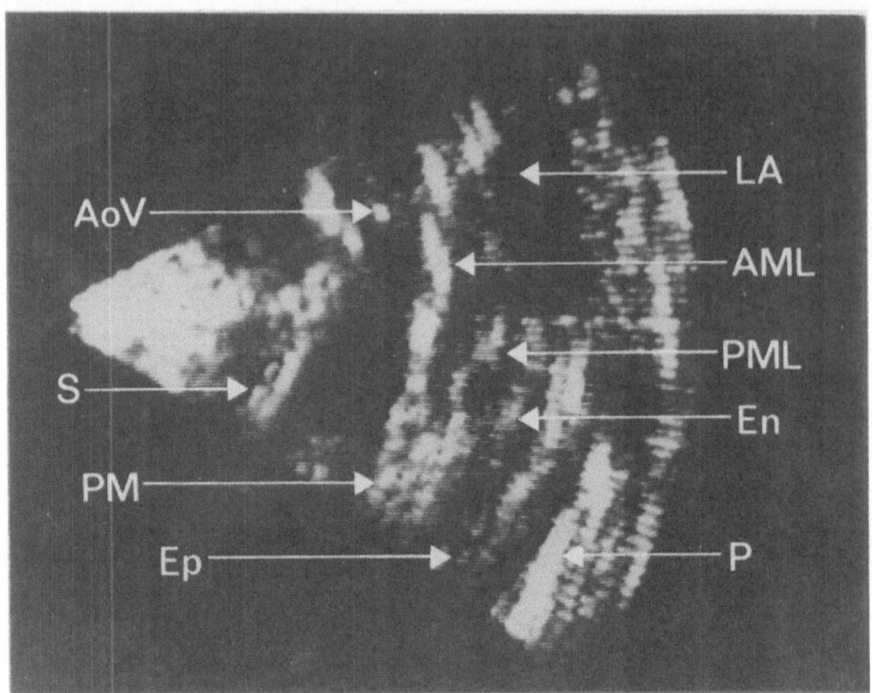

fig. 6. Long axis of left ventricle. AoV = aortic valve cusps, S = interventricular septum, PM papillary muscles, Ep = epicardium, P = pericardium, En = endocardium, PML = posterior mitral leaflet, AML = anterior mitral leaflet, LA = left atrium (courtesy Dr. von Ramm).

delay elements. This makes it very convenient for digital control.

The computer control, although expensive, is very flexible in a sense that more complicated delay patterns can be achieved. This makes it possible to superimpose spherical or aspherical delay functions on the linear delay functions necessary for beam deflection. In this way fixed focusing at transmission and variable focusing at reception is possible. These features already cause a considerable improvement of the lateral resolution.

This may further be improved by the non-linear processing of received signals that has been applied.

In contrast to the Electroscan and the Echostat here all receiver channels contain logarithmic amplification before adding the pertinent signals. As a result a dynamic range compression has been achieved for each channel and therefore also for the resulting sum. Of even more significance, however, is the fact that this sum (or resulting signal) is the sum of logarithms of individual signals and therefore the logarithm of the product of all channels. Here we have a special kind of multiplicative processing.

It is known of multiplicative processing in general that it results in smaller beams and side-lobe reduction. On the other hand, however, the so called multiple target problem may be introduced. This means that phantom-images may occur when cross-products of different targets appear on the screen.

The system described above, seems not to suffer too much from this phenomenon.

Conclusion

In addition to the multi-element switched array systems now also phased-array systems have become available for cardiac work. The most outstanding difference is the size of the probe. Since its dimensions are comparable with convential single transducers, the energy is radiated through a very small coupling area into all directions within a sector of maximally 90 degrees. This implies that the probe can be placed at practically all desired intercostal spaces for viewing the heart without the difficulty of shadowing by the ribs.

Another very important advantage is the possibility of focusing both at transmission and at reception; in the latter case with tracking focus.

A third advantage that seems to be very promising is the fact that at reception directional information is available in amplitude and phase in the respective channels. Therefore it is in principle possible to realize matched filtering or deconvolution techniques for improving particularly lateral resolution. This may be accomplished either by digital or by optical computers.

In the latter case it will be possible to perform such techniques in real time. Thus preserving the paramount feature of real time imaging of dynamic phenomena within the body, especially in cardiology.

References

1) Somer JC: *Instantaneous and continuous pictures obtained by a new two-dimensional scan technique with a stationary transducer.*
   In: Proc. in Echo-Enceph. Intern. Symp. on Echo-Encephalography, Ed. E. Kazner, W. Schiefer, K.J. Zülch, Publ. Springer-Verlag, New York, p. 234-238 (1967).

2) Somer JC: *Electronic sector scanning for ultrasonic diagnosis.*
   Ultrasonics, Vol. 6, Nr. 3, p. 153-159 (1968).

3) Somer JC: *Electronic sector scanning with ultrasonic beams.*
   In: Ultrasonographia Medica Vol. 1, Proc. 1st World Congress on Ultrasonic Diagnostics in Medicine and SIDUO III, Ed. J. Böck and K. Ossoinig, Publ. Verlag der Wiener Medizinischen Akademie, Wien, p. 27-32 (1971).

4) Kamphuisen HAC, Somer JC, and Oosterbaan WA: *Two dimensional echo-encephalography with electronic sector scanning (clinical experiences with a new method).*
   J. of Neurology, Neurosurgery and Psychiatry, Vol. 35, nr. 6, p. 912-918 (1972).

5) Freund HJ, Somer JC, Kendel KH, and Voigt K: *Electronic sector scanning in the diagnosis of cerebrovascular disease and space-occupying processes.*
   Neurology, Vol. 23, nr. 11, p. 1147-1159 (1973).

6) Thurstone FL, and von Ramm OT: *A new ultrasound imaging technique employing two-dimensional electronic beam steering.*
   In: Acoustical Holography Vol. 5, Proceedings of the Fifth International Symposium, Ed. P.S. Green, Publ. Plenum Press, New York and London, p. 249-259 (1973).

7) von Ramm OT, Thurstone FL, and Kisslo J: *Cardiovascular diagnosis with real time ultrasound imaging.*
   In: Acoustical Holography Vol. 6, Proceedings of the Sixth International Symposium, Ed. Newell Booth, Publ. Plenum Press, New York and London, p. 91-102 (1975).

8) Kisslo J, von Ramm OT, and Thurstone FL: *A phased-array ultrasound system for cardiac imaging.*
   In: Proceedings of the Second European Congress on Ultrasonics in Medicine, Ed. E. Kazner, M. de Vlieger, H.R. Müller, V.R. McCready, held in Munich 12-16 May 1975, Publ. Excerpta Medica, Amsterdam-Oxford and American Elsevier Publishing Co., Inc., New York, p. 67-74 (1975).

9) Somer JC: *Electronic sector scanning in cerebral diagnosis.*
   I. Principle and technical development p. 304-308. Ultrasonics in Medicine, Eds. M. de Vlieger, D.N. White, V.R. McCready. Proceedings of the Second World Congress on Ultrasonics in Medicine, Rotterdam, 4-8 June 1973.

Acknowledgement

Part of the illustrations used in this article has been published before. Figure 1a, 1b, 2, 3, 4 and 6 were published respectively in references 2, 9, 1, 2, 2 and 7.

Data processing of time-motion information in Echocardiography.

by J.A. Vogel, G. van Zwieten, N. Bom,
Thoraxcenter, Erasmus University, Rotterdam, Netherlands.
W.J. Gussenhoven, Interuniversitair Cardiologisch Instituut,
Amsterdam, Netherlands.

Introduction

Echocardiography has proved to be an important technique for real-time visualisation of the heart in motion. In complement to the conventional M-mode recordings, two dimensional moving cross-sections of the heart are obtained with the multiscan principe as described by Bom 1), 2) and Roelandt 3), 4).
Information revealed in this way is considerably more than can be digested immediately. Therefore automation in acquisition and processing of clinical data can be
helpful. Work in this direction has already been reported by Griffith 5); McSherry
6); Waag 7) and others.
In this article the time-motion information as available in an M-mode recording and
information obtained with a multi-element real-time system, will be analysed (fig. 1).
Then attention will be paid to acquisition and processing of data presented in an M-
mode recording. Also a technique for reconstruction of time-motion information
from a real-time series of cardiac cross-sections will be discussed.

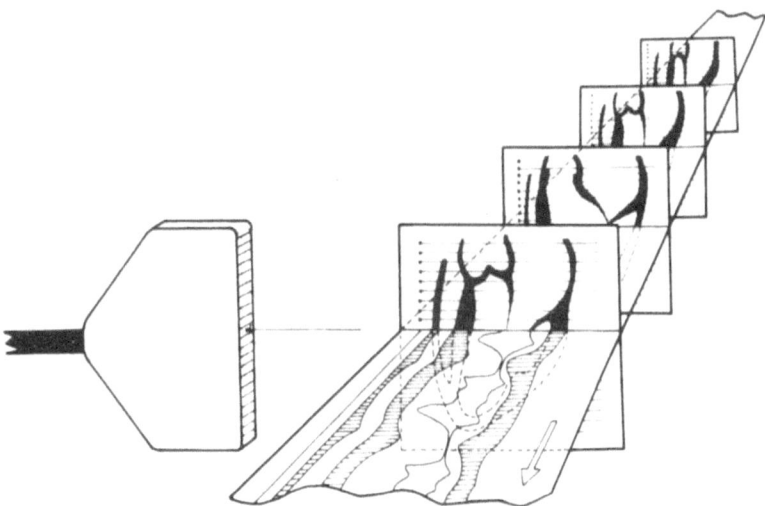

fig. 1. Schematic drawing of information obtained by real-time visualisation of the heart in
motion. Anatomic information is shown in the two dimensional cross-sections. Dynamic and
functional information is preserved in the time motion relations, as represented by the reconstructed M-mode recording.

335

Echocardiology, N. Bom editor, published by Martinus Nijhoff, the Hague 1977.

Analysis methods

Time-motion analysis

The well-known M-mode as obtained in the single element routine is a time-motion recording and each echo can be described in two dimensions by its position in depth and time. Movement of structures in a direction perpendicular to the soundbeam is not recorded. Consequently only a selected narrow portion of the heart in depth is studied as a function of time. Calculation on two or three dimensional geometry such as volume studies, based on M-mode, suffers from severe limitations.

The cardiac chamber may contract irregularly and the uni-dimensional soundbeam essentially yields the motion pattern of two chamber points only. Differences between the echo axis of the left ventricle and the true minor axis will also diminish the reliability in obtaining true information about the entire chamber.

In cardiac parameter estimation based on M-mode recordings attempts have been made to incorporate the missing dimension by making an assumption.

Volume calculations are normally carried out with the assumption of an ellipsoidal model of the left ventricle (LV) in which the major axis is assumed to be twice the minor axis (V = volume = $\pi/3$ m^3, m = minor axis). Circumferential fiber-shortening rate is calculated by estimating the first derivative of the LV dimension and by normalizing for the end diastolic dimension. This calculation is based on knowledge of diameter changes in only one direction.

The validity of the assumptions as mentioned in the above calculations is under discussion. An ellipsoidal model may be reasonably valid in cases of heart disease with a symmetrical contraction of the ventricle.

However, if part of the ventricle is diseased it is unreasonable to suppose the heart to contract normally. In coronary artery diseases, for instance, akinetic and dyskinetic segments of the ventricular walls may deform the ventricle. In dilatated hearts the shape of the ventricle may change from ellipsoidal into spherical shape.

It seems more appropriate instead of introducing errors caused by assumptions, to just base the useful parameters which indicate ventricular performance on accurately observed dimensions as may be obtained with ultrasound techniques. In this article calculated parameters have been derived from direct ultrasonically observed data only.

Cross-sectional analysis

A cross-sectional image of the heart can be obtained by a scanning technique with a linear array system.

In real-time systems a Polaroid photograph is a well-known example of a two-dimensional representation of a cross-section. This kind of presentation has also disadvantages. Specific echoes are difficult to identify since their characteristic motion pattern has been lost.

Real-time study of the heart with the multi-element system provides the following information in the diagnosis of heart diseases:

336

- visualisation of the dynamics of cardiac contraction
- qualitative valve motion analysis in valvular heart diseases
- information on size and shape of structures.

Although a global impression may be obtained directly, it is obvious that it is impossible to digest all this information immediately. It is also questionable how to introduce this information in some way in a patient file. The computer can be helpful in extraction of useful data. Processing of the different types of echo information, as described here, can result in a useful presentation of cardiac dynamics and dimension variations.

Processing of time-motion recordings

A growing patient load and an increasing emphasis on extraction of useful quantitative data necessitates uniform and efficient acquisition and processing of echo data. This has led to the development of a computer assisted system for analysis of M-mode recordings. See fig. 2.

The described system employs the following devices:
1. PDP11/10 minicomputer (16K words memory, disk and decwriter)
2. digitizing tablet (.3 mm resolution)
3. video scanned computer memory and TV monitor
4. video hard copy device
Most programs are written in the Fortran IV language.

The system has been developed for:
1. Standardized analysis of routinely acquired echocardiograms.
2. Experimental analysis of M-mode recordings.

processing equipment for analysis
of M mode echocardiograms

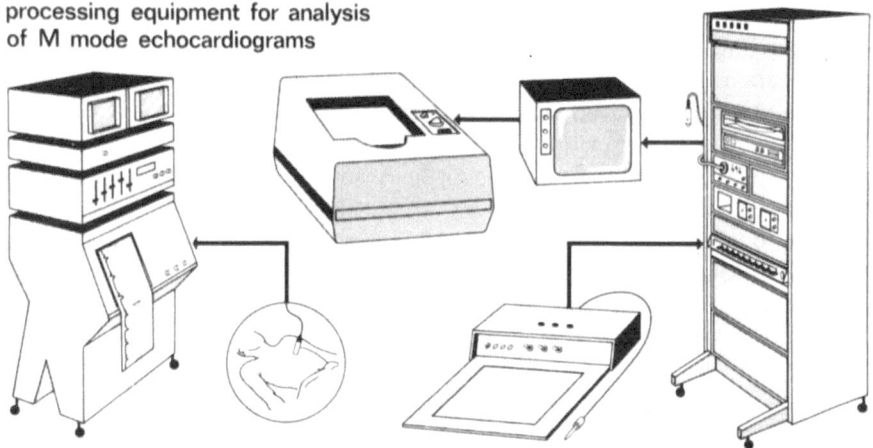

fig. 2. A schematic drawing of the echocardiographic data equipment. The ultrasound system is shown to the left. The digitizing tablet and video hard copy device are shown in the middle and the computer configuration to the right.

The computer analysis of routine echocardiograms is an ideal tool to enforce a uniform and standardized analysis of echocardiograms. A program for this type of analysis guides the operator through a prescribed sequence of all measurements and judgements to be made of the routine echocardiogram and provides the user with an immediate echo report.

Another advantage is that acquired data can be stored directly on disk for later retreaval.

The experimental analysis is mainly directed to study and derivation of not easily obtained cardiac parameters in an efficient way.

To facilitate the use of the system by the clinician or echo technician, the following approach has been chosen:

all programs are comprised in a single program system with a simple "start up" procedure. After start up all program initiation and data handling is done in an interaction between the user and the program via the digitizing tablet and the TV display. To this end a small part of the digitizing tablet is used as a key board. A template marked with alpha numeric characters and special function boxes is fixed on the tablet and data can be entered by touching the appropriate boxes with the digitizing pen. All program messages and questions are displayed on the TV monitor and all operator responses are entered via the digitizing tablet.

In the dialogue and data entry phase of each program, data validation and error checking is carried out. This is to avoid program crashes during processing of the acquired data. If any error is encountered after data entry, the question is repeated and the data must be entered again. Some errors will result in a restart of the running program (except for fatal system errors which might destroy the operating system structure).

After start up of the system, a master control program is initiated which is used for the entry of patient identification data and selection of the program for the analysis to be performed.

Patient data once entered are available for all programs. On exit of a selected program the master control program is automatically started again. The patient data acquisition phase of the master control program can be skipped so that for a given patient any combination of analysis programs can be used without the re-entering of patient identification data.

However, one must realise that there must be a correct tracing that allows for justifiable extraction of the parameters which are computed by the selected program. In the following two examples of programs are given according to the two types of analysis methods mentioned before.

Standardized analysis

After entry of patient identification data such as name, date of birth, length, weight and so on via the master control program, the report or standard analysis program may be selected. This program asks first for the clinical question and the technical

338

quality of the recording. The technical quality of the recording is included as an indication for the reliability of the measurement.

Next the quantitative analysis of the tracing is performed. The operator must select a suitable portion of the tracing on which the structures to be measured are identifiable. First the end diastolic ventricular dimensions are measured by touching off the RV (RV = Right Ventricle), RV/IVS, (IVS = Interventricular Septum) IVS/LV, (LV = Left Ventricle), LVPW endocardial (LVPW = Left Ventricular Posterior Wall) and LVPW epicardial echoes at end diastole; preceded by one calibration by touching two depth markers at 5 cm distance. This is repeated for the end systolic ventricular echoes. Secondly the mitral valve echoes are entered and then the aortic and left atrial echoes.

Structures which can not be identified are omitted by tipping the enter box on the key board part of the tablet. From the available echo points, all distances and related parameters are computed and a measurement summary is displayed for acceptance by the operator. It is also possible to reenter a selected portion of the echo points if the operator is not convinced of the correctness of his own measurements.

The computed dimensions and related parameters are the following:
- right ventricular inner diameter
- septal thickness
- left ventricular inner diameter (LVID)
- left ventricular posterior wall thickness, both for end diastole and end systole
- aortic diameter (AO)
- left atrial diameter (LA)
- mitral valve amplitude
- mitral valve EF slope
- ratio IVS/LVPW, ratio LA/AO, fractional shortening of LVID during contraction.

After acceptance of the quantitative data a qualitative analysis of the echocardiogram is performed. For each structure or condition to be judged a multiple choice table of standard phrases is displayed and the operator must indicate one or more appropriate entries of the tablet. If the standard phrases are not sufficient to describe the condition, lines of free text may be entered.

The standard phrases cover most of the usual conditions seen on the echocardiogram. These include for example mitral valve abnormalities, behavior of ventricular walls, absence or presence of pericardial effusion, absence or presence of asymmetrical septal hypertrophy. Some 120 phrases are included. The numbers of the indicated phrases together with the free text progenerate a qualitative report on the echocardiogram. This procedure forces the investigator to carry out a complete and standardized review of the echocardiogram and also allows for efficient storage of a routine echo report. After completion of this part of the program both the quantitative and qualitative data are stored on disk for print out at the end of the analysis session (fig. 3).

```
AZR Dykzigt                          Erasmus University
Thoraxcenter                         Echocardiography

Patient data:        Name: G. van Doorn        Sex: M
                     Birth date: 12-11-49       Echo nr. 760001
                     Weight: 69 kg              Code: 23-41
                     Length: 1.80 m             Date: 05-06-76

Reason of consult:

Quality of tracing:
                     ---------------------------------------------
Interpretation:      Diast. mov. ant. mitr.    normal
                     Syst. mov. ant. mitr.     normal
                     Post. mitr.               "W" (normal)
                     Syst. septum thickening   normal
                     Pericard. effusion        no
                     ---------------------------------------------
                         E.D.           E.S.            Normal

Ventricle            RVID  24.4 mm    19.3 mm       22 mm
dimensions:          LVID  55.6 mm    34.8 mm    30-50 mm (E.D.)
                     IVS   11.1 mm    14.1 mm     5-13 mm (E.D.)
                     LVPW  13.0 mm    15.2 mm     8-12 mm (E.D.)
                     ---------------------------------------------
                     IVS/LVPW (E.D.)   0.86
                     LVID shortening   0.37
                     ---------------------------------------------
Aorta + L.A.         Ao diameter      28.8 mm    20-38 mm
dimensions (E.S.)    L.A. dim         36.8 mm    20-40 mm
                     L.A./Ao           1.28
                     ---------------------------------------------
Mitral valve         Amplitude        30.2 mm     > 17 mm
                     Slope            67.6 mm/sec > 70 mm/sec
                     ---------------------------------------------
Conclusion:          No signs of ASH
                     Good contractions of LV
                     Normal Echocardiogram.
```

fig. 3. Print out of a complete standardized analysis report of a routine echocardiogram.

Experimental analysis

A computer-assisted system with a digitizing tablet may also be used for extending the quantitative interpretation of M-mode echocardiograms. After retracing of the essential features of an M-mode recording a computing system can determinate parameters and plot curves of change in cardiac parameters during one or more cardiac cycles. In this field of M-mode evaluation a number of programs has been developed for general use or scientific purpose.

340

As an example of the experimental analysis a description of the program for analysis of the left ventricular inner diameter is given.

The analysis starts with a command for calibration. Calibration is possible by indicating three points with the pen in a rectangular coordinate system: the origin (free choice); the corresponding point 1 second later and the point 5 cm above the origin. After calibration, the posterior and anterior endocardial left ventricular wall echoes are traced for at least one cardiac cycle. The digitized data are translated, rotated and scaled according to the calibration points. The data are filtered by a low-pass filter to remove hand-tracing errors and are stored in a fixed element array in memory. The sampling points in this array are equally spaced in time. After indication of two successive R-waves from the simultaneously recorded ECG the following parameters are calculated:

- heart-rate
- R-R time interval
- ejection time
- end systolic dimension
- end diastolic dimension
- fractional shortening.

Ejection time (EJCTIM) is calculated as the time difference between the first indicated R-wave and 50 msec (for correction of isovolumic contraction) and the minimum posterior-anterior dimension.

End diastolic dimension (EDD) is calculated as the dimension at begin ejection time and end systolic dimension (ESD) is the minimum posterior-anterior dimension.

Fractional shortening (FS) is calculated by

$$\text{FS (percent)} = \frac{\text{EDD - ESD}}{\text{EDD}} \times 100 \text{ percent}$$

In all these calculations no assumptions about a volume model have been made according to the previously mentioned arguments.

Velocity information (shortening rate = SR) is obtained by instantaneous calculation of rate of change as the first derivative of left ventricular dimension (D):

$$\text{SR} = \frac{dD/dt}{\text{EDD}}$$

Mean shortening rate (SRMEAN) is calculated by:

$$\text{SRMEAN} = \frac{\text{EDD - ESD}}{\text{EJCTIM} \times \text{EDD}}$$

Peak shortening rate in contraction is SRMAX and the peak relaxation rate is SRMIN.

$$\text{SRMAX} = \text{MAX (SR)}, \text{during contraction}$$
$$\text{SRMIN} = \text{MIN (SR)}, \text{during relaxation}$$

Velocity information is an indication for left ventricular performance. However, it has to be realised that only a small area of the LV is considered, so accurate differentiation between normal and abnormal ventricles depends on knowledge of the behavior of the left ventricle as a whole. This knowledge can be obtained by observing the patient with a two dimensional real time system before recording the M-mode which will be analyzed. Velocity information may have value in follow-up studies where the patient serves as its own control.

The final patient report includes, besides general patient information and calculated parameters, continuous plots of the left ventricular diameter and shortening rate versus time.

An example of the report is shown in fig. 4.

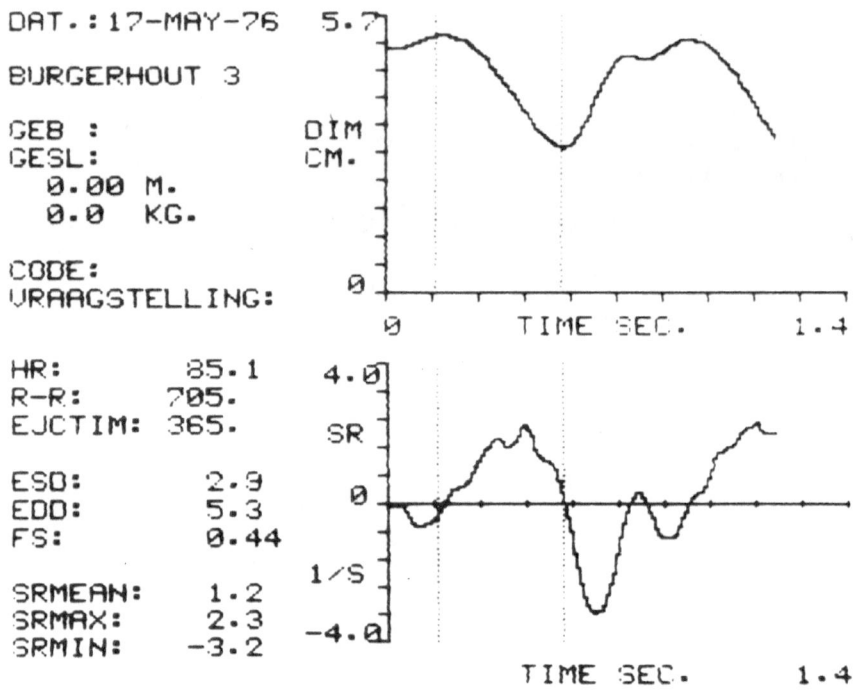

fig. 4. The results of an experimental analysis program. This shows an example of the output of a normal individual.

Processing of all the data is carried out in about one minute. This report is displayed on the TV screen and a hardcopy can be made. Statistical experiments, described earlier by Brower 8) and Vogel 9), have shown that the computer system adds no significant systematic or random error in parameter estimation.

The type of processing, described here, offers new possibilities in information extraction from M-modes. Continuous plots of estimated cardiac parameters may be provided and the processing may be extended to several heart beats (study of arr-hythmias), so large quantities of data can be obtained now in investigations which are otherwise time consuming.

Processing of real-time recorded 2D images

A digital recording system has been developed for direct storage of the time series of two dimensional multiscan images.

In this system cross-sectional information as well as time-motion information is present and advanced possibilities in processing of echo data become available.

The processing equipment consists of a PDP11-E10 computer; interfacing modules and TV display facilities. In recording the analog multiscan images are converted to digital computer words in the, so called, line convertor as described by Ligtvoet 10). In one second 50 digitized images are transferred to computer memory and stored on a digital disk. The storage capacity of the disk is about 18 sec of real-time recording. This recording system has been described in detail by Vogel 11).

ECHO PROCESSING DATA FLOW

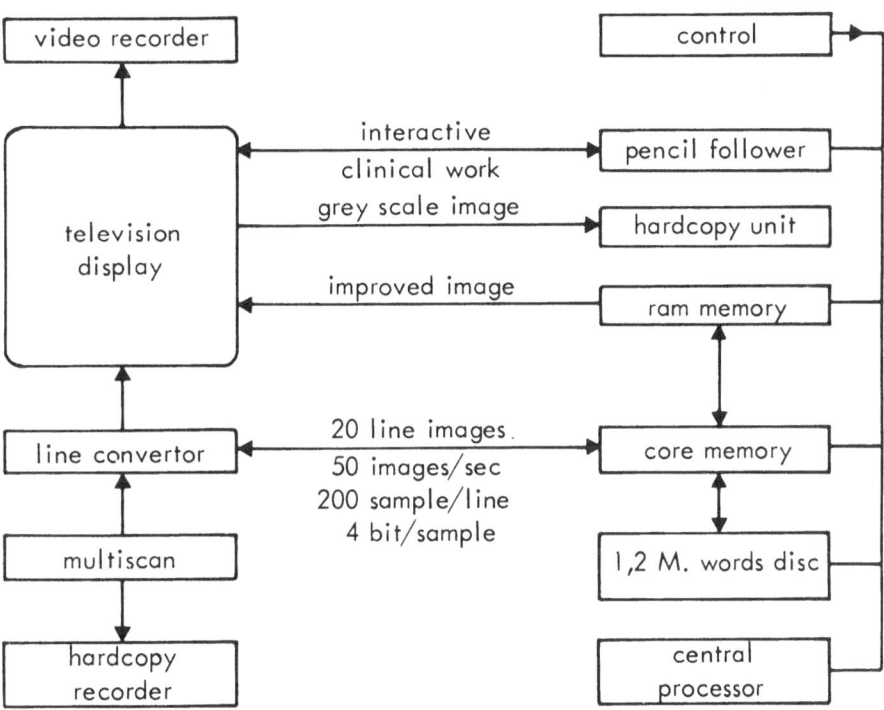

fig. 5. A block diagram of the echocardiographic data processing equipment. The two-dimensional echocardiographic system with video facilities is shown to the left. The computer configuration with video scanned RAM memory and pencil-follower is shown to the right.

A block diagram of data flow in the system is shown in fig. 5. During recording the images are displayed on a TV monitor. Replay of the images is possible with the same line convertor. The most important display facility of the system is a video scanned memory device. This device acts as normal computer memory and the contents of this memory is, by use of a scanning technique, directly visable on the TV monitor with full line density and 16 grey levels. A grey-scale video hardcopy unit and an interactive pencil follower complete the video section of the equipment.
Reduction of image distortion, image enhancement and structure recognition have been described elsewhere 12).

Here a method of effective use of the time-motion information will be described. Movements of the structures are preserved in this real time recording system. Registration of this movement is possible by a time-motion reconstruction technique. This technique is applied to the complete series of 2D cardiac images. After study

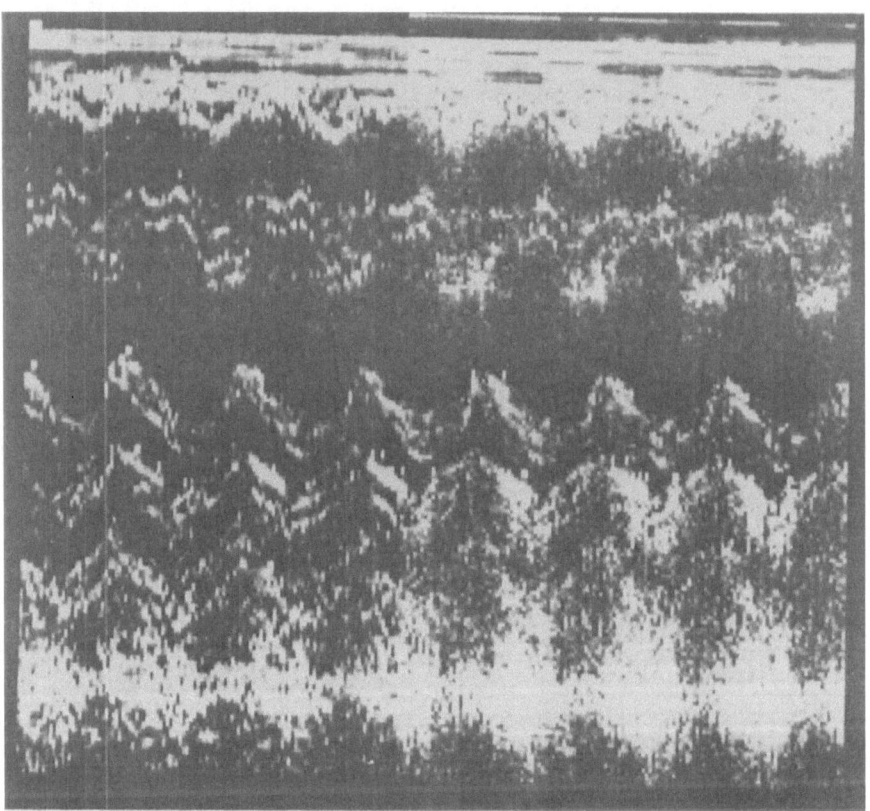

fig. 6. Reconstruction of an M-mode from a patient with mitral stenosis and pericardial effusion. To the right the unprocessed part and to the left the processed part of the recording is shown. Note the improved quality in registration of septum and endocardium and the visualisation of the effusion (anterior and posterior).

of the 18 sec sequential 2D image recording one image is selected and displayed on TV monitor. With a pencil follower a line through a structure of interest is indicated. Along this line an M-mode is constructed by calculation of this line in the sequential images.

The video scanned memory device enables display of the M-mode in grey scale on TV monitor. Programs are available for afterwards processing of the M-mode. A result is shown in fig. 6.

On TV screen a multiscan image may be displayed together with a time-motion reconstruction along a line in that image. Structures can be recognized now by their anatomic relationship as shown in the multiscan image and by their motion in time. This new type of display will be helpful in proper structure recognition and analysis of the dynamics of the heart.

The M-mode can be reconstructed in any desired direction, so M-modes can be obtained from positions and directions which are otherwise impossible to produce.

Extension of this reconstruction method is possible by repetition of the process in different directions. In this multiple M-mode reconstruction there is an exact time-relation between all the M-modes since all M-modes are obtained from the same cardiac cycles. Multiple M-mode reconstruction is useful in timing studies of opening and closure time of the various valves.

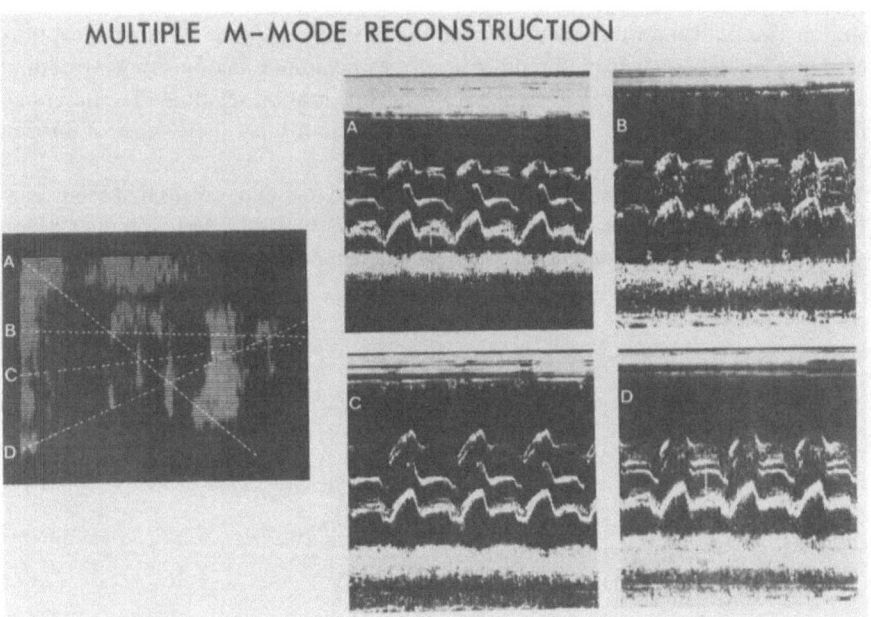

fig. 7. Multiple M-mode reconstructions from the same time series: aorta and left atrium. The registration shows a remarkable difference by the reconstruction in various directions.

345

A limitation of a single element M-mode is the fact that only the axial motion component will be recorded.

Multiple reconstruction of M-modes in different directions yields an overal impression of motion of structures.

An example of multiple M-mode reconstruction is shown in fig. 7.

Multiple reconstruction is also useful for education purposes in echocardiography. Incorrect aiming of the single element transducer or false interpretation of the tracing may lead to an incorrect diagnosis.

In fig. 7d the apparent separation of the leaflets of the aorta is only caused by variation of the aiming through the aorta.

Discussion

Processing of echocardiographic data is directed towards proper presentation and efficient handling of diagnostic information by means of display methods and parameter determination. Data analysis of real-time series of cross-sectional images beyond the important immediate observation may result in all required information but is extremely complicated and time consuming. In complement to real-time 2D observation of the heart, which yields important qualitative information, in normal clinical routine the essential quantitative information is obtained from standard single element tracings in time motion. It seems apparent that for further and more wide introduction and appreciation of Echocardiology the introduction of a standard analysis and reporting method as discussed in this paper is essential. Real-time recording of two dimensional multiscan images combines anatomic and structural information with the dynamic information in time motion relations. The described time motion reconstruction technique is a method to display these types of information together.

The data processing unit described here for standard and experimental M-mode analysis and the M-mode reconstruction from 2D images, may lead to a more systematic approach in echocardiographic analysis and can contribute to the improvement of knowledge of the moving heart in the patient.

References

1) Bom N, Lancée CT, Honkoop J, and Hugenholtz PG: *Ultrasonic viewer for Cross-Sectional Analysis of Moving Cardiac Structures.*
Biomed Engng 6/11, 500 (1971).

2) Bom N, Lancée CT, van Zwieten G, Kloster FE, and Roelandt J: *Multiscan Echocardiography I. Technical Description.*
Circulation 48, 1066 (1973).

3) Roelandt J, Kloster FE, ten Cate FJ, Bom N, Lancée CT, and Hugenholtz PG: *Multiscan Echocardiography; description of the system and initial results in 100 patients.*
Hart Bulletin 4, 51 (1973).

4) Roelandt J, Kloster FE, ten Cate FJ, van Dorp WG, Honkoop J, Bom N, and Hugenholtz PG: *Multidimensional Echocardiography an Appraisal of its clinical usefulness.*
British Heart J, 36, 29 (1974).

5) Griffith JM, and Henry WL: *Video scanner-analogue computer system for semi-automatic analysis of routine echocardiograms.*
Am J. Cardiol. 32, 961 (1973).

6) Mc Sherry DH: *Computer processing of diagnostic ultrasound data.*
IEEE Trans Sonics Ultrasonics 21, 91-97 (1974).

7) Waag RC, and Gramiak R: *New concepts for acquiring, processing and imaging cardiac ultrasound data.*
Proc. 2nd World Congress on Ultrasonics in Medicine, June 1973.
Excerpta Medica, Amsterdam (1974).

8) Brower RW, van Dorp WG, Vogel JA, and Roelandt J: *An improved method for the quantitative analysis of M-mode echocardiograms.*
Eur. J. Cardiol. 3, 171 (1975).

9) Vogel JA, Brower RW, Bom N, van Zwieten G, and Roelandt J: *Automation in Processing of echocardiographic data.*
Computers in Cardiology (1975).

10) Ligtvoet CM, Vogel JA, van Egmond FC, and Vletter WB: *Direct conversion of real time two dimensional echocardiographic images.*
(In press).

11) Vogel JA, Ligtvoet CM, Bom N, van Zwieten G, and Hugenholtz PG: *Processing Equipment for Two-Dimensional Echocardiographic data.*
Ultrasound in Med. & Biol. Pergamon Press (1975).

12) Vogel JA, Theunissen JMH, Ligtvoet CM, van Dorp WG, and Lancée CT: *Data Processing in two-dimensional echocardiography.*
Proc. WFUMB (1976).

AUTHOR INDEX

SUBJECT INDEX

351

Two-dimensional imaging
see imaging

Ultrasound

Valve
see pulmonary-, tricuspid-, mitral valve and aorta

Wall motion
see left ventricle